Narrative Research in Health
and Illness

D1342237

Narrative Research in Health and Illness

Edited by

Brian Hurwitz

Professor of Medicine and the Arts, Department of English, King's College London, UK

Trisha Greenhalgh

Professor of Primary Health Care, University College London, UK

Vieda Skultans

Professor of Social Anthropology, University of Bristol, UK

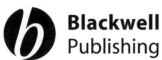

Published by Blackwell Publishing Ltd
Blackwell Publishing, Inc., 350 Main Street, Malden, Massachusetts 02148-5020, USA
Blackwell Publishing Ltd, 9600 Garsington Road, Oxford OX4 2DQ, UK
Blackwell Publishing Asia Pty Ltd, 550 Swanston Street, Carlton, Victoria 3053, Australia

First published in 2004

Library of Congress Cataloging-in-Publication Data

Narrative research in health and illness / edited by Brian Hurwitz, Trisha Greenhalgh,
    Vieda Skultans.
    p. ; cm.
  Includes bibliographical references and index.
  ISBN 0-7279-1792-7 (pbk.)
  1. Physician and patient. 2. Narration (Rhetoric) 3. Discourse analysis, Narrative.
4. Medicine—Research—Methodology.
  [DNLM: 1. Narration. 2. Physician-Patient Relations. W 62 N2346 2004]
I. Hurwitz, Brian. II. Greenhalgh, Trisha. III. Skultans, Vieda.

  R727.N27 2004
  610.69′6—dc22   2004013970

ISBN 0-7279-1792-7

A catalogue record for this title is available from the British Library

Set in India by Siva Math Setters, Chennai
Printed and bound in Spain by GraphyCems

Commissioning Editor: Mary Banks
Development Editor: Nic Ulyatt
Production Controller: Kate Charman

For further information on Blackwell Publishing, visit our website:
http://www.blackwellpublishing.com

The publisher's policy is to use permanent paper from mills that operate a sustainable
forestry policy, and which has been manufactured from pulp processed using acid-free
and elementary chlorine-free practices. Furthermore, the publisher ensures that the
text paper and cover board used have met acceptable environmental accreditation
standards.

Contents

Contributors

Annabelle Auerbach
Head of Content at mykindaplace.com

Clive Baldwin
School of Health Studies, University of Bradford, UK

Paul Bate
University College Hospital, London and University College London Medical School, London, UK

Catherine Belling
Department of Preventative Medicine, Stony Brook University School of Medicine, New York, USA

Petra M Boynton
Department of Primary Health Care and Population Sciences, University College London, UK

Robin Bunton
Community Evaluation and Research Group, University of Teeside, UK

Rita Charon
College of Physicians and Surgeons of Columbia University, New York, USA

Arthur W Frank
Department of Sociology, University of Calgary, Alberta, Canada

Yiannis Gabriel
The Business School, Imperial College, London, UK

Peter Goldie
Department of Philosophy, King's College London, UK

Trisha Greenhalgh
Department of Primary Health Care and Population Sciences, University College London, UK

David J Harper
School of Psychology, University of East London, UK

Andrew Herxheimer
Emeritus fellow, UK Cochrane Centre, Oxford, UK

Brian Hurwitz
Professor of Medicine and the Arts, Department of English, King's College London, UK

Kip Jones
Centre for Evidence in Ethnicity, Health and Diversity, De Montfort University, Leicester, UK

Lesley Jones
Institute of Medical Genetics, University of Wales College of Medicine, UK

Marilyn Kendall
Centre for Public Health and Primary Care Research, University of Edinburgh, UK

James Le Fanu
The Telegraph Newspaper

Cheryl Mattingly
Department of Anthropology and Department of Occupational Science and Therapy, University of Southern California, Los Angeles, California, USA

Scott Murray
Department of Community Health Services, University of Edinburgh, Scotland, UK

Thomas B Newman
Division of Clinical Epidemiology, University of California, San Francisco, USA

Frances Rapport
Swansea Clinical School, University of Wales, Swansea

Catherine Kohler Riessman
Department of Sociology, Boston College, USA

Ruth Richardson
Medical Humanities Unit, Wellcome Trust Centre for The History of Medicine, University College, London, UK.

Vieda Skultans
Department of Sociology, University of Bristol, UK

Gareth Williams
School of Social Sciences, Cardiff University, Wales, UK

Eugene Wu
Prince of Wales Hospital, Chinese University, Hong Kong

Allan Young
Department of Social Studies of Medicine, McGill University, Quebec, Canada

Sue Ziebland
Department of Primary Health Care, University of Oxford, UK

Introduction

Narration is as much part of human nature as breath and the circulation of blood.

(As Byatt, 2000)[1]

Narrative studies hail from widely differing territories within the humanities and social sciences,[2] but they share, at their core, both a teller and a tale. Storytelling invokes words uttered and heard or written and read, images depicted and deciphered or gestures enacted and understood. Once closely aligned with the spoken or written word, narrative studies today embrace a wealth of other expressive media, including dance, film, mime, comic strips, song, and painting.

Polymorphous in content, malleable in form and dynamic in expression, narratives are compositions of unfolding meanings which can be discerned and followed by an audience.[3,4,5] Narrative thinking and imagining therefore embody temporal and causal frames of reference manifest in myths, cave art, fables, fiction, and drama. Closely synonymous with humanity itself, narrative capabilities such as imagining, hypothesising and plotting have offered marked evolutionary advantages to humans over thousands of years.[6]

This book takes forward and extends a number of themes set out in *Narrative-based medicine*,[7] an earlier volume published at a time when many practitioners in health care sensed the narrowness of the prevailing rationalist framework in medicine and were beginning to take note of the "narrative turn" in the social sciences and humanities. We were not by any means the first writers to recognise the importance of narrative in clinical practice (see, for example, the earlier major contributions of Balint,[8] Kleinman,[9] Brody,[10,11] Mishler,[12] and Montgomery Hunter).[13] We saw our objective at that time as building a bridge between this somewhat sparse, specialist literature and the practitioner at the bedside who was drawn to the concept of "narrative health care" and was looking for the linguistic and intellectual tools with which to describe and analyse his or her experience.

Seven years on, we were asked to produce a second edition of *Narrative-based medicine* and realised that we needed to do more than ask the chapter authors of the previous book to update their contributions. By this time, narrative in health care was developing its own corpus of research and had a thriving network of scholars drawn variously from the health professions, anthropology, philosophy, and other primary disciplines, who were debating its conceptual, theoretical, and methodological basis, and who came together regularly in conferences, seminars, and the virtual reality of email communities, to present their empirical work and discuss contemporary problems and challenges.

Any new book on the narrative basis of health care, we felt, would need to reflect its new found maturity as a field of interdisciplinary study, should set out its emerging evidence base, and critically explore its methods of enquiry. We have therefore structured the book to reflect the current theoretical and empirical landscape of narrative studies, and in particular to indicate how narratives mediate between subjective and objective points of view and between the personal, institutional, and social dimensions of health and illness. We have also included one or two more radical chapters that question some generally accepted assumptions, expose controversies, and suggest alternative perspectives for future enquiry.

Structure of the book

We have divided the book into three sections, though it should be noted that some chapters straddle the following taxonomic categories. **Section 1: Narratives** includes ten chapters, mostly based on empirical research, that present the voice of the patient, carer or companion. Together they illustrate the range of knowing that is generated by a narrative approach. They demonstrate important differences in the methodology of research that seeks to collect stories from the ill, vulnerable, dying, and bereaved or that seeks to explore the dynamic interactions between teller, tale, and listener. **Section 2: Counter-narratives** addresses the rhetorical, subversive, and creative roles of narrative. The first chapter of this section delineates two contrasting narratives of deafness identity and affiliation, while the following three present a lesser-known story as a challenge to another, more dominant or accepted story. The final chapter in this section shows how new counter-narratives can arise and begin to hold sway despite facing opposition from scientifically based counter-narratives concerning how best to contain a very small risk of a very serious danger eventuating. **Section 3: Meta-narratives** considers the grand narratives of society, history, and ideology within which our individual life stories (as citizens, risk takers, health service users, researchers, scientists, or policy makers) are enacted. The remainder of this introduction sets out some of the key theoretical issues covered in these three sections. It is not necessary to read the introduction in full before sampling the chapters, but you may like to return to this section periodically as you work through the book.

Section 1: Narrative

The need to reconcile the subjectivity and uniqueness of human experience with the physical reality of the body and a larger impersonal picture besets all the human sciences.[14] But it poses a special challenge for clinical practice, perched as it is between the singularity of personal experience and the generalities of biological structure and mechanism.[15] Howard Brody, contributing to the predecessor to this volume, formulated the problem in this way:

> To deal with the part of medicine which treats everyone as the same, we must extract the narrative from the patient and recast it as a "case history" or as a medicalised retelling of the story. If we do not do this we can never bring to the patient the undoubted benefits of modern medical science. If we do only this, we dehumanise the patient, fail to address him or her as an individual, and ultimately may very well increase the patient's suffering.[16]

The philosopher Richard Wollheim, in *The Thread of Life,* unravels subjectivity in terms of viewpoint, arguing that: "the subjectivity of a phenomenon is how the phenomenon is for the subject".[17] Much of Western science has promoted objectivity at the expense of subjectivity – to describe a view as "subjective" has become a way of discrediting that view. Both as individuals and more particularly as scientists, we learn to impose an artificial, impersonal order on the world and to equate that with reality.[i] But as the philosopher Thomas Nagel makes clear in discussing the importance of human experiences, our lives are not lived through the mediation of an external observer: "Life is lived from inside, and issues of significance are significant only if they can be raised from inside"[22] (p 197). "Insideness" cannot therefore be ignored, Nagel argues, for there is something irreducible about subjectivity, which cannot be captured by causal or functional explanations. He illustrates this non-reducibility with the example of the bat: "Even without the benefit of philosophical reflection anyone who has spent some time in an enclosed space with an excited bat knows what it is to encounter a fundamentally alien form of life" (p 168). No amount of understanding of the brain mechanisms of the bat will tell us what it *feels like* to be a bat, or to see the world through bat ears. There is an explanatory gap because any account based on observation and measurement leaves out subjectivity. As Nagel asks, "What would be left of what it was like to be a bat if one removed the viewpoint of the bat?" (p 173).

The chapters in Section 1 illustrate a key contribution of the narrative perspective: the requirement that human subjectivity should no longer be seen as the devalued opposite of scientific objectivity, linked in some assumed zero-sum relationship whereby more of the one must necessarily mean less of the other. Rather, objective assessment (for example, medical diagnosis) and objective intervention (for example, medical treatment or palliation) provide but one important dimension of knowing. However complete the objective dimension, if we exclude subjectivity and its narrative expression through dialogue, we remove diversity of viewpoint and impoverish the knowledge we can gain about human suffering and the impact of our efforts to care.

In Chapter 1 Rita Charon begins the Narrative section by portraying a patient – seen two days before she penned the chapter – who was "profoundly depressed, non-English-speaking, with a discouraging list of ailments including atrial fibrillation [an irregular heart beat] with its attendant need for chronic anticoagulation, and disabling back pain unresponsive to conservative management". The core challenge in the encounter was not to complete the various biomedical checks and decisions (complicated though they were), but to find a way – through the depression, through the language barrier, through the profound social distance that poverty generates – to engage with this woman as one human to another. Once Charon could achieve this, the biomedical encounter became straightforward and the various medical interventions could be efficiently arranged. She comments: "The satisfaction I felt was the satisfaction of an *internist* – not of an ethicist and not of a narratologist although I am those things too – in my having found a way, today anyway, to be her doctor."

The Italian philosopher Cavarero distinguishes two key questions about the nature of human beings: "The first asks 'what is man?' The second asks of someone 'who he or she is'".[23] Who-questions are often superficially collapsed into what-questions because it seems easier to describe oneself in role (as a teacher, parent or Bristolian, for example) than to address the question of who we actually are. To fully address a who-question requires a story to be told about how we have come to be the person we are. Instead, schematic "stick figure" characterisations come to stand in for the narrative of personal identity.[24] But understanding human beings requires more than characterisation, as Goldie makes clear, when considering an actor preparing to play a part[25] (p 198). The actor not only needs to study the script, but to learn also about the biographical and subjective background of the individual he or she is playing.

Clinicians, like their academic colleagues, may feel more at home with characterisation than with narrative. Characterisation ("a housewife", "a drug user", "a social worker") encompasses the shared aspects of experience and the generalisable. Narrative, on the other hand, expresses the uniqueness of each person and addresses the listener, not as a professional, but as a fellow human. Rita Charon's chapter eloquently evokes and explains the nature of this human-to-human engagement.

In Chapter 2 Eugene Wu and colleagues provide two contrasting views on the SARS epidemic in Hong Kong. Wu was a front-line clinician treating patients with this new and often fatal disease; later, he became a victim of SARS himself. His published scientific account of his own unusual complications of SARS (reproduced from *The Lancet*) is contrasted with his very personal account of being admitted to his own ward by a colleague, watching his fellow doctors and nurses dying in adjacent beds, and contemplating a drastically changed future for himself. A commentary considers the different contributions of the objective (scientific) perspective and the subjective (phenomenological) perspective.

Wu's two very different accounts of his own SARS illness – one as a scientist and the other as a patient – vividly illustrate how personal identity is created through subjective narrative. Richard Rorty argues that human selves emerge at the intersection of old and new uses of language. Wu's scientific case report is reassuringly structured and predictable in form, and uses words in established and agreed-upon ways. His personal narrative account, on the other hand, is much less predictable and uses literary devices such as surprise, suspense, and metaphor, which take us into the domain of the less known: "To have meaning is to have a place in a language game. Metaphors by definition do not"[26] (p 18), although they clearly carry meaning. Quinn comments that "Metaphor is the quintessential challenge to the objectivist account, according to which only literal concepts and propositions can describe the real world".[27]

One reason why some people find medical encounters bruising is precisely because the institutional and professional use of language central to medical practice leaves little room for the personalisation and creative use of language essential to the development of a sense of self. The patient's illness narrative is more than an account of symptoms: it is a form of self-creation through autobiographical literary expression. In Chapter 3 Marilyn Kendall and Scott Murray provide a charming example of the way in which poetic meaning is arrived at in accounts of severe personal illness. Their transposition of recorded narratives in poetic form supports Mishler's argument[12] about the futility of attempting to establish exact correspondences between speech and writing. Meaning is not to be nailed down in ever more exact rules of transcription. Rather, meaning emerges through interpretation and in this study the researchers' finely tuned ears allowed them to discern a poetic structure in narratives of heart failure.

In Chapter 4 Cheryl Mattingly addresses another aspect of severe illness, describing how narratives are used to create and enact hope in the face of it – at a time when the expected narrative may be one of despair and hopelessness. She describes the mother of an African-American child who died at the age of 6 of a brain tumour, but whose various enacted performances during the period of dying, and after the child's death, spoke continually of hope.

Hope, says Mattingly, "is not something discovered or wished. It is painfully created; it is performed", and because healing is so intimately connected to hope *how* hope comes to be performed bears strongly on how healing can be achieved. She draws upon the anthropological work of Victor Turner on healing rituals to show that such rituals have a dramatic or narrative quality that both intensifies personal experience and sets it in the context of a shared story[28-29]. Above all, healing rituals are powerfully emotive, and embody performative or enactive qualities. Mattingly emphasises the importance of "small moments" and the clinician's power to transform routine clinic time into experientially important time. Narrative research, she concludes, concerns not just recording stories perfectly told and structured. It must also acknowledge, and make room for, incomplete fragments and fumblings toward storied forms.

In Chapter 5 Petra Boynton and Annabelle Auerbach offer an analysis of the fragmentary narratives sent as postings to a teenage health website which ran an online feature on self-injury and invited responses from readers. The 260 postings, most of which were from teenagers who actively self-injured, offered a very different picture of this behaviour (and of the sort of person who engages in it) from that provided in standard psychiatric textbooks. Once again, the subjective voice provides insights that more conventional scientific enquiry had failed to uncover.

In Chapter 6 Andrew Herxheimer and Sue Ziebland describe how the Database of Personal Experiences of Health and Illness (DIPEx), an online database of people's narratives of becoming ill, receiving treatment, and – in some cases – dying, adds to "objective" knowledge in more conventional medical databases such as the Cochrane Library. Drawing on the unparalleled experience of the DIPEx team in collecting over 750 narrative interviews, the authors raise and discuss some methodological challenges of this type of research. Their observations about common themes from widely differing narratives illustrate a well-described tension in moving from the individual illness narrative to a more generalised (and generalisable) interpretation. John Berger, in his memorable account of a doctor friend's work in the Forest of Dean, describes the movement between the particularity of illness experience and the universalising dynamic within diagnosis and treatment. He notes that illness and unhappiness both exacerbate a sense of uniqueness.[30] But it is not just diagnosis and treatment that are predicated on comparative exercises: the experience of illness creates a need to compare and share stories. The DIPEx database opens new opportunities for the ill – and those who care for them – to compare and to share their individual stories.

The DIPEx project points to the cardinal role of the listener in narrative, for as Jackson points out, "When storytelling loses its dialogical dimensions it becomes not only self-referential and solipsistic, but pathological"[31] (p 40). Without interpreting audiences, without social affirmation, stories wither. Both Kleinman and Frank have written previously of the critical role of the listener when an illness narrative is being recounted.[9,32] This intersubjective element of narrative is particularly apparent in narratives of dying. In Chapter 7 Arthur Frank describes the way in which accepted ideas about a "good death" (implicitly, common to all who die) can distort the idiosyncrasy and particularity of final experience. The "good death" as lived in reality must tap into individual subjectivity through active dialogue between patient, carers and clinicians. In Chapter 8 Catherine Belling addresses a similar theme and makes a persuasive case for the indispensability of dialogue. In order to complete the story, a witness is needed. "The patient-author, then, cannot tell the end of life in isolation. One more verbal act is essential to establishing narrative closure: told by the physician, this is the account that along with diagnosis, begins the story of dying: prognostication."

For the Russian literary theorist Michael Bakhtin, true dialogue means not cutting off the idea from the voice.[33] It involves being sensitive to the lived experience of the other. In analysing narrative there is a tendency to reify it rather than recognise the evolving and dialogic nature of narrative. For Bakhtin narrative is by its very nature both polyphonic and dialogic, rather than single voiced. In telling a story we not only use words in the way that others have used them before us, we add *our* meanings to theirs and thus build up a jointly authored narrative.[34,35]

In Chapter 9 philosopher Peter Goldie focuses on the central importance of viewpoint to narrative: "If being objective is contrasted with being perspectival, then narrative discourse is not objective, for it is essentially perspectival." Nevertheless, he argues narrative can be objective in the sense of conveying an appropriate evaluation of, and emotional response to, what is recounted.

Goldie's chapter reflects a contemporary shift in the way philosophers conceptualise emotion, seeing it as the means we use to indicate what is important to us. Rather than emphasising the control which culture exercises over shaping feelings, and its power to evoke the same feelings through ritual, this approach finds in emotion recognition of the vulnerability and non-repeatability of human life. Nussbaum has reiterated the role emotions play concerning things that "elude the person's complete control".[36] In this context, the conventional socio-anthropological perspective which invites us to see feelings as reiterated social creations may be misguided, since it seeks to impose a shape on human experience that arguably distorts its essential nature. Feelings are particularly involved where we confront loss and the non-repeatability of human experiences. Nussbaum puts this well:

> [T]o imagine the recurrence of the very same circumstances and persons is to imagine that life does not have the structure it actually has ... Aristotle suggests that a certain sort of intensity will be subtracted; for he holds that the thought that one's children (for example) are "the only ones one has" is an important constituent of the love one has for them, and that without this thought of non-replaceability a great part of the value and motivating force of the love will be undercut.[37] (p 39)

On this account, emotions arise from (are embedded in) unique narrative particularities, and they mark some of our profoundest aspirations and vulnerabilities[37] (p 41). Emotions help to situate where we stand in relation to the world in a way that beliefs, by themselves, cannot easily do. Goldie elsewhere has developed a theory of the emotions as cognitive, intentional, and narrative in structure; despite their association with irrationality, they have their origins in purposeful frameworks.[25] Emotions punctuate fears for, and failures in, life projects. According to this reading, rather than being blind and irrational, emotions can offer the most illuminating insights into an individual's standpoint: "Feeling towards is thinking of with feeling" (p 19).

This first section ends with a warning from Yiannis Gabriel in Chapter 10: as narrative becomes the epistemological backlash against the extreme rationalism that was popular in medicine at the turn of the twentieth century, we should beware of reifying the patient's narrative and according it ultimate credibility. Subjectivity, he argues, has an ambivalent relationship to narrative and does not automatically confer authenticity or representational fidelity. Rather, he contends, narratives need to be interrogated (something also emphasised by conventional clinical method) in much the same way as any other claims to truth. He concludes:

> Deception, blind spots, wishful thinking, the desire to please or to manipulate an audience, lapses of memory, confusion, and other factors may help mould a story or a narrative. It is the researcher's task not merely to celebrate the story or the narrative but to seek to use it as a vehicle for accessing deeper truths than the truths, half-truths, and fictions of undigested personal experience.

Section 2: Counter-narratives

An early observation about narrative, and one that has been repeatedly confirmed by the publication of individual accounts of illness,[38-45] is the role of the personal illness narrative in presenting an alternative voice from that offered in the standard biomedical account. Several chapters in this book take up the specific theme of counter-narrative. In Chapter 11 Lesley Jones and Robin Bunton consider stories of deafness. Echoing a contemporary ideological controversy, they tell two deafness stories – "wounded" and "warrior". The wounded are a group of deaf people who despair about their disability, feel outcast from society, and wish that they could hear. The warriors are a minority with their own language and identity, misunderstood and victimised by mainstream society, and fiercely proud of their unique culture. The wounded (mostly those with partial hearing loss or who have lost their hearing late in life) view deafness as a deficiency ("lack of hearing"); the warriors (mostly those who were born profoundly deaf or, as the activists term it, were born Deaf) seek recognition, citizenship, and, in some cases, segregation. This group, argue Jones and Bunton, would view the offer of a cochlear implant (to restore hearing) as an insult, not a cure. A commentary by Philip Zazove, himself congenitally deaf, presents yet another counter-narrative: the overwhelming majority of people with a hearing loss have a partial loss acquired late in life and seek integration with, not segregation from, wider society. Even those who are totally deaf from birth would generally view themselves as deaf, not Deaf. Zazove makes the important observation that despite the fact that what might be called the "Deaf Pride" community are in many ways unrepresentative of deaf people in general, "The warrior mentality of the Deaf community provides enormous support for these individuals by giving them a sense of community and self worth that they otherwise wouldn't get."

In Chapter 12 Clive Baldwin develops the counter-narrative theme by addressing the medical "syndrome" – Munchausen syndrome by proxy (MSbP). His chapter, based on detailed empirical work on the narratives of both parents and doctors, highlights the complex issue of determining any simple notion of "truth" from narratives. As he says (p 219):

> The medical encounter is one of narrative translation and as such is open to mis-hearings and misunderstandings. Patients do not present their symptoms in a clinical manner; they present only those symptoms they think important; can respond to the same question differently depending upon their relationship with the questioner and so on. This translation process is fraught with difficulty and can be used, if uncritically accepted as neutral and benign, against the mother in allegations of MSbP.

In Chapter 13 medical journalist James LeFanu presents the story of parents whose infants were diagnosed as suffering from shaken baby syndrome (SBS). The biomedical account – of a classic collection of injuries caused by a particular form of trauma inflicted by a malign adult who subsequently lies about the sequence of events – was once thought authoritative, objective, and (allegedly) "evidence-based". However, some parents' accounts offer a powerful alternative narrative: a plausible account of accidental trauma, faithfully recounted, followed by a series of humiliating and distressing interviews with professionals characterised by suspicion, distrust, and partial disclosure.

In Chapter 14 Ruth Richardson describes parents' responses to the traumatic experience of finding out about the unconsented removal of their dead child's organs. She recounts that parents perceived pathologists as "quarrying", "ransacking", and "abusing" their children's bodies. As an author, she uses language and metaphor in a new and original manner, to express parents' perspectives. Rorty has noted that "Metaphors are unfamiliar uses of old words, but such uses are possible only against the background of other old words being used in familiar ways"[26] (p 40). In Rorty's account, the innovative use of language is the essence of narrative expression (p 28). Richardson's use of language, however, should not be seen as the rhetorical craft of a creative narrator, but rather as the words of a narrator who adopts the perspective of those who feel wronged. The immediacy, allegiance, and emotion in the voice of her account contrasts with the more detached and effaced voices of the social scientist in Baldwin's chapter and the investigative journalist in LeFanu's contribution, who both utilise verbatim quotes as a surrogate voice. Differences in narrative voice show how powerfully nuanced narrative accounts can be, and the many semantic levels at which they can operate.

The second section ends with paediatrician and epidemiologist Tom Newman presenting, in Chapter 15, two stories that "hit the media" in the United States – concerning a baby who developed brain damage following high plasma bilirubin levels at birth (neonatal jaundice), and another baby who died in an air crash after travelling unrestrained by a seat belt. In both cases, an official, scientific narrative argued that these infants were merely the unlucky victims of million-to-one risks. But in both cases the emotive personal story of the mother overshadowed the measured advice and codified evidence of the experts. Something, each mother argued, must be done – and it was. Brian Balmer, a philosopher specialising in public understanding of scientific knowledge, offers a commentary on why stories can be more powerful than statistics.

Section 3: Meta-narratives

In *The Postmodern Condition*,[46] Jean-François Lyotard defines meta-narratives as the grand narratives of wider society within which we interpret our personal world and experiences. Christianity, Marxism, feminism, modernist science, and the various historical diaspora of displaced groups are all examples of over-arching stories that provide perspectives on the nature of the social world, where it came from, and where it is going. Because, as Jackson says[31] (p 16), *"storytelling tends to interdigitate and reinforce extant social boundaries"*, personal narratives inevitably reflect and incorporate wider social meanings.

Gareth Williams in Chapter 16 describes the way in which personal narratives of ill health incorporate a lay understanding of the prevailing social forces that bear upon ill health. He refers to the way in which these "knowing narratives" not only help construct auto-biographies of ill health, but also relate personal to social inequalities. In a very different example, in Chapter 17 Vieda Skultans writes autobiographically of her experience as an infant refugee in post-war Germany. The chapter highlights how very early narrative memories are shaped by the historical circumstances of refugeedom – specifically, the need for connectedness and a sense of belonging to a wider community in the face of disconnection from a known and secure world.

The social world is not merely reflected in personal narratives: it constrains and impoverishes our interpretation of them. In Chapter 18, for example, Cathy Riessman reinterprets an illness narrative she collected in a field study some twenty years ago, and identifies a particular social world contained within the personal illness narrative of her narrator, Burt, who suffered from multiple sclerosis in the early 1980s. In her present-day reflections, Riessman couches Burt's perceptions of "being alone" in the particular historical and geographical context of a United States before disability rights had begun to emerge as a movement. Disabled people then spent their time at home, contemplating (and accepting as inevitable) their damaged bodies and lost social roles. A contemporary re-reading of her field interview notes highlights something that was curiously inapparent to her as a researcher at the time: Burt's narrative lacks any perspective on the social injustice of his situation.

Riessman's chapter illustrates an important principle: that even though narrative is a uniquely creative form, we never have an entirely free hand in its lived construal. MacIntyre elaborates this point:

> We are never more (and sometimes less) than the co-authors of our own narratives. Only in fantasy do we live what story we please. In life, as both Aristotle and Engels noted, we are always under certain constraints. We enter upon a stage which we did not design and we find ourselves part of an action that was not of our making. Each of us being a main character in his own drama plays subordinate parts in the dramas of others, and each drama constrains the others.[47]

The notion of the narrator as the living bearer and shaper of language, and as an independent actor in life's drama, challenges the more conventional notion of the passive patient seeking advice, help and sympathy from the health professional. Goffman (quoted by Cathy Riessman on page 312 of this book) puts it thus: "what talkers undertake to do is not to provide information to a recipient but to present dramas to an audience". Paul Bate, an organisational anthropologist, describes in Chapter 19 the story of a facilitated and researched quality improvement initiative in a UK NHS hospital trust. The conventional narrative of organisational change, he argues, is couched in "the vocabulary of coercion, competition, tyranny, hegemony, control, subjection, engineering, manipulation, domination, subordination, resistance, opposition, diversity, negotiation, obedience, and compliance". A different approach uses different vocabulary: *"cooperation, convergence, coherence, integration, and consensus"*, for which the development of a shared story can prove the critical mechanism. In emphasising the critical role of enacting stories as a vehicle for collective action, he cites Kling on p 337 of this book:

> Social movements are constituted by the stories people tell to themselves and to one another. They reflect the deepest ways in which people understand who they are and to whom they are connected ... They are constructed from the interweaving of personal and social biographies – from the narratives people rehearse to themselves about the nature of their lives ... The construction of collective action, therefore, is inseparable from the construction of personal biography, from the ways, that is, we experience the imprecation of our individual and social selves.

This notion of a social world constraining and shaping the unfolding of narrative is given a different twist by two authors who write on how science itself takes a storied form and of how its emplotment is shaped by social forces. In Chapter 20 Trisha Greenhalgh reinterprets the writing of philosopher Thomas Kuhn, who developed the notion of paradigmatic research traditions. She argues that the unfolding of scientific research within any particular tradition is an inherently narrative phenomenon. Using a detailed example from a recent cross-disciplinary systematic review, she argues:

> If research unfolds historically over time (with one study leading directly, though never with mechanistic predictability) to the next study; if research traditions often (and perhaps always) follow a common plot; if the unfolding of the tradition depends on a cast of different characters (with experimenters, gurus, faithful footservants, obsessional puzzle-solvers and doubting Thomases all having their accorded parts to play in different phases); if negotiated (and, necessarily, shared) meanings and models are a prerequisite for focused, directed scientific activity – we surely have the makings of an important new hypothesis: that no research field can be understood without attention to the over-arching storylines that describe its progress.

On a similar theme, Allan Young in Chapter 21 offers a hypothesis that the "illness" of post-traumatic stress disorder is less a scientific "fact" than a social construction by researchers. Furthermore, he argues, the cognitive techniques that scientists unconsciously use to further their research have extraordinary similarities to the abductive reasoning used by characters in fictional detective stories: constructing a (somewhat artificial) puzzle and then solving it. Abductive reasoning, he argues, involves five key logico-literary devices: analogy (using a well understood phenomenon as a model for explaining a poorly understood one), synecdoche (depicting the whole by one of its parts), metonym (implicating one feature by reference to another which is contiguous in time or space), induction (a generalisation inferred from multiple instances or observations), and deduction (inferring a particular instance from general principles). These are all, Young argues, devices grounded in literary techniques, and we should recognise the ultimately subjective and arbitrary influences they bring to science.

One characteristic of meta-narratives is that, unlike the particular individual story being recounted, they are not immediately apparent to the listener or reader. Indeed, the meta-narrative embraces (and assumes) a particular world view and ideology, which teller and listener tend to take for granted. The first task of those who seek to challenge a particular meta-narrative is to deconstruct it and lay bare these various assumptions and the communicative and literary devices used to perpetrate them, as Young has done with one particular scientific research tradition.

In Chapter 22, David Harper offers a similarly detailed and critical exposition of the meta-narrative that both drives and seemingly justifies healthcare policy making in relation to the seriously mentally ill. Using a recent UK government White Paper on compulsory detention of people with mental illness[48] he demonstrates how metaphor, rhetorical devices, and implicit emplotment are used to present a particularly polarised view of the dangers of one policy option (caring for people with psychosis in the community) and the benefits of another (locking them away). The over-arching discourse of this particular White Paper, Harper argues, is not one of the provision of care for a particular group of patients but one of protecting the public from a group of dangerous individuals who are a menace to "normal" people. Quantitative data on actual risk of harm from such individuals are overlooked through a rhetorical device known as narrative accounting – that is, offering qualitative estimates such as "most people" or "the risk is substantial". This, argues Harper, reflects a deeper ideological meta-narrative in contemporary policy making circles, which is inherently normative, coercive, and dismissive of individual liberty.

The book concludes with a chapter by Brian Hurwitz which considers narrative temporality in stories, clinical relationships, and case histories.

Medical processes generally unfold in a linear fashion over time. In part, this results from their depiction within a biological rather than an experiential order, and from a convention that edits out many of the twists and turns of patients' ill health experiences, particularly those thought to carry no clinical (that is, causal) significance. But as Peter Brooks has pointed out, plotting – an activity which is common to graphic and narrative depiction – links what happens (in the future) with causal determinations in reality, imagination or fiction.[49] Linear temporal unfolding, a feature of first person pathographies however richly textured, as much of case histories, is usually revealed by segmentation of the story into medico-biographical eras – before, at the beginning, during, and at the end of an illness – the tempo of each varying. Time is unevenly compressed, stretched, and gaps are created in order to generate an appropriate "bird's eye, after-the-fact version" of what happened.[50] Pathographies and case histories instantiate Paul Ricoeur's observation that "to narrate a story is already to 'reflect upon' the event narrated".[51] The narrative of fact is never a simple mirror of events. It is a recounted version of what happened.

Narrative voices

This volume demonstrates the need (and the justification) for a re-valuing of the subjective, the perspectival, and the personal in medicine and health care. But whilst there is a strong theoretical basis for promoting the principles of narrative more widely in clinical medicine, we should recognise just how profound is the change required. Byron Good, the Harvard anthropologist, has painstakingly demonstrated the difficulty medicine has in *not* excluding, let alone in coming to terms with, the subjective. Indeed, he argues that medical history taking should be seen as providing lessons in the exclusion of the subjective: "The central speech acts in medical practice are not [about] interviewing patients but presenting patients"[52] (p 78). Categories and concepts emerging in medical interviews fashion the written case history, but "the write-up is not a mere record of a verbal exchange. It is itself a formative practice, a practice that shapes talk as much as it reflects it, a means of constructing a person as a patient, a document and a project"[52] (p 77). Thereby, traditional medical education teaches students to shape and take control of the patient's oral contribution.

Howard Waitzkin sees the medical encounter as "a micro-political situation, in which the control of information reinforces power relations that parallel those in the broader society, especially those related to social class, gender, race and age".[53] In "prescribing" particular behaviours for a healthy life, for example, medical practitioners can strengthen and re-articulate particular social institutions and ideologies – most obviously by couching the possibility of future illness in terms of individual risk behaviour rather than in terms of (say) socioeconomic inequalities, gender roles, or political inaction. Simon Sinclair's ethnographic study of medical students and their education adopts a similar view. In *Making Doctors: An Institutional Apprenticeship,* he describes the important business of clerking a patient: "The history as 'given' by the student to the doctor is, in effect, a reconstruction of the patient's experience as if the patient were a doctor".[54]

Through standardised questioning and a cut and paste technique, the patient's experiential account is transformed into a medical case, consisting of presenting complaint and history. In the process of history taking and case presentation much that gave meaning to the patient's narrative is thereby eliminated. But Gilbert Lewis, a medically trained anthropologist, views the clinical case history and medical record not as "a narrative of illness, nor a description of the encounter between the doctor and the patient, but rather as a statement which combines what the patient complained of with answers to some directed questions and observations made by the doctor".[55] In his account of the case history, "the patient's own words" are on an equal footing with the doctor's questions and observations.

What Lewis' account appears to ignore is the politics of language and quotation. How much of the original meaning of what the patient says is preserved when re-sited amongst the words of others? Mishler describes the way in which doctors maintain control and continuity of discourse, by relocating patients' talk to a different semantic world.[56] In the medical interviews which Mishler analysed, the interlocutor exercises total control over both the questions asked and the shape of acceptable answers.[56] Similarly, in the composing of questions, certain kinds of structured and semi-structured interviews determine the shape of possible answers. Mishler terms this approach, the "stimulus response model" of interviewing;[57] it leaves no space for attempts by patients or ethnographic subjects to seek to renegotiate the terms of interviews, or to introduce new priorities for discussion.

Barrett, a psychiatrist turned anthropologist,[58] who has a finely tuned ear for taken-for-granted truths and metaphorical turns of phrase, sees the case history as a "segmented object", in which the distinctive contributions of nurses, social workers, and psychiatrists are hierarchically organised and welded into a "testament to consensus". His discussion of the written construction of schizophrenia shows how case notes systematically eliminate subjectivity, excluding common sense understandings and empathy, which come to be replaced by an objective distance between interviewer and interviewed.

Katherine Montgomery Hunter makes out a far more radical case for the narrative structure of medical knowledge. It is because "the imperfect fit between biological knowledge and the expression and treatment of disease in the individual leaves room for variants, surprises, anomalies"[13] (p 67) which find narrative expression in clinical anecdotes, that medical degrees have typically been divided between the biological sciences and clinical apprenticeships organised around the narrative presentation of illness as case studies. But narratives of doctors are structured by a different narrative logic from those of patients: "The determination of the diagnosis and the consequent choice of treatment bring the medical plot to a close. ... In the patient's story, closure is governed by a different plot, one which has a structure almost as invariant as the medical one. The restoration of health or its inalterable loss will close the story, just as loss of health real or foreshadowed was its genesis" (p 127). It is not that the patient's story is irrelevant to the medical story but it is swallowed up and given a new meaning by the medical story: "Once it has yielded its information, the patient's version of the events of illness, as well as the life out of which it is told, is often ignored. Like the Old Testament in the reign of the New, the patient's story has been superseded – not by being forgotten or denied or controverted but by being interpreted" and transformed (p 131). This retelling of the story affects the patient's life in different ways, "sometimes leaving scarce a mark, sometimes altering it with earthquake force" (p 132).

Despite ethnographic studies which demonstrate how far much of medicine is still removed from the principles set out in this book, the medical meta-narrative is itself changing. Once paternalistic, autocratic, and segregationist, the medical profession increasingly seeks to democratise its own ranks, work with (and learn from) other professional groups (notably nursing, sociology, economics, and ethics) in seeking to develop and promote "patient-centred" clinical care. Doctors and medical students are encouraged to adopt open-ended questioning techniques and thereby to elicit storied responses and reports (see, for example, Byrne and Long's 1976 study of doctors talking with patients[59] and, more recently, Moira Stewart et al[60]).

In his recent book *Narrative Based Primary Care*, John Launer points to the growing acceptance by doctors and health carers "that professionals do not have a monopoly on describing people's experiences when they are ill, or on telling them what to do about it"[61] (p 3). The claim to a monopoly on the truth in the past reflected a monopoly on power as much as it may have reflected a privileged method (science) for accessing a persuasive version of the truth.[62] Just as the centre of power in healthcare relations is shifting away from the grasp of professionals and towards the control of patients,[63] so the notion of healthcare truth is becoming more pluralistic and perspectival.

David Morley's collection of memoirs, poems, and short stories by patients, health carers, and writers springs from these realisations.

Commissioned and paid for by Birmingham Health Authority, which distributed 25 000 copies to its entire work force, its contributors powerfully contest the institutional, medical, authorial control of healthcare narratives. The book exemplifies an emerging dynamic of resistance to conventional institutional, professional linguistic forms of depiction in health care.[64]

In reading this volume many voices are heard. Voice draws attention to the timbre, expressiveness, and tone with which a story is told, to the presence, involvement, and moral position of its author. Voice also links to the idea of unity and control of a literary work, and to the individuality of narrators. But much as voice owes to literary and film studies, its meaning in healthcare is invigorated with politics, where it stands for the assertion of interests of previously ignored experience and points of view.[65–68] In the chapters that follow we encounter the raw presence of narrators, as in Mattingly's account of a mother's reaction to her daughter's diagnosis of a terminal illness; in a researcher's reflective voice in dialogue with earlier speakers, as in Riessman's chapter; in the effaced presence of the empirical investigator who gives focused attention to the voices of mothers accused of MSbP, as in Baldwin's chapter; in the author who *speaks out* and *speaks up* for a cause, as in Richardson's chapter; and in the voice of the frightened child-adult caught up in a disconnected world, as in Skultans' chapter.

In presenting the creative diversities of subjective and objective viewpoints that pervade healthcare practice, today, *Narrative Research in Health and Illness* engages many personal, moral, institutional, and social aspects of health, and touches on issues of power and empowerment. In the variety of interdisciplinary methods and conceptual frameworks which the volume encompasses, we venture to hope that it properly and comprehensively displays the state of narrative studies in health at the start of the twenty-first century.

Endnotes

i   Daston points out that objectivity, rather than being an unchanging benchmark for human knowledge, has a history of shifting meanings[18] (p 597). For example, objectivity refers not to attempts to eliminate the subjective idiosyncrasies of observers but also to eliminate the idiosyncrasies of the natural world in order to produce standardised working objects. The atlas became the paradigm for this kind of object in the late nineteenth century. "The atlas aims to make nature safe for science; to replace raw experience – the accidental, contingent experience of specific individual objects – with digested experience"[19] (p 85). Pictures and atlases created through mechanical techniques of reproduction came to be regarded as "the words of nature itself" (p 116). The association of standardised imagery with objectivity had important implications for the understanding of human behaviour and promoted the pictorial representation of deviant categories such as the insane and the criminal.[20] In other words, knowledge of other people was to be obtained through observation, preferably aided by mechanical standardising techniques. But the visual representation of others tells us more about the root metaphors and stereotypes of a culture than it does about lived experience.[21]

References

1   Byatt AS. *On histories and stories: selected essays.* London: Chatto & Windus, 2000, p 166.
2   Krieswirth M. Trusting the tale: the narrativist turn in the human sciences. *New Literary History* 1992;**23**:629–57.
3   Mitchell WJT, ed. *On narrative.* Chicago and London: University of Chicago Press, 1981.
4   Scholes R, Kellogg R. *The nature of narrative.* New York: Oxford University Press, 1966.
5   Chatman S. *Story and discourse: narrative structure in fiction and film.* Ithaca, NY and London: Cornell University Press, 1978.
6   Argyros A. Narrative and chaos. *New Literary History* 1992;**23**:659–73.
7   Greenhalgh T, Hurwitz B. *Narrative-based medicine: dialogue and discourse in clinical practice.* London: BMJ Books, 1998.
8   Balint M. *The doctor, the patient and his illness.* London: Pitman, 1959.
9   Kleinman A. *The illness narratives: suffering, healing and the human condition.* New York: Basic Books, 1988.
10 Brody H. *Stories of sickness.* New Haven, CT: Yale University Press, 1987.
11 Brody H. *Stories of sickness.* Oxford: Oxford University Press, 2003.
12 Mishler E. Representing discourse: the rhetoric of transcription. *Journal of Narrative and Life History* 1991;**1**(4):225–80.
13 Montgomery Hunter K. *Doctors' stories: the narrative structure of medical knowledge.* Princeton, NJ: Princeton University Press, 1991.
14 Smith R. *The human sciences.* London: Fontana, 1997.
15 Hurwitz B. *Medicine and subjectivity.* Inaugural Lecture, King's College, London, 2003.
16 Brody H. Foreword. In: Greenhalgh T, Hurwitz B, eds. *Narrative-based medicine dialogue and discourse in clinical practice.* London: BMJ Books, 1998, p xiv.
17 Wollheim R. *The thread of life.* New Haven, CT: Yale University Press, 1984, p 38.
18 Daston L. Objectivity and the escape from perspective. *Social Studies of Science* 1992;**22**:597–618.
19 Daston L, Galison P. The image of objectivity. *Representations* 1992;**40**:81–128.
20 Gilman SL. *Seeing the insane.* New York: John Wiley, 1982.
21 Radley A. Portrayals of suffering: on looking away, looking at, and the comprehension of illness experience. *Body and Society* 2002;**8**(3):1–23.
22 Nagel T. *Mortal questions.* Cambridge: Cambridge University Press, 1991.
23 Cavarero A. *Relating narratives: storytelling and selfhood.* London and New York: Routledge, 2000, p 13.
24 Davis D. Rich cases: the ethics of thick description. *Hastings Center Report* 21 July/Aug 1991:12–17.
25 Goldie P. *The emotions: a philosophical exploration.* Oxford: Clarendon Press, 2000.
26 Rorty R. *Contingency, irony and solidarity.* Cambridge: Cambridge University Press, 1989.
27 Quinn N. The cultural basis of metaphor. In: Fernandez J. *Beyond metaphor: the theory of tropes in anthropology.* Stanford, CA: Stanford University Press, 1991, p 57.
28 Turner V. *The ritual process: structure and anti-structure.* Chicago: Aldine, 1969.
29 Turner V. *The anthropology of performance.* New York: PAJ Publications, 1986.
30 Berger J. *A fortunate man: the story of a country doctor.* London: Allen Lane, 1967, p 74.
31 Jackson M. *The politics of storytelling violence, transgression and intersubjectivity.* Copenhagen: Museum, Tusculanum Press, 2002.
32 Frank A. Just listening: narrative and deep illness. *Families, Systems and Health* 1998;**16**:197–216.
33 Bakhtin MM. *Problems of Dostoevsky's poetics.* Minneapolis, MN: University of Minnesota Press, 1984, p 279.

34 Bakhtin MM. *The dialogic imagination: four essays* (trans C Emerson, M Holquist). Austin, TX: University of Texas Press, 1981.
35 Bakhtin MM. *The dialogic imagination: four essays* (trans C Emerson, M Holquist). Austin, TX: University of Texas Press, 1992.
36 Nussbaum M. *Upheavals of thought: the intelligence of emotions.* Cambridge: Cambridge University Press, 2001, p 41.
37 Nussbaum M. *Loves knowledge: essays on philosophy.* New York and London: Oxford University Press, 1990.
38 Diamond J. *C: because cowards get cancer too.* London: Vermillion Books, 1998.
39 Crossley ML, Crossley N. 'Patient' voices, social movements and the habitus; how psychiatric survivors 'speak out'. *Soc Sci Med* 2001;**52**:1477–89.
40 Dean RG. Stories of AIDS: the use of narrative as an approach to understanding in an AIDS Support Group. *Clinical Social Work Journal* 1995;**23**:287–304.
41 Frank A. *At the will of the body: perspectives on illness.* Boston, MA: Houghton Mifflin, 1991.
42 Frank A. *The wounded storyteller: body, illness, and ethics.* Chicago and London: University of Chicago Press, 1995.
43 Gould SJ. The median isn't the message. In: Greenhalgh T, Hurwitz B, eds. *Narrative-based medicine: dialogue and discourse in clinical practice.* London: BMJ Books, 1998.
44 Mattingly C, Garro LC. *Narrative and cultural construction of illness and healing.* Berkeley, CA: University of California Press, 2000.
45 Weinbren H, Gill P. Have I got epilepsy or has it got me? Narratives of children with epilepsy. In: Greenhalgh T, Hurwitz B, eds. *Narrative-based medicine: dialogue and discourse in clinical practice.* London: BMJ Books, 1998.
46 Lyotard J-F. *The postmodern condition: a report on knowledge.* Manchester: Manchester University Press, 1984, p 7.
47 MacIntyre A. *After Virtue. A Study in Moral Theory.* London: Duckworth, 1981.
48 Department of Health/Home Office. *Reforming the Mental Health Act.* White Paper. London: The Stationery Office, 2000.
49 Brooks P. *Reading for the plot: design and intention in narrative.* Oxford: Clarendon Press, 1984.
50 Davidoff D. *Who has seen a blood sugar?* Philadelphia: American College of Physicians, 1996, p 5.
51 Ricoeur P. *Time and narrative,* vol 2 (trans K McLaughlin, D Pellauer). Chicago: University of Chicago Press, 1985, p 61.
52 Good B. *Medicine, rationality and experience: an anthropological perspective.* Cambridge and New York: Cambridge University Press, 1994, pp 77, 78.
53 Waitzkin H. *The politics of medical encounters: how patients and doctors deal with social problems.* New Haven and London: Yale University Press, 1991, p 54.
54 Sinclair S. *Making doctors: an institutional apprenticeship.* Oxford and New York: Berg, 1997, p 201.
55 Lewis G. *A failure of treatment.* Oxford: Oxford University Press, 2000.
56 Mishler EG. *The discourse of medicine: dialectics of medical interviews.* Norwood, NJ: Ablex, 1984, p 123.
57 Mishler EG. *Storylines: craftartists' narratives of identity.* Cambridge, MA and London: Harvard University Press, 1999, p 150.
58 Barrett R. *The psychiatric team and the definition of schizophrenia: an anthropological study of person and illness.* Cambridge and New York: Cambridge University Press, 1996.
59 Byrne PS, Long BEL. *Doctors talking to patients: a study of the verbal behaviour of general practitioners consulting in their surgeries.* London: DHSS/HMSO, 1976, pp 143–59.
60 Stewart M, Brown JB, Weston WW, McWhinney IR, McWilliam CL, Freemna TR. *Patient centred medicine: transforming the clinical method.* London: Sage, 1995.
61 Launer J. *Narrative-based primary care.* Oxford: Radcliffe, 2002.
62 Harré R. Some narrative conventions of scientific discourse. In: Nash C, ed. *Narrative in culture.* Routledge: London and New York, 1994, pp 81–101.
63 Tattersall R. The expert patient: a new approach to chronic disease management for the twenty-first century. *Clinical Medicine* 2002;**2**:227–9.
64 Morley D. *The gift: new writings for the NHS.* Exeter: Stride Publications, 2002.

65 Robinson J. *A patient voice at the GMC*. London: Health Rights, 1988.
66 Branigan E. Story World and Screen. In Onega S, Garcia Landa A, eds. *Narratology*. Essex: Longman, 1996, p 234–248.
67 Nichols B. The voice of documentary. In: Nichols B, ed. *Movies and methods: an anthology*, vol 2. Berkeley, CA: University of California Press, 1985, pp 260–1.
68 Department of Health. *The expert patient: a new approach to chronic disease management in the twenty-first century.* London: DoH, 2001;www.ohn.gov.uk/ohn/people/expert

Section 1:
Narratives

1: The ethicality of narrative medicine

RITA CHARON

Sickness calls forth stories. Whether in the patient's "chief complaint", the intern's case presentation, the family member's saga of surgery, or the coroner's death note, patients and health professionals recognise problems, gauge progress, and lament defeat, in part, through telling about illness and having others listen. Medical ethics is no different from other aspects of clinical practice in having been found to have deep and consequential narrative roots. Those who assist individual patients to navigate the moral channels of illness have discovered that training in health law and knowledge of moral principles do not suffice to fulfil ethical duties toward the sick. They are learning that they also must equip themselves with sophisticated skills in absorbing and interpreting complex narratives of illness – the better to hear their patients, to accompany them on their journeys, and to honour what has befallen them. And, true to transformative form, narrative theory and practice have renewed and redefined the very enterprise of what used to be called bioethics.

The contemporary field of medical ethics arose in the mid-1960s in response to wrong-doing and potential wrong-doing by health professionals. Harvard anaesthesiologist Henry Beecher blew the whistle on biomedical scientists who were experimenting on patients without their consent.[1] Around the same time, medicine's growing technological ability to prolong life in the face of organ failure, starting with renal dialysis, triggered the public's anxious realisation that doctors might be in a position to decide which of us would live and which would die. From Beecher's 1966 essay in the *New England Journal of Medicine*, bioethics was conceptualised as a means to protect the patient from the doctor/scientist.[i] The bioethicist arose to intervene on the side of the patient in an adversarial relationship between doctor and patient. Hence, the early concerns of medical ethics – informed consent, safeguarding patients' autonomy, and resource allocation – arose from the formulation that doctors, left to their own devices, will exploit patients or in some way harm them and that patients need defence against them.

The assumption that the doctor–patient relationship is an adversarial one has governed the development of bioethics' agenda, training, professionalisation, and world view, in North America at least. The extreme focus on patient autonomy, for example, can only be understood if the doctor is seen as poised to take advantage of a patient for unscrupulous reasons. The middlemen and middlewomen who populate the bioethical field between doctor and patient have tended until recently to be adversarially trained in either law or juridically inflected moral philosophy. David Rothman's "strangers at the bedside" have not only been "strange" to medicine: they have been downright hostile.[2]

Once the doctor–patient dyad was conceived as an adversarial one, contractual safeguards emerged to protect the one from the other. Ethical care became governed by negotiated instruments – advance directives, Institutional Review Board protocols, informed consent processes, conflict of interest disclosures. Bioethicists joined licensing boards, insurance company functionaries, and hospital admissions privilege overseers in building a tort-based, law-enshrining enterprise for controlling doctors and protecting patients. Now, many of these protections were needed to control the abuse of power and the avarice of some within medicine and bioscience, and medicine as a whole is safer than it otherwise would be. Nonetheless, thinking of medicine as an adversarial enterprise has hurt us all deeply in unrecognised ways.

Bioethics suffered a perilous restriction of its vision and influence once it accepted – often implicitly and seemingly unconsciously – the assumption that patients must be protected from their doctors. In some ways, bioethics achieved a caricature of its own mission. Again, the example of autonomy is most telling. In their zeal to protect patients' autonomy, bioethicists designated as paternalism any expression of personal opinion or clinical counsel on the part of health professionals. So as not to manipulate patients, some doctors have ended up withholding their own viewpoints from confused patients, leaving patients and families to make their treatment choices alone. Protecting patients' autonomy, in the extreme, constitutes abandonment.

But doctor–patient relationships are *not*, or at least need not be, adversarial ones. Certainly, there can be disagreement or disappointment or defeat within these dyads. There can be misunderstandings that lead to such polarised points of view that doctor and patient see different realities. There can be, and very usually are, lapses in generosity and failures to be attuned to all of a patient's concerns. There is, more often than we realise, greed. There is sometimes, we hope rarely, sadism. And there are always differences of opinion on what, clinically, to do about any medical situation. But, with exceptions, the doctor–patient dyad is not hostile and exploitative, and to treat it as such limits tremendously its growth toward true caring.

What impresses clinicians is the tremendous range of what, most fundamentally, to do during office hours. I saw a middle-aged woman two days ago in my internal medicine practice.[ii] She was relatively new to me: profoundly depressed, non-English-speaking, with a discouraging list of ailments including atrial fibrillation with its attendant need for chronic anticoagulation, and disabling back pain unresponsive to conservative management. She lived alone in an apartment in the city with no income except a little public assistance, poverty-level rent forgiveness, and state-program coverage for her medical care. In the interval since her last visit to me, I had succeeded in appointing her to a Spanish-speaking psychiatrist – no easy task in an overburdened clinic system! – to replace the prior clinic that had treated her so demeaningly that she felt the worse for going and had lapsed from treatment. With the interpreter sitting with us in the office, we set about our work. Was I ever tempted to start right in on the anticoagulant and the clotting time and leave it at that! The woman's dense depression was so menacing, so overpowering, that I had to *force* myself to dwell in her presence. I had to quite literally sit on my hands so as not to busy myself checking her latest coagulation test results on the computer or scanning the pill bottles for their prescription renewal dates.

She did not need me to do those mechanical things, at least not at the start of our visit. She needed me to bear witness to her despair. Although there was another doctor responsible for treating her depression, I had to acknowledge the reality of her life – its painful and suffusing darkness. I knew from a previous visit that she had recently been to Latin America for the funeral of her mother. I learned on this visit that a young cousin had just died of the complications of diabetes, raising great fears in the patient that she, too, had diabetes. As a corollary, I discovered that fears of illness, realistic and not, added tremendously to the patient's burden of depression. I also learned that she liked the new psychiatrist and that attending the twice-weekly therapy group helped her.

So I began to find some solid ground for myself in relation to her, some ground, that is to say, upon which to stand that would not cave in and drop me defenceless into the morass of her depression. I could appreciate with her our success in finding a new psychiatry clinic that seemed an improvement over the last one. I could ask her straightforwardly about her mood, the acknowledgement of her depression now possible without eliciting my panicky helplessness because we had done something practical to address it. I could listen as she mourned the deaths that seemed to have occurred all around her. I could offer, quickly and with great optimism, a blood test to prove she did not have diabetes. At the same time, I could behold the tremendous courage she demonstrated by living in the face of her punishing depression. Despite the depression, she got dressed in the morning, she left the apartment, she kept her appointments, she took her medicines. What a commitment to life she demonstrated. I tried to voice my awe at her strength during our conversation.

And only then could I turn the corner toward the management of her heart disease and back pain, having not sought refuge in the body from the terror of the soul. As it turned out, our conversation about the blood tests, electrocardiographs and pills was much more brisk and efficient by virtue of our having started with her life and her mood and her fears. In effect, our medical business, by being informed by her overwhelming fears about illness and death, could proceed more effectively because I now knew how desperately she feared illness, and I could offer some aspects of her on-going treatment as a talisman for keeping well. More important in developing an effective therapeutic alliance than any technical skill was, I believe, my ability to tolerate Mrs M's profound depression and not to flee from it *because, of course, to flee from her feelings is to flee from her*.

In retrospect, as I collected myself in private in preparation for the next patient, I realised with a great sense of satisfaction that I had not abandoned her, however strong had been the temptation to do so. I had found a way to *be* with her – despite not speaking her language and despite my own experiences with depression that she forced me, briefly, to relive – so as to fulfil the duties I incurred by virtue of having heard her (or even more simply and instrumentally, the duties I incurred by virtue of having been assigned as her physician by the Medicaid bureaucracy). The satisfaction I felt was the satisfaction of an *internist* – not of an ethicist and not of a narratologist, although I am those things too – in my having found a way, today anyway, to be her doctor.

I think this picture of my office hours helps to convey what I mean to say about the doctor–patient dyad. I mean to draw attention to the tremendous benevolence available to us to do every day, the acts of goodness we can choose to perform or to omit in our clinical transactions. Not mere kindnesses, these acts contribute directly to our clinical effectiveness, and omitting them risks clinical failure. *These* are the acts of ethical medicine – not only signing the advance directive or talking about futility in the Intensive Care Unit – but these private acts that require courage and clinical common sense. What a privilege for me that, in the course of an ordinary day in practice, I am offered the chance to give this woman what I believe she needs clinically, to do so at some minor cost to myself (the sinking reminder of impending doom that surrounds us all), and to emerge from our visit feeling better than I did before it.

What would happen to bioethics if the doctor–patient dyad were to be conceptualised as an occasion for such clinically relevant goodness; if it were seen not as a contractually governed hostile relationship of exploitation but as an intersubjective personal relationship of vulnerability and trust? How would one practise bioethics if medical practice were understood as an enterprise in which one subject enters relation with another subject, both participants in the intersubjectivity illuminating one another's goals, hopes, desires, and fears, and contributing regard, trust, and courage?

Over the past decade, conventional bioethics has struggled to find its way among its chosen principles and has found itself too thin to really address actual values conflicts that arise in illness.[3] Although so-called principlist bioethics might be equipped to adjudicate appropriate surrogacy for the incapacitated terminally ill patient or to assess the risk to human subjects of a clinical research trial, it is ill equipped to guide an internist in caring for a depressed woman with heart disease or to help a paediatrician to tell parents the meaning of their 2-year-old boy's autism. Because, in part, principlist bioethics arose to deal with oppositional clinical relationships, it cannot be expected to support or to augment caring relationships.

Any number of alternative approaches to addressing the ethical problems in health care – feminist ethics, communitarian ethics, liberation ethics, phenomenological ethics, casuistry, and virtue ethics – have altered the conceptual geography of bioethics. With their foundations not in law and Anglo/continental moral philosophy but in the particularities of individuals, the singularity of beliefs, the perspectival nature of truth, and the duties of intersubjectivity, these complexly differing approaches share a commitment to narrative truth and to the power of telling and listening. They share a realisation that meaning in human life emerges not from rules given but from lived, thick experience and that determinations of right and good by necessity arise from context, plot, time, and character. These approaches do not start with an assumption that patients must be protected from their doctors. Instead, they all, in somewhat different ways, locate patients and their families *near* to those who care for them. Rather than emphasising – and therefore intensifying – the divides between patients and health professionals, these methods seek congress among human beings limited by mortality, identified by culture, revealed in language, and marked by suffering. It is not the case that some are sick and some are well but that all will die.

Although these approaches emerged quite spontaneously and simultaneously, around the mid-1980s, from such traditions as feminist studies, post-colonial studies, phenomenology, and liberation theology, they can be seen from this historical vantage point to constitute a family of narrative ethics. Indeed, the system that has ended up being called narrative ethics has borrowed tremendously from all these efforts, finding in their commonalities a core for practice.[4,5] What characterises these approaches as "narrative" is that they take as given that each sick person enters sickness singularly, that each disease signifies differently, and that each death connotes the end of its life particularly. It is the ethos of narrative ethics that one must tell of what one undergoes in order to understand it and that, as a consequence, the health professionals who accompany one through illness have a responsibility to hear one out. Among the tenets of narrative ethics are the requirements to hear all sides, to contextualise all events, to honour all voices, and to bear witness to all who suffer. Training for such practice, it follows, is textual and interior – developing the skills of close reading, reflective discernment, self-knowledge, and absorptive and accurately interpretive listening. Deriving from narrative theory as it is articulated in literary studies, phenomenology, anthropology, psychoanalysis, and qualitative social sciences, these notions join bioethics to many seemingly unrelated human enterprises like the practice of law, the profession of faith, and the understanding of human psychology. These fields, too, have been inflected by the knowledge of how stories are built and what happens when one tells or listens to them.[6,7,8]

Bioethics has been the lucky recipient of narrative dividends from intellectual and clinical developments far afield itself. Independently from any developments in bioethics, new knowledge from narrative theory and practice has made its way into medicine. Narrative studies have gradually found welcome readers and adherents among doctors, nurses, social workers, patients, and those who study medical care (indeed, this book that you are holding in your hands is one testament to the major influence narrative ways of knowing have had of late on health care).[9,10] Narrative contributions to medicine have influenced bioethics, if only by having equipped some clinicians with narrative methods of making sense of their clinical and ethical duties toward patients, methods that turn out to be more helpful than those available from principlist or legalistic bioethics. Bioethics, then, is doubly informed by narrative theory: through the developing narrative competence of its "bio" sphere (the practice of medicine) and the increasing narrative commitments of its "ethics" sphere (the practice of ethics).

Narrative influences from outside bioethics have amplified voices within bioethics that have respected stories all along. The work of religious scholar Stanley Hauerwas, for example, took on new authority once the narrativist turn was noted elsewhere in the academy.[11] Richard Zaner's phenomenology has become saturated with a respect for and insistence on narrative methods and interests.[12] Lawyer-ethicist George Annas has turned to writing plays. Inspired by such seminal texts as Alasdair MacIntyre's *After Virtue* and Bernard Williams' *Moral Luck*, philosophical bioethics has been challenged to grasp the storied elements of moral thought and the irreducibility of human plights.[13,14] Although principlist bioethics is still distantly taken up with autonomy, incapacity, and informed consent, its local practitioners have realised that they are *not* judges but listeners, *not* measuring capacity or next-of-kinhood but measuring the depth of loss.

The place of narrative in medicine and in ethics can be illuminated by recognising the place of narrative in life (and, *pari passu*, this move helps us to recognise how medicine and ethics are but instances of life). In writing about the Iranian Islamic revolution and its attendant losses of freedom, especially by Iranian women, literary scholar Azar Nafisi explains how fiction sustained her and her students through ordeals of repression.[15] Nafisi kept alive empathy, the imagination, and courage by teaching such works as *Pride and Prejudice* and "Daisy Miller," works that require their readers to inhabit alien spheres and to adopt and respect contradictory points of view, works whose protagonists develop the courage to choose freedom. Fiction's critical and irreplaceable consequences are to force readers to recognise the storied shape of reality, to understand in the most basic way that there is no meaning outside of the plots into which one weaves the fragments of life, and that one *must* choose one's plots. We make it up; in the most primal and primitive and primary way, we make it up. We do not "capture" the truth that exists around us through scientific measurements or through controlled experiments. We do not represent that which is external to us detachedly and objectively and replicably. No. Instead, we incorporate our sensations and perceptions and desires and ideas into a form which we first tell to ourselves and then might tell to others.[16,17,18] Identity itself – one's sense of being a self – arises from the crib narratives we tell as infants, the entries we hide in our adolescent diaries, the associations we voice to our analysts, and the accounts we give of ourselves when befriended, when ill, when accused, when reflecting, or when imagining.[19,20] These stories we tell merge with those we hear – in fiction, in fairy tales, in family legends, in sacred texts – in great banks of plot, great plots of grounds for knowing, for rooting, for cultivating the self.[21,22] Telling and listening to stories are as organically necessary as are the circulation of blood or the respiration of oxygen to establish and maintain a self by metabolising into it that which is non-self and then contributing products of the self back into that alien domain, thereby making it home.

I have written elsewhere about what I consider to be the most salient contributions of narrative theory to medical practice – the means to probe, honour, represent, and live in the face of temporality, singularity, intersubjectivity, causality/contingency, and ethicality.[23] What is lacking in medicine – and, I suggest here, in bioethics too – is precisely the mode of vision made possible through sophisticated narrative practice, especially in relation to these five broad areas. It is with narrative temporality that we mark the passage of time, providing those who live amid illness with the urgency and the patience to claim our numbered days and to see forward and backward toward their meaning.[24] It is with the narrative tools of description and dialogue and trope that we can render – and therefore recognise and admire – singular individuals and situations, not as instances of general phenomena but as irreducible and therefore invaluable particulars.[25] It is only with narrative effort that we achieve first the subject position and then, with luck, the intersubjective bond between ourselves and others, thereby inaugurating the therapeutic relationship.[26] It is with narrative emplotment that we attempt – often against all odds – to make causal sense of random events or humbly acknowledge the contingent nature of events that have no cause, enabling us both to diagnose disease and to tolerate the uncertainty that saturates illness.[27] Finally, it is with narrative acts and skills that we recognise and live up to the ethical duties incurred by having heard one another out and the indebtedness we sustain by having been heard by another.[28]

I run the risk of ethereality. Let us descend to 6 Garden South, the hospital floor on which, some months ago, I was ward attending, caring with my residents and medical students for severely ill patients admitted to Presbyterian Hospital with terminal cancer, end-stage renal failure, heart failure, liver failure, failure to thrive. Throughout the month we came across and found ways to live with serious ethical conflicts.

Mrs M was admitted for terminal care of Stage 4 breast cancer.[iii] Only 48 years old, she wanted badly to live, and yet the oncologists had nothing left to try. The resident complained that the patient's unrealistic sons wanted "everything done". The sons' obdurate demands for intensive medical care inflamed the resident's searing guilt that there was nothing more to do, and so he was very angry at them. I gently suggested that he ask the social worker to convene a family meeting to clarify the goals of care. The very next day, the social worker sat with both sons, their wives, the resident, the intern, and the medical student caring for the patient. With the safety of the social worker's presence, my resident was able to put into words the hopelessness of continuing treatment. He emphasised his commitment to the patient's freedom from pain and discomfort. The sons, it almost goes without saying, were exquisitely aware that their mother was dying. Their insistence that the doctor "do everything" was just the only means available to them, up until then, to register their undying loyalty and unswerving commitment to the well-being of their mother. Once my resident asked them to join with him in acknowledging that the end was near, they could surrender their stance of hostility and blame and could begin their long road of mourning.

Mr A, a middle-aged man with a long history of alcoholism, was admitted to hospital in liver failure. Another resident and intern adeptly deployed powerful diuretics, tapped fluid from the patient's abdomen, and replenished nutrients, often deficient in alcoholics. And yet the patient sank further and further into encephalopathy and coma. His mother was at his bedside, rocking and praying, even when the patient could no longer hear her. My resident and intern did not flinch, even in the face of the suspicion that their rather aggressive treatment had made matters worse, from consulting with the liver specialists, thinking through the deranged physiology involved in end-stage liver failure, and devising new approaches when the standard ones failed. What impressed me was that they did not give up. Every morning at rounds they meticulously reported all the patient's ins and outs, the results of his blood tests and scans. One morning, he woke up. He had been over a week in deep coma with all the earmarks of an irreversible vegetative state, and yet he rose. As I spoke with him that first morning, I said something in my little broken Spanish that I hoped translated to "Thank God you're alive!" And the patient winked. He winked! Imagine had we given up.

A woman was admitted as an emergency from a nearby dialysis centre with fever and evidence of bacterial sepsis, probably from an infected dialysis access graft. Another woman suffered complications from needed surgery, resulting in pulmonary and neurological compromise. These two cases made our team brood on the dangers of medicine as we know it. My young doctors were forced to ask themselves, "Are patients better off with us or without us?" When a complication occurs, however well understood and accepted its risk, one cannot help but feel responsible. The residents and interns caring for both these patients had to display enormous tact and professionalism to convey the clinical truth to the patients and their families while dealing with their own confusing calculus of benefit and risk.

What did my team learn about bioethics? We learned that the words one says – like "do everything" – can have multiple contradictory meanings and that ethical medicine requires an active intersubjective process, working against a gradient of complacency or convention or detachment, to discover the meaning of words. We learned about duty – duty in the face of self-inflicted disease, duty in the face of our own shortcomings, duty in the face of the inevitable complications of our yet-primitive medicine. Such duties are not prescribed by oversight committees or specialty boards but are discerned, over time, through a life lived humbly around illness and the consequences of trying to intervene in it. Surrendering neither to nihilism nor to deceit, my house officers fulfilled the ethical duties that accrue to their knowledge, to their loyalty toward their young science, and to their constancy in the care of individual patients.

Over the course of the month, we became all the more able to behold the singular, the mystery, the marvel. Why did Mr A wake up?

We will never know. And yet, we can celebrate, as miracle, his resurrection. We can learn from his course how to do even better with the next case of end-stage liver failure, while we can let ourselves *wonder* what happened as he slowly awakened, from how far away he travelled to open his eyes and then to wink. "I had a guy," my intern will say years from now, "who was encephalopathic even longer than your guy but he woke up. Keep giving him lactulose; diurese him gently, don't give up." We all learned about the savage contingency implicit in our work – in the occurrence of aggressive breast cancer, in the success or failure of diuresing or tapping the alcoholic, in the ways that we and our patients responded to the sickness all around us. As they told me stories at attending rounds – "This is the fourth CPMC admission for this 54-year-old chronic alcoholic with a history of DTs, positive family history of alcoholism, and multiple failed attempts at detox" – making sense in our own little way of the events of others' lives, we understood the capricious nature of our emplotment, and we recognised the artificial process by which, for our sakes alone, we impose on the contingent our sense-making plots, realising full well that as new pathophysiological explanations replace the faulty ones we live with now, the stories which we tell of what befalls our patients will change along with them.

On 6 Garden South, we did not address the ethicality of our clinical situations separately from their temporality or causality or contingency or singularity or intersubjectivity. *It happens all at once.* The ethical dimension is one facet of a narratively competent medicine, or narrative medicine for short, that occurs *while* the intersubjectively linked participants (some well, some ill) behold the singularity of one another and their situations, while they fathom where in the arc from birth to death they might be now, while they search for causes amid the random and the unfair. What humans owe to one another is not excisable, as a discrete concern, from the whole texture of how they reach one another, how they place themselves in time, how they emplot the events that occur to them, how they tolerate ambiguity or uncertainty, or how they recognise the absolute uniqueness of one another (and, in reflection, of themselves too), how they hear one another out. As a result of all these things, they perform for one another acts of goodness, their benevolence the full enactment of their science, of their justice, of their art.

We begin, then, to contemplate the consequences of choosing a new plot within which to consider medicine and its ethics. If ethics recognises medicine not as an adversarial process but rather as an on-going intersubjective commitment in the face of vulnerability and trust, what becomes of its practice?

To practise such ethics requires that practitioners, be they health professionals to begin with or not, must be prepared to offer the self as a therapeutic instrument. The ethicist must enter the clinical situation, willing to suffer in the process. If another kind of ethicist could fulfil his or her duty by hearing, in the safety of a conference room, the report of a patient's predicament and somehow making judgments from afar about the proper action to pursue, the narrative ethicist must sit by the patient, lean forward toward the person who suffers, and offer the self as an occasion for the other to tell and therefore comprehend the events of illness. This ethicist does his or her work by absorbing and containing the singular patient's plight, soliciting others' perspectives on the situation, being the flask in which these differing points of view can mingle toward equilibrium. Not all things dissolve, and so solutions are not the only end points craved by this ethics. Instead, we choose to live with the tensions of all things being said, all things being heard, sedimenting toward stillness. What the person practising narrative ethicality knows for sure is that he or she will be transformed by contributing benevolence and courage to another person's plight. Revolutionary, consequential narrative once again enacts its truth that nothing remains unchanged by story.

Let me close by reproducing for you a story written by Rose Susan Cohen, MD during her third year of medical school.[iv] We have learned that reflective writing is a powerful method for developing the textual and interior skills required of narrative ethicality. Years ago, I invented the Parallel Chart as a place where health professionals can write in non-technical language about critical aspects of their care for patients, aspects that cannot be written in the hospital chart. Clinicians and students write in the Parallel Chart about what they witness patients to endure in illness and what they themselves undergo in caring for the sick. This is an excerpt from Dr Cohen's Parallel Chart:

Altagracia. I am obsessed with her first name ... I imbue her name with spiritual, romantic, and mysterious overtones.

"Yo se que yo voy a morir en el hospital." I know that I am going to die in the hospital. Clutching her wrinkled face, which droops on the left, with her tendinous, wasted hands with papery dry purple skin, she looked at me through her claw-like fingers. She's childlike, hidden.

Failure to thrive. She won't eat. She kicks, she hits, she clutches and bends your fingers. No, you can't open her eyes to shine a light, and you can't open her mouth. She's hiding from me, deep inside her body.

Slowly, she's dying ... Her brain is 79 years old, infarcted, probably demented, but I want to believe that there is a complicated, dignified sadness in her mind that she is sequestering from the world. She lies in bed lamenting, suffering, crouching on her side, mourning mysterious and not so mysterious losses of her life.

We all shuffle into her room and peer at her. "Hola, hola," I call softly. She swats her arms and covers her face. I keep thinking about her premonition, "Yo se que yo voy a morir en el hospital." Did I really hear her say that? Did I imagine that she could speak? The attending spoke. "We need to peg her and place her."

Altagracia, graceful and seemingly out of touch, pretends we aren't there.

This beautiful, if doomed, clinical act of beholding the human mystery of this woman with humility and absorptive grace *means* something – for the student/writer and also, perhaps, for the patient. By writing this description of Altagracia, Dr Cohen takes the measure of her own awe, her loyalty to the patient, and her hopes for her own and her patient's futures. She exposes her own desires – to believe in the patient's dignity, to grant her her mystery, to distinguish herself from the insensitive attending physician, the only one in the story consigned to the past tense. The author's muscular imagination "fills in" that which dementia has erased, enabling her to treat her patient with reverence. By searching for (or by being open to) and choosing the words, the images, the time course, and the plot of this story, the author gives birth to a particular way of comprehending the events of this hospitalisation. This patient, whom the attending physician dismisses as a transfer to a nursing home once a stomach tube is placed, emerges by virtue of the writing as a mysterious, powerful, complicated woman whose difficult behaviour can be interpreted as complexly determined and connotative. She of the highest grace is the heroine and not the victim of her story, knowing that which others do not know, hiding in her wasted husk a life of great ambition. Only by having apprehended such a vision of the patient can the student care for her with benevolence and, therefore, effectiveness.

The ethics I have described in this chapter and that are teachable through narrative training are within-medicine ethicality, not without-medicine bioethics. This ethicality is not one that one can "contract out", that one can surrender to another to perform. Nor is it applied only when certain topics arise – futility of treatment, for example, or protection of human research subjects. Governing clinical actions at all times, narrative ethicality endows the practitioner with an eternal awareness of the vulnerability and the trust of self and other. A narrative ethicality saturates the doctor, nurse, social worker, or ethicist with the sensibility and the skill to recognise and to fulfil the duties incurred by intersubjective nearness, by mutual singularity, by knowledge of causes, and by the sense that time, by its nature, runs out. If sickness calls forth stories, then healing calls forth a benevolent willingness to be subject to them, subjects of them, and subjected to their transformative power.

Endnotes

i The term "bioethics" was coined around the same time by two persons. Sergeant Shriver came up with the word to denote the new ethics-for-medicine institute being established by the Kennedy family at Georgetown University. What Shriver meant by the term was the rather instrumental application of legal and philosophical principles to solve dilemmas in medical research and practice. Physician Van Rensselaer Potter also created the word, but in his hands it denoted a "science for survival", that is, an environmentally inclusive effort to live, as humans, in concert with the universe with a recognition that the biological life interacts with the moral life. Evidently, the first definition ascended, although the second may be emerging from the cosmic shadows. See Martensen R. Thought styles among the medical humanities: past, present, and near-term future. In: Carson RA, Burns CR, Cole RG, eds. *Practicing the medical humanities: engaging physicians and patients.* Hagerstown, MD: University Publishing Group, 2003, pp 99–122.

ii I have merged the descriptions of several patients I saw during one morning in practice to make my point, and so I have not elicited consent to publish this description, as it does not actually "belong" to any one of the several men and women who are part of this portrait.

iii These patients are unrecognisable composites of many patients my team cared for over the month.

iv Dr Cohen has consented, in writing, to my publishing this excerpt of her writing.

References

1 Beecher HK. Ethics and clinical research. *N Engl J Med* 1966;**74**:1354–60.
2 Rothman D. *Strangers at the bedside: a history of how law and bioethics transformed medial decision making.* New York: Basic Books, 1991.
3 Dubose ER, Hamel RP, O'Connell LJ, eds. *A matter of principles? Ferment in US bioethics.* Valley Forge, PA: Trinity Press International, 1994.
4 Charon R, Montello M, eds. *Stories matter: the role of narrative in medical ethics.* New York: Routledge, 2002.
5 Nelson HL, ed. *Stories and their limits: narrative approaches to bioethics.* New York: Routledge, 1997.
6 Bruner J. *Making stories: law, literature, life.* New York: Farrar, Straus & Giroux, 2002.
7 Hauerwas S, Jones LG, eds. *Why narrative? Readings in narrative theology.* Eugene, OR: Wipf and Stock, 1997.
8 Sarbin TR. *Narrative psychology: the storied nature of human conduct.* New York: Praeger, 1986.
9 Charon R. Narrative medicine: a model for empathy, reflection, profession, and trust. *JAMA* 2001;**286**:1897–902.
10 Greenhalgh T, Hurwitz B. *Narrative-based medicine: dialogue and discourse in clinical practice.* London: BMJ Books, 1998.
11 Burrell D, Hauerwas S. From system to story: an alternative pattern for rationality in ethics. In: Engelhardt HT, Callahan D, eds. *The foundations of ethics and its relationship to science: knowledge, value, and belief,* vol 2. Hastings-on-Hudson, NY: Hastings Center, 1977.
12 Zaner R. Sisyphus without knees: exploring self-other relationships through illness and disability. *Literature and Medicine* 2003;**22**:188–207.
13 MacIntyre A. *After virtue: a study in moral theory,* 2nd ed. Notre Dame, IN: University of Notre Dame Press, 1984.
14 Williams B. *Moral luck: philosophical papers, 1973–1980.* Cambridge and New York: Cambridge University Press, 1981.
15 Nafisi A. *Reading Lolita in Tehran: a memoir in books.* New York: Random House, 2003.

16 Aristotle. *Poetics* (trans GF Else). Ann Arbor: University of Michigan Press, 1970.
17 James H. *The art of the novel* (ed. RR Blackmur). New York and London: Charles Scribner's Sons, 1934.
18 Forster EM. *Aspects of the novel*. New York: Harcourt, Brace & Company, 1927.
19 Eakin PJ. *How our lives become stories: making selves*. Ithaca, NY: Cornell University Press, 1999.
20 Kerby AP. *Narrative and the self*. Bloomington, IN: Indiana University Press, 1991.
21 Bruner J. *Actual minds, possible worlds*. Cambridge, MA: Harvard University Press, 1986.
22 Trilling L. *The liberal imagination: essays on literature and society*. New York: Viking Press, 1950.
23 Charon R. *Narrative medicine*: Honoring the Stories of Illness. New York: Oxford University Press, (forthcoming).
24 Ricoeur P. *Time and narrative*, 3 vols (trans D Pellauer, K McLaughlin). Chicago: University of Chicago Press, 1984–1988.
25 Rimmon-Kenan S. *Narrative fiction: contemporary poetics*, 2nd ed. New York: Routledge, 2003.
26 Levinas E. *Entre-nous: on thinking-of-the-other*. New York: Columbia University Press, 1998.
27 Brooks P. *Reading for the plot: design and intention in narrative*. New York: Knopf, 1984.
28 Booth W. *The company we keep: an ethics of fiction*. Chicago: University of Chicago Press, 1988.

2: Soldiers become casualties: doctors' accounts of the SARS epidemic

EUGENE WU, FRANCES RAPPORT, KIP JONES, TRISHA GREENHALGH

Box 2.1 Extract from *The Lancet* 2003;361:1520–1

Haemorrhagic-fever-like changes and normal chest radiograph in a doctor with SARS, by Eugene B Wu and Joseph JY Sung, Departments of Medicine and Therapeutics, Prince of Wales Hospital, Shatin, New Territories, Hong Kong, People's Republic of China

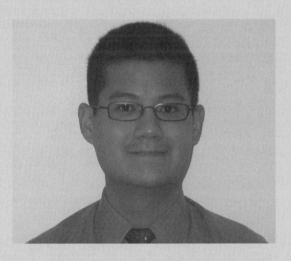

The index case of severe acute respiratory syndrome (SARS)[1] was admitted to ward 8A in the Prince of Wales Hospital, Hong Kong, on March 4, 2003. [2] On March 10, 2003, a 33-year-old doctor (EBW) working on ward 8A developed a fever of 39·6 °C. He was examined by JJYS. His fever had gone by March 12, and his chest radiograph was normal. His platelet count was 94×10^9/l and white-cell count was $3·4 \times 10^9$/l (monocytes $0·4 \times 10^9$/l). A nasopharyngeal swab grew no pathogens. He was admitted to the SARS triage

(Continued)

Box 2.1 *(Continued)*

ward on March 13, and was started on oseltamivir phosphate 75 mg twice a day and levofloxacin 500 mg daily. Further blood tests showed disseminated intravascular coagulopathy (platelets 61×10^9/l, D-dimer 630 ng/ml, prothrombin time 11·1 s, activated partial thromboplastin time (APTT) 43·3 s). His white-cell count was $1·8 \times 10^9$/l (neutrophils $1·1 \times 10^9$/l, lymphocytes $0·5 \times 10^9$/l, and monocytes $0·2 \times 10^9$/l. His chest radiograph showed a prominent right hilum. CT of his thorax showed an ill-defined opacity with an air bronchogram in the apical posterior segment of the right lower lobe and diffusely in the right middle lobe. He was started on oral ribavirin 1·2 g thrice daily and intravenous methylprednisolone 500 mg daily. His fever settled the next morning and his coagulopathy improved (APTT 40·7 s, platelet count 105×10^9/l, and D-dimer of 564 ng/ml). On March 19, 2003, oral prednisolone 1 mg/kg was started.

On the evening of March 20, he had a fever of 38·9 °C. His white blood cell count rose to $15·7 \times 10^9$/l (predominantly due to an increase in neutrophils). A secondary bacterial chest infection was suspected, and cefipime 2 g was given intravenously. Over the next 2 days he became increasingly breathless and his coagulopathy became worse (D-dimer 716 ng/ml, prothrombin time 11·9 s, platelets 199×10^9/l). The patient was given a single dose of methylprednisolone 500 mg intravenously and 4 l/min of oxygen. After this, he began to get better. Coagulation parameters returned to normal, he was weaned off of oxygen, and was discharged from hospital on March 31, 2003, on 0·3 mg/kg prednisolone and ribavirin 600 mg orally three times a day. On April 7, his chest radiograph showed worsening consolidation of the consolidation of the right middle zone and the prednisolone was increased to 0·5 mg/kg.

References

1 Centres for Disease Control and Prevention 2003. Severe acute respiratory syndrome (SARS). Atlanta: http://www.cdc.gov/ncidod/sars/ (accessed April 8, 2003).
2 Anon. Updated interim case definition. Update: outbreak of severe acute respiratory syndrome – worldwide, 2003 *MMWR* 2003;**52**:241–8.

In the early days of the SARS (severe acute respiratory syndrome) epidemic, a young Hong Kong physician, working on an emergency ward that was rapidly filling with patients suffering from a new, obscure, and (as it emerged) often fatal chest infection, himself developed symptoms of the disease. His duty colleague, Dr Joseph JY Sung, examined him, confirmed the diagnosis, and admitted him to his own ward – where he developed some unusual complications before making a protracted recovery. The two doctors subsequently wrote up their experience as a "research letter" and published it in *The Lancet* (Box 2.1).[1]

In the same issue of *The Lancet*, Professor Brian Tomlinson and Dr Charles Cockram wrote an account of the epidemic from the perspective of the medical director of a modern, well-equipped teaching hospital whose staff faced a real risk of dying from this illness at a time when its pathological basis was still a mystery and its treatment highly experimental (Box 2.2 below).[2] Both accounts were strikingly dispassionate and written in an impersonal, telegraphic style, lacking emotion as required by modern scientific journals. The underlying story of professional heroism, altruism, and fear for personal safety was conspicuous by its absence. We invited Dr Wu to provide a more personal account of his own illness (Box 2.3 below), and, with the authors' generous consent, analysed the three pieces from a narrative perspective.

The narrative in Box 2.1 (Drs Wu and Sung's article in *The Lancet*) is constructed as a linear journey from health to life-threatening illness and back to health, mapped in relation to diagnosis, illness pathway, and treatment. It is a sobering story, following the route of high fever, rise in white blood cell count, increasing breathlessness, medication, and eventual recovery – somewhat against the odds. The story in Box 2.2 (Professor Tomlinson and Dr Cockram's discussion of the epidemiology of SARS) is, similarly, a story of precise factual detail, focusing on the number of people presenting, manifestations of presentation, spread of disease, and efforts to treat and contain the epidemic.

Both stories are delineated by the facts offered up. Tomlinson and Cockram's story, for example, concentrates on the rapidity with which the epidemic took hold, the proportion of cases with high fever, the speed of physical deterioration in victims' health, and the sense of an overwhelming lack of knowledge surrounding the disease's natural history and possible curtailment. Also striking is the impersonal manner in which the stories are portrayed – matter-of-fact and devoid of sentiment. Given the implicit human drama of the events, both these factual accounts lack an element of knowing that must have surely been recognised and considered by the writers involved. Consequently, each begs the identity of a narrator who, if present, would enable us to "know" the story more keenly and relate to the illness experience more readily.

When writing their articles for *The Lancet*, Drs Wu and Sung, Tomlinson and Cockram were inevitably influenced by conventions of journal style and the "medical template" for reporting diseases. They chose an empirical approach, nothing more but nothing less. No narrative of grief, portent, anxiety, fear, pain, suffering, despair or hope for these writers, even though (and this is the rub) this may be what the reader most wishes to hear. The smiling photograph of Dr Wu, published in *The Lancet* (much against its usual editorial conventions), makes a silent announcement: "here I am". The image reaches out to the reader in a way the text pointedly resists doing.

Gergen[3] argues (p 6) that the words and stylistic conventions used in medical journal reports "derive their meaning from the attempt of people to coordinate their actions within various communities". Furthermore, as the biochemical data and other test results presented in Box 2.1 illustrate, these linguistic conventions evolve over time into codified symbols with the ability to compress large amounts of assumed knowledge and background information and deliver it for their intended audiences (and, by intention or coincidence, to withhold such information from others). The members of different groups of scientists, policymakers, campaigning communities and so on go through a lengthy socialisation process to enable them to produce and understand papers comprised of a kind of "shop talk" that heightens participation in the language game, enabling them to ring-fence their areas of expertise.

This professional "codification" produces icons with the accumulated power to persuade, convince, establish authority, and represent authenticity, but which through this very process carries the inevitability of skewing and/or stifling wider community discourse and input. Left out of the mix in the standard scientific report is a consideration by authors and publishers of their own participation in, and communication with, the larger community to which we all claim membership. The extreme restraints on exposing the personal that have been self-imposed by and superimposed upon Drs Wu and Sung in their article in *The Lancet* are presumably intended to illuminate a particular scientific discovery. At the same time, their absence leaves the reader oddly dissatisfied.

Two things heighten the reader's sense of anxiety about the piece: First, it is written in the third person, yet written in part by the very person to whom these events happened. Second, it is presented at a time when the general public know very little about SARS and its consequences. Although doctors at the time perceived a palpable desire for "facts" about SARS, the need for emotional consensus was arguably just as compelling, but less readily expressed by the medical community.

These authors gave crisp scientific accounts that clearly met the expectations of *The Lancet's* editor and readership for style and "storyline". Those who submit papers to medical journals do not generally expect these aspects of their work to be challenged beyond the benchmark of the journal's "instructions to authors". But when we considered their published work – with their permission – through a more critical lens, we found much revealed in the very style and storyline. Alphonso Lingis, discussing "exposure through presentation", says "to enter into a conversation with another is ... to throw open the gates of one's own positions; to expose oneself to the other, the outsider; and to lay oneself open to surprises, contestation, and inculpation ...".[4] If we follow Lingis' argument, it is through our surprise and questioning of the style taken by the authors that we find the missing person in the tale.

The issue of "personhood" is central to the phenomenological school of philosophy, which is interested more in the person who writes or paints, reads the tale or views the painting, than in the act of writing or painting itself. In the words of Merleau-Ponty, "Perception is not a science of the world … it is the background from which all acts stand out, and is presupposed by them." From a phenomenological perspective, the focus of the story is (in Box 2.1) the absent person who wonders, for example, if and when he will die, and whether his family will be spared, and (in Box 2.2) the absent person who feels acutely that his hospital is under the world's gaze and wonders who of his devoted staff will lose their young lives to this illness.

Phenomenological analysis is based on the precept that any phenomenon must be "placed concretely in the lifeworld so that the reader may experientially recognise it". Van Manen[5] (p 351) talks of understanding as a "lived throughness". "Lived throughness" illustrates the subject's desire to really experience the phenomenon from a personal perspective.

But what of our perception of these two articles? How can we experience a "lived throughness" of these stories, when we ourselves may have no experience of the SARS phenomenon and when the perceiving subject has been so expertly edited out? Phenomenology argues that all perception is embodied. Merleau-Ponty[6] comments that intentions cannot be separated out from that which is perceived and Dahlberg and Dahlberg[7] comment (p 7): "the perceiving and the perceived are inseparable". We project ourselves subjectively, yet the process of projection intertwines us with our object, "just as the sleeping is one with [our] slumber" (p 7). Consequently, through perception the possibilities of the world are shown to us as we use our bodies as "the vehicle of being in the world" (p 82), making sense of possibility through perceived embodiment with the world. Offering an example of embodied perception, Dahlberg and Dahlberg suggest: "when I see the front of the house, it tells me that I am able to walk around the house. My body is the non-perceived center towards which all objects turn their sides" (p 6). Thus our consideration of these articles, through embodied perception, encourages us to walk around the edges of the stories, to see beyond factuality to the humanism hidden on the other side. Phenomenology would account for this drive as an aspect of our integrality with the lifeworld. It is our need to experience, because "Being-in-the-world" in this way is the fundamental ontology that suggests we can do no other.[8,9]

The person who reads the article by Dr Wu, who survived to provide his account of SARS, unconsciously seeks, through embodied perception, to be integrally at one with the person belying the tone of the text. We recognise the personal in all its richness and poignancy though it was never told and never need be told, and through an imagined humanistic interpretation of events, appreciate more fully the facts under scrutiny. Though the personal may never be forthcoming, by extracting the story we find most lacking, we make of it our own, creating the story we are most longing to hear.

Box 2.2 Extract from *The Lancet* 2003;361:1486–7

SARS: experience at Prince of Wales Hospital, Hong Kong, by Brian Tomlinson and Clive Cockram, Department of Medicine and Therapeutics, Chinese University of Hong Kong, Prince of Wales Hospital, Hong Kong SAR, People's Republic of China

... The first cases probably occurred in Guangdong Province in southern China in November, 2002. The term SARS appears to have been first used for a patient in Hanoi who became ill on Feb 26, 2003, and was evacuated back to Hong Kong where he died on March 12. The physician who raised the alarm in Hanoi, Carlo Urbani, subsequently contracted SARS and died. The first case in Hanoi had stayed at a hotel in Kowloon, Hong Kong, at the same time as a 64-year-old doctor who had been treating pneumonia cases in southern China. This doctor was admitted to hospital on Feb 22, and died from respiratory failure soon afterwards. He was the first known case of SARS in Hong Kong and appears to have been the source of infection for most if not all cases in Hong Kong as well as the cohorts in Canada, Vietnam, Singapore, USA, and Ireland, and subsequently Thailand and Germany.

The index patient at PWH was admitted on March 4, 2003, and had also visited this hotel. He had pneumonia which progressed initially despite antibiotics, but after 7 days he improved without additional treatment. On March 10, 18 health-care workers at PWH were ill and 50 potential cases among staff were identified later that day. Further staff, patients, and visitors became ill over the next few days and there was subsequent spread to their contacts. By March 25, 156 patients had been admitted to PWH with SARS, all traceable to this index case. One important factor in the extensive dissemination of infection appears to have been the use of nebulised bronchodilator, which increased the droplet load surrounding the patient. Overcrowding in the hospital ward and an outdated ventilation system may also have contributed.

... Procedures causing high risk to medical personnel include nasopharyngeal aspiration, bronchoscopy, endotracheal intubation, airway suction, cardiopulmonary resuscitation, and non-invasive ventilation procedures. Cleaning the patient and the bedding after faecal incontinence also appears to be a high-risk procedure.

... Long hospital stays, even in less ill patients, are required, and the high proportion of patients requiring lengthy intensive care, with or without ventilation (23% in the 138 cases from PWH), and the susceptibility of health-care workers bodes ill for the ability of health-care systems to cope. Even when the acute illness has run its course, unknowns remain. Continued viral shedding and the possible development of long-term sequelae, such as pulmonary fibrosis or late post-viral complications, means that patients will require careful surveillance.

This Commentary is dedicated to the frontline health-care staff who have shown courageous devotion to duty throughout this epidemic.

Our examination of multiple commentaries around the same theme reveals not only the many layered patterns of understanding that can be acquired through the process of telling and experiencing, but also an appreciation of each commentary as an end in itself. Each stands alone in its aspect, offering the factual, the emotive, the "human", the autobiographical – neither more nor less revealing, more nor less precise, more nor less integral to our overall understanding of the SARS epidemic than the commentary that came before it. Grouped together as these commentaries are in this chapter, we are provided, not with a single revelation, but with a plurality of revelations, experiences and opportunities and as such, are encouraged to bear witness to the uniqueness of the parts and the solidarity of the whole.

Tomlinson and Cockram's editorial in *The Lancet* (Box 2.2) was one of the first scientific overviews of the SARS epidemic, and appeared as something of a refreshing counterpoint to prevailing media stories which had hit the airwaves with a vengeance in early 2003.

Media reports were notable for their lack of objective truth and their heavy and often inappropriate use of imagery and metaphor. One of the most startling images was the picture of quarantined patients in Taiwan threatening to throw themselves from the windows of the hospital building where they were "imprisoned". Visually, the SARS epidemic seemed to have taken on the dynamics of a hostage situation, and the image of patients attempting to escape from their doctors, even if death ensued, poignantly illustrated the confusion and terror surrounding its management.

In a BBC programme televised in the spring of 2003 entitled, "SARS – The True Story", produced for Horizon, the programme-makers wonder if SARS would be "worse than Aids". The programme is replete with military metaphors: "borders closed", "containment", "battles won", "WHO war plan", "WHO's most powerful weapon", "defence mechanisms", "the full force of scientific might", and so on. The disease is imbued with its own military tactics: it is "on the loose" and it "penetrates, takes over and reproduces", and that "rumours are deadly". Interestingly, viewers were also told that SARS was now an "official threat" because WHO had "named the demon".[i]

Susan Sontag, in her exquisitely written book, *Illness as metaphor: Aids and its metaphors*,[10] used examples from literature and the arts to place a historical perspective on how we talk about illness and death and how such talk often uses military metaphors. In the twenty-first century, where illness itself can become a weapon of warfare, the metaphor seems to have come full circle.

In narrative terms, these two accounts present us with what Wengraf[11] (p 232) and others refer to as the "lived life" (Boxes 2.1 and 2.2) as opposed to the "told story" (Box 2.3), both components of any "good" story. The lived life presents us with plain facts: the "who, what, when and where" that are the skeleton of any report, even dispassionate media stories. Nonetheless, possible outcomes can be induced from the bare bones of the "lived life" apparatus of a story, just as the Tomlinson and Cockram editorial in *The Lancet* (Box 2.2) demonstrates. It is in the "told story", however, that narrators create their own individual gestalt or world view woven from the facts and accounts of what they have to say about the "who, what, when and where". The *"told story"*, or thematic ordering of the narration, involves the construction of the narrators' systems of knowledge, their interpretations of their lives, and their classification of experiences.

One or the other leads to audience dissatisfaction. In the end, told stories and lived lives always come together. They are continuously dialectically linked and produce each other; this is the reason why we must hear both levels no matter whether our main target is the lived life or the told story.[12] It is by "listening" to Eugene's told story through his diary entries that these links are finally made, satisfying the audience.

Box 2.3 SARS – a personal account by Dr Eugene Wu

10 March 2003
The secure familiarity of my usual Monday morning ward round is disrupted when I notice many of the nurses on the ward wearing facemasks. The ward sister informs me that a number of patients with undiagnosed chest infections have spiked a fever this morning. Since I have been working on the ward for several months, I figure I am probably already infected by this presumed viral illness. Sure enough, that evening I become pyrexial.

12 March 2003
I return to the hospital for review and as I walk onto the observation ward, I am shocked to find almost half my colleagues in our cardiac team sitting in hospital beds. They all look reasonably well at this stage and the atmosphere is one of optimism about our health and scepticism about the necessity of our admission. Today, my temperature has settled and my chest X-ray is clear and so I am allowed home. I leave gleefully, under the envious gaze of my bed-bound colleagues, feeling that I have probably escaped more serious problems.

14 March 2003
Following an abnormal blood test, I am called back to the hospital for review and am admitted from casualty. As I walk onto the triage ward for SARS, I have a strong sense of déjà vu. Although the ward is very familiar to me, everything seems different as I am in a different role. Lying in the bed is a lot more frightening than standing at the end of it in a white coat! In all those years doing ward rounds, I never realised that it was so frightening for the person in the sickbed. I wonder whether the reassurance I tried to give as a doctor was enough to overcome their fear. On the other hand, I realise that many of the

patients I usually see have chronic illnesses or are in hospital for a simple procedure and their fear is probably less. I find it very hard to express my own fear to the doctors who see me. They are excellent doctors, but the doctor patient encounter on a busy ward round seems an inappropriate context for the expression of fear. If I recover and am able to resume my practice of medicine, I hope to use the ward round as an opportunity to pick up an inkling of fear in my patients, and then return to these patients at a different time, outside the ward round situation, to try to comfort their fears.

15 March 2003
A fellow doctor from my team is admitted onto our ward. When we go to welcome his arrival, we see with alarm that he is extremely short of breath, managing only 88% oxygen saturation on 100% oxygen. He is cold, clammy, disorientated, hypoxic, and basically at death's door. A decade of admitting medical patients from accident and emergency has instilled in me an alarm bell that sounds out loud in my mind: "This man needs intensive care immediately." This disease can make a perfectly healthy young man into an ICU candidate in a matter of days.

17 March 2003
It's now the seventh day since the onset of my symptoms and things are not looking good. My blood test results are worsening day by day and my temperature chart resembles a mountaineer's dream! Over the past few days there has been a change of mood on the ward. The earlier optimism has been replaced by terror. Every day, one or more of our colleagues on the ward becomes more breathless. We watch from our beds as one after another is transferred to intensive care, much like prison inmates watching others taken to execution.

Like a man whose taste buds are hit by a hot curry, we are becoming painfully aware of the contagiousness and ferocity of this virus as more and more staff fall ill to it while looking after those who are already infected. Soldiers became casualties, aid workers became victims. A sense of helplessness combines with fear. Many of us are thinking, will we get through this?

I am getting more and more concerned about my own survival. I try to think of what things I have left undone in my life, but am too feverish to make any sense. I have been waiting to do final corrections on my MD thesis from the University of London, and I figure if I die, they might grant me the degree out of compassion. On the other hand, what would I do with a MD after death?

A new drug combination – steroids and ribavarin – was suggested to us today. This treatment was apparently what the doctors in China used to treat atypical pneumonia. In the absence of a better option we agree to use this cocktail. As I sit looking at the methylprednisolone dripping into my arm, I can't help wondering whether this is a bad mistake, or good therapy.

18 March 2003
In most known causes of fever, the temperature would diminish with steroids. So the downward trend of fever this morning offers little confirmation about the therapeutic value of the drugs we took yesterday. On the other hand, after seven straight days of high fever, it is some relief to find myself awakening fever free. With a more alert mind and symptomatic improvement, I turn to read from the Bible on my bedside cupboard. "He allowed no one to oppress them; for their sake He rebuked kings. 'Do not touch my anointed ones; do my prophets no harm'" (Psalm 105:14–15).

(Continued)

Box 2.3 *(Continued)*

The image of God protecting His people and pushing away those who may harm them replaced my fears with a sense of security. At this stage, the feeling that God is attending to my illness is more important than how my illness appears to be progressing on paper.

23 March 2003
Yesterday the nurses kept telling me that my oxygen saturation was not good – around 92%. I felt fine. I don't see how a healthy 33-year-old should need oxygen, but if it makes the nurses happier, I will go along with the treatment. Today, I take off my oxygen to go to the bathroom and on returning I feel very dizzy – almost collapsing. A nurse comes to my aid and records my saturation to be 88%. Since then, I have been banned from coming off oxygen. I never realised oxygen dependency was such a bind. You are tied to the wall supply like a dog on a leash. Anywhere I want to go, I must justify getting a porter and a wheelchair with tanked oxygen. It's easier to stay put.

26 March 2003
After four days on oxygen, tied to the leash, frustration is beginning to dominate my emotional horizon. Thankfully, today I finally manage to wean off oxygen with a saturation of 94%.

A young doctor in our department, whom I have known since he was a third year medical student, is admitted with SARS today after looking after us on the ward. I feel a little guilty, although I am not sure I was "the one" to infect him. Fortunately, he seems totally well and is walking around the ward, but from my own experience, I know that this disease tends to do its worst damage in the second week.

28 March 2003
It is amazing how quickly frustration and fear turn to boredom once you are well. The last few days in hospital have been mind numbing. Watching the news for the seventh time today was a highlight in itself. There is only so much reading, thinking, pondering, and chatting on the phone one can do. Tomorrow, the first cohort of doctors and nurses who were infected will leave, many of them from this ward. I am not keen to be left behind here, so have opted to go to a rehabilitation hospital to sit out my remaining three days.

1 April 2003
O Joyous day! Discharge day. One of the most difficult things about this illness has been the complete isolation. From the first day of my illness, I knew that this was contagious and had already asked my wife to sleep in a separate bedroom and to wear a facemask. During the first half of my hospital stay, only spouses were allowed to visit with full protective gear. In the latter half, no visitors were allowed whatsoever. So for almost three weeks, I have had no outside contact apart from my masked wife. Even so, every time she came in to visit, I was worried that she would become infected and so asked her to stay only for a short while. On top of the physical isolation, there was also profound emotional isolation. I was aware that my family was on the edge of not coping with the whole situation. How does one tell a very anxious mother that you have DIC? How does one tell one's wife that one is requiring more oxygen today when she is already on the brink of tears? I chose not to, but felt increasingly like I was standing alone upon a tall growing pole in the desert.

On going home today, the isolation situation remains uncertain since we do not know how infectious we are. We have been advised to remain in isolation at home for a week. So instead of the happy reunion hugs, my family and I shared a 3 metre distanced masked chat, which felt distinctly incongruous.

10 April 2003

The curtain of fear about my family's health is finally removed when my viral culture results return clear. However, the physical gap that protected my wife has left behind a shadow of itself, much like a phantom limb. I am not sure whether this is due only to the long period of separation, or whether part of it is also about my change in body image. The long period of steroid use has produced a classical "lemon on sticks" look. I first noticed this after I came off oxygen in hospital when I went for a shower. I was struck by how odd my shape has become. I somehow cannot believe that these thin limbs belong to me. Even though I have never put much of my self-esteem upon my physical appearance, this dramatic change has made me feel that I have become very odd.

Postscript

On discharge, we all thought that our chest X-rays would clear up within a week. Of course, this did happen to some, but many of us had residual shadowing. Three and a half months out from my first symptom, my right lower lobe is still hazy. Every clinic feels like Groundhog Day – a rerun of last visit – "your lungs are still not clear – go take more steroids – see you in x weeks again". Frustration with the tedious nature of this disease is worsened as the euphoric side effect of the steroids diminishes as the dose is reduced. There is quite a lot to come to terms with. The cushingoid "lemon on stick" look is not exactly in fashion right now. Muscle wasting that does not respond to weight training will no doubt win me the slowest progress award at my gym. The combination of facemask and steroids do wonders for acne. Fortunately, we can cover them up with ever increasing size facemasks.

My residual worries over my younger colleague who caught the illness while looking after us were confirmed. He became more breathless and was admitted into ICU. He suffered a long and horrible period during his second week. I spoke to him briefly on the phone, but he was too breathless to carry much of a conversation. I rang up several of our fellow Christian doctors and we prayed for his healing that evening. Many others were seriously ill at this stage and I felt really helpless. Many doctors, nurses, and health care assistants who were ill at the same time as myself have not made good progress and remain in ICU. As time passed, their condition became more and more irreversible and their prognosis increasingly grim. It seems there was no way out apart from going through the mortuary. The death of the first staff nurse in Hong Kong was a harsh blow upon the already low morale of the staff. As more doctors and nurses died, I felt a combination of sad loss and anger. Something ought to be done to stop the continuing infection of staff. For this loss of life, doing everything to prevent further infection will not be enough, for the death itself is already too much to bear.

In the 10 years of being a doctor, life has been running on a very hectic schedule. On calls, clinical work, research projects, MRCP exams, MD thesis, training, altogether keeps one very busy indeed. For once, I have three months of sick leave. The sudden and dramatic amount of time and space seem to worsen the vacuum left by this illness. I felt helpless and useless and spent my time writing articles, doing research, visiting, and encouraging others who

(Continued)

> **Box 2.3 (Continued)**
>
> *were recovering. I long to return to work, if only to relieve the boredom, but also to see how resuming the opposite role is like. Several recovered doctors met for lunch today and I raised the question as to whether they would consider continuing in medicine if they caught SARS again next year. Some said they would, some said they would not. I think being a doctor is a calling, a calling to help those in need. A calling is not something we give up on in the face of adversity. Yet I admitted, perhaps by the third time I caught SARS, I might reconsider my "calling".*

Eugene Wu's diary entries provide the human story so necessary in making sense of SARS that was so strikingly lacking in *The Lancet* pieces and in the early media reports. Part of being human and engaging as a storyteller's audience is our need for a "good" story, ie, one that has a beginning, a middle, and an end; that has coherence and "moral order" (for example an appropriately happy or tragic ending); that has authenticity (events and reactions "ring true"); and in which we ourselves can identify strongly with the narrator or one of the characters.[13] There also needs to be a storytelling lexicon and history shared between the narrator and the listener. Without these things, stories can fall flat because they fail to satisfy the emotional needs and storytelling requirements of the human listener.

Eugene's follow-up diary entries fill this gap. They tell a story in his own words of disruption, shock, worry, frustration, helplessness, pain, and fear. The reader, alerted to SARS and its devastation by the media, immediately identifies with these emotions in Eugene's diary entries and can imagine her/himself experiencing the same reactions if she or he were faced with the disease personally. All this said, Eugene's is also a story of optimism and diminished fear through spiritual strength. The story tells how one man experiences SARS and tries to make sense of it through the irony that "soldiers became casualties, aid workers became victims".

Eugene takes us on a journey from his beginnings in the security of his familiar role as healer, reporting on the envious gaze of his unwell peers around him, through the point where he joins them in this unwanted mutual experience. He presents himself "suddenly, in a different role" – a lesson that could have benefited *The Lancet* audience had it been presented in that forum. He wonders, "Will we get through this?" This Parsifalian[ii] transformation of the hero represents the key moment when the audience becomes transfixed by the story, identifying with the narrator in his abrupt metamorphosis. It is the point in the story where the reader joins the narrator on his journey. When the narrator exclaims, "Will we get through this?" it is an invitation to the reader to join him – the situation is, in Van

Manen's words,[5] "placed concretely in the lifeworld" (p 351), so that the reader may experientially recognise it. The reader responds, "Yes, I understand your fear and uncertainty and join you, but we *must* continue on." Such collusion between storyteller and audience is necessary if we are to find the experience (as extraordinary as it may be) "ordinary" and, therefore, believable as shared experience. Its "ordinariness" is not in the details, but rather our shared response to them. From this point on the audience is won over and identifies with the narrator, win or lose.

Eugene's diary is brought to life through metaphor, simile, and imagery. His "chart resembled a mountaineer's dream". The awareness of the ferocity of the virus hits him "like a man whose taste buds are hit by a hot curry". The dehumanising impact of being attached to oxygen is like being "a dog on a leash", and his illness hangs over his altered relationship with his wife "like a phantom limb". Through such imagery, Eugene becomes the adventurer of many of the stories we have read, facing whatever adversity and challenge is waiting for him in his epic journey. As he describes the various therapies he wonders, as any patient might, "whether this is a bad mistake, or a good therapy". As his fever subsides and his fears diminish, he now begins to gain strength from his Bible reading as well. The reader breathes a sigh of relief at this point, but the story's postscripted dénouement reminds us that even once the immediate dangers are over, serious illness leaves a long legacy of frustration and boredom, as well as a permanently altered relationship to what used to be normal and taken-for-granted (the daily routine of work; the assumption of a particular professional career ladder; a youthful, healthy body; and a circle of healthy friends and colleagues).

Eugene's diary offers us a story of optimism and courage in the face of death, described through a journey of doubt and fear sustained by faith. In some ways, Eugene's chronicle is a retelling of so many of the Bible stories that may have comforted him throughout his ordeal (the Exodus, the trials of Job, the temptation of Christ, for examples). By not couching his narrative in the language of fear and conflict (that construct and personify a disease as "other", "foreign", "the enemy") and highlighting instead the common ground of *shared* illness experience, the mutual metaphors of daily life and the collective stories of adversities overcome, Eugene enables his audience to reach catharsis through personal identification with its main character's drama of recovery. Because the story's conclusion presents the reader with Eugene's frustration and fear turning to boredom, this too becomes a crucial identifying moment for readers, many of whom may have witnessed or overcome an illness and/or confinement themselves. Even in the most devastating of stories, after danger has passed the ordinary returns transfixed and transformed. By capturing this, Eugene's epic comes full circle.

Without a proactive request from the editors, the story in Box 2.3 would never have been told before a public audience. It was the compelling nature of Eugene's first factual account (Box 2.1), as well as the reserved but poignant tribute added as a footnote to Tomlinson and Cockram's article (Box 2.2) that prompted us to "ask for more story" (a phenomenon well described in qualitative research, and discussed by Wengraf[11] – see pp 119–20). Thus, the three pieces together provide an audience with thick description of both Eugene's lived life and told story, allowing the reader to participate in developing fully the case history of the experience of this particular complication of SARS.

Acknowledgements

Box 2.1 Reprinted with permission from Elsevier (The Lancet, 2003; 361:1520–1).

Endnotes

i One of the first proactive decisions made by the WHO in relation to the emerging epidemic was to assign the objective-sounding acronym "SARS" to the ill-defined and uncertain phenomenon "severe acute respiratory syndrome". This has parallels with the early days of the Aids epidemic. Spelled "AIDS" initially, the first major illness known mainly by its acronym was declared a proper noun ("Aids") in 1986 – well before the main features and course of the disease had been properly documented. Naming things (constructing new words), it seems, helps in the "fight" against disease.

ii In Wagner's opera *Parsifal* the main character, is asked: "Do you know what you have seen?" But Parsifal cannot answer, as he is overcome by the suffering he has seen, and this requires more than just a vision of things. He must first acquire knowledge on the physical plane. This alone will enable him to internalise what he has seen and make it part of his consciousness. Wagner remarked that a strong awareness of suffering *can raise the intellect of the higher nature to knowledge of the meaning of the world*. Those in whom this sublime process takes place, it being announced to us by a suitable deed, are called heroes. *Collected Writings of R Wagner*, vol 10. (*Gesammelte Schriften und Dichtungen*, 10 volumes, Leipzig 1871–83. Now in eight volumes, reprinted by the University of Nebraska Press.)

References

1 Wu EB, Sung JJY. Haemorrhagic-fever-like changes and normal chest radiograph in a doctor with SARS. *Lancet* 2003;**361**:1520–1.
2 Tomlinson B, Cockram C. SARS: experience at Prince of Wales Hospital, Hong Kong. *Lancet* 2003;**361**:1486–7.
3 Gergen KJ. Social theory in context: relational humanism. Draft copy for J Greenwood (ed.), *The mark of the social*. New York: Rowman and Littlefield, 1997. Available from http://www.swarthmore.edu/SocSci/kgergen1/web/printer-friendly.phtml?id=manu9.

4   Lingis A. "The murmur of the world". In: W Brogan, J Risser, eds. *American Continental Philosophy.* Bloomington, IN: Indiana University Press, 2000.
5   van Manen M. From meaning to method. *Qualitative Health Res* 1997;7(3):345–69.
6   Merleau-Ponty M. *The primacy of perception* (trans J Edie). Evanston, IL: North Western University Press, 1964.
7   Dahlberg H, Dahlberg K. To not make definite what is indefinite: a phenomenological analysis of perception and its epistemological consequences in human science research. Paper presented at the 21st International Human Science Research Conference, 2002.
8   Heidegger M. *Being and time.* Oxford: Blackwell, 1962.
9   Honey MA. The interview as text: hermeneutics considered as a model for analysing the clinically informed research interview. *Human Development* 1987;**30**:69–82.
10 Sontag S. *Illness as metaphor: Aids and its metaphors.* London: Penguin, 1991.
11 Wengraf T. *Qualitative research interviewing.* London: Sage, 2001.
12 Rosenthal G. Reconstruction of life stories: principles of selection in generating stories for narrative biographical interviews. In: Josselson R, Lieblich A, eds. *The narrative study of lives.* London: Sage, 1993.
13 Launer J. *Narrative-based primary care.* Oxford: Radcliffe, 2002.

3: Poems from the heart: living with heart failure

MARILYN KENDALL, SCOTT MURRAY

When you are in the middle of a story, it isn't a story at all, but only a confusion; a dark roaring, a blindness, a wreckage of shattered glass and splintered wood; like a house in a whirlwind, or else a boat crushed by the icebergs or swept over the rapids and all aboard powerless to stop it. It's only afterwards that it becomes anything like a story at all, when you are telling it, to yourself or to someone else.

(Margaret Attwood, *Alias Grace*, 1999)

Introduction

Stories are no longer unexpected in illness accounts, as any general practitioner who is running 30 minutes late will tell you. Patients often clearly feel that they can explain things best via a story, and even in a busy surgery will preface their accounts with, "Well, Doctor, so as you can understand, what happened was ..." At the same time a growing interest in narrative, across many disciplines has focused attention on storytelling as a universal human activity and never more so than at difficult times in our lives[1-5] such as when we experience illness.

This chapter draws on a large qualitative research study (see Box) which aimed to construct a patient- and carer-centred account of people's changing physical, psychological, social, spiritual, and information needs when living with, and dying from, severe heart failure or lung cancer.[6]

The research study

Objective: To compare prospectively the illness trajectories, needs, and service utilisation of two groups of patients, one with cancer, and the other with advanced non-malignant disease.

Design: Serial, three-monthly, qualitative interviews for up to one year with patients, their carers, and key professional carers. Two multidisciplinary focus groups. Data were tape recorded, coded, and examined using techniques of narrative analysis.

Setting: Community.

Participants: Twenty patients with inoperable lung cancer, and 20 patients with advanced cardiac failure (New York Heart Association Grade IV) identified in hospital by their consultants, and their main informal and professional carers.

Main outcome measures: The perspectives of patients, their informal and professional carers about their needs and available services.

Results: We conducted 219 qualitative interviews. Cardiac failure patients had a different illness trajectory from the more linear and predictable course of lung cancer patients. In contrast to lung cancer patients, those with cardiac failure had little information about, and a poor understanding of their condition and prognosis. They were less involved in decision making. Facing death was the prime concern of lung cancer patients and their carers. Frustration, progressive losses, social isolation, and the stress of balancing and monitoring a complex medication regimen dominated the lives of cardiac failure patients. More health and social services including financial benefits were available to lung cancer patients, although not always utilised effectively. Cardiac patients received less health, social, and palliative care services and care was often poorly co-ordinated.

Conclusions: The experience of dying from these two common conditions was contrasting. Care for people with advanced progressive illnesses is currently prioritised by diagnosis rather than need. Patients, carers, and professionals perceive the need to address this inequity. End-of-life care for patients with advanced cardiac failure and other non-malignant diseases should be proactive and designed to meet their specific needs.

The research approach that we adopted ensured participants had time and space within the interviews to tell their stories, if they wished. Almost invariably patients and carers themselves chose narrative accounts, and resisted attempts to view their illness apart from, or as an isolated episode in, their wider life story. It was apparent from the interview accounts that both patients and carers found living with severe heart failure difficult and demoralising.[i] Little wonder then that people, when given the chance in a leisurely research interview, endeavoured to make some sense of this experience, and of themselves, in story form.[14,15,16] Consequently, we felt we should continue to honour their preferences in our approach to analysis, by retaining these stories as whole narrative units.

Two narrative poems

Narrative poem 1: Mr HH "What's going to happen next?"

Now this happened only
About a month ago.

One day I was up
At the centre

And my leg,
My left leg,
Was really sore
And it was swollen up.

And then my arm
Was really killing me,
You know?
Really pain!

And of course
With the swelling
And everything
That's the first thing
You're going to tell them
Is that you've got
This swelling
Because they keep
Asking you
"How are your ankles?"
And various things
You know,
For water retention
And that.

So my wife phoned the doctor
And she came
And of course
When she looked at me
She said,
"I think you've got
Gout."

And of course
I just laughed it off
You know?
I thought
"Gout??
No, no"
Because normally
You associate that
With the feet and that
You know?

So anyway
She took a blood sample

And went away
And a couple of days later
I got a phone call
Telling me
I had to go to
The hospital
To see
The specialist.

And I went down
And
Lo and behold
It was gout.

But seemingly it's something
To do with the amount of,
It's something
To do with the,
Something in the blood
I think.
And it could be to do with
The water tablet
I was taking.

So what they did was
They extracted fluid
Off the knee
And then injected
My wrist
Because it was absolutely
Killing me
You know
All the way
Up my arm
And they gave me this support
To wear.

And of course
When I got this
The chap says to me,
"I'll put you on
These tablets
For gout."
So that's more tablets
I'm on.

Then last week
I was at the doctor
And I told her
My wrist was killing me
And she said
They'd arrange for me
To go back
To the hospital
At the end
Of the month.
And then she phoned me back
To tell me
That I had to increase
The tablets
Again.

They gave me
Another
Tablet
A day!!

So you get
You just keep wondering
What's going to happen
Next?

And this
Is what gets you.
You know?
You say,
"What's
Going to happen next?"

You sort of
Get deflated
A bit
Because you feel
As though,
Well.
One minute
You're feeling
It's bad enough
Because somewhere
During the day
There's times when you've got

To go and lie down
Because you just feel
Sort of jaded
And tired.
Then when something like this
Happens
You sigh
And you say,
"It's another,
Another step
backwards."

And this is what I feel.
I just feel
That I've never really
Since the by-pass,
I've never really
Had any benefit.

I mean,
I know they had to do
What they had to do.
But I'm just one
Of these
Unfortunate ones.
The heart was in
Such a state
That they couldn't
Do anything
For me
Other than the by-pass,
And these are
The kind of things
You've just got to live with.

And it's hard.

It is hard.

I mean the doctors
They see you
Like maybe,
Well,
I'll see the
Hospital doctor

In a couple of weeks.
Now I see him
And it maybe
Another four, five months
Before I see him
Again.
And I've been doing that now
For the best part of
Three years.

But it all fell
Sort of pear shaped.
Och, it's just been
One thing
After another.
I'm just
An old crock really.

Narrative poem 2: Mrs N "If you were a horse...": a carer's story

[Mr N in square brackets]

Well, he's the same again,
Started, you know,
The swelling up.

And the doctor
Didn't put off,
Any time,
This time.

It wasn't a case of
Trying this,
And trying that,
And trying,
The next thing.

She said,
Before she had spent,
So much time,
On phone calls,
To the doctor,
At the hospital,
It was much better,
Just to get him in.

So he went in,
At the beginning of December
And he actually had been having,
Some rather strange turns.

[She had wanted me
In the hospital,
For the sole reason that,
She could try things
Today,
And at the latest,
Have the results by,
Tomorrow.
Instead of all this,
Backwards and forwards.]

But he had been having,
These very strange turns.
Very dizzy turns.
It just seemed to be
Something that
Came over him.

But we realised
How bad they were
After they had him
On the heart monitor,
Because every time he took one
On that
It went
Absolutely crazy.

Oh yes.
It went
Absolutely crazy.
And it's one
Of the tablets,
That he has
For his asthma,
Which they say
Is a very
Dangerous drug.

He's been on it
For many years,

And it's affecting
His heart,
And they are trying
To stop it
But they can't
Stop it
Because
He can't breathe
Without it.
The hospital doctor said,
The last time we were in,
Which was three weeks ago,
That it had
To be stopped,
Because it was affecting
The rhythm
Of his heart.

And we did try
To stop it
And I had to phone
Our own doctor
Because he was struggling
And she came in
And she said to him,
"Which would you rather have,
You know,
The heart out of rhythm,
Or not able to breathe?"

He said,
"Well,
If I'm going to die,
I'd rather die
With my heart stopping
Than gasping
For breath."

The strange thing is,
He's not aware of it,
Being irregular.
He didn't feel
Anything there.
It was just
In his head.

Well anyway,
They took him in
And they had him
On the heart monitor,
Then they had him
On a pump thing,
To get the fluid off,
Which they always seemed to manage
To shift quite quickly.

So he was hooked up to things
And couldn't get
Moving around
At all,
But they decided
They were going
To let him home
For Christmas.
He was to
Get home.

[They promised they would have me
Better
By Christmas,
But the test didn't run
As well
As they'd expected.

See the likes of every morning
The blood lady
Would come round
And she would always take,
Three samples,
And then the next morning,
Or even that night,
I could have a change
In the tablets.

So some days
With the Warfarin
I was on three
Some days
I was on four
Some days
I was on two

And some days
I didn't
Have any at all.]

But anyway,
He was to get home
On Christmas Eve
And he was to go back in
On Boxing Day.
But then they just changed
Their minds
Again
And said,
"You can take him home
And keep him home
And we will just get him in
Next week
And check him out
Again."

But he got home
On Christmas Eve
And he had
Christmas Day
And he took ill
The next day
And he has not really
Picked up
Very well
Since then.

And because
Of his chest problems
And everything else
You know
I got the doctor in

And I was quite disappointed
Actually
At the lack of support
The lack
Of back up
Because she came in once
And said,
"Oh, get him out of bed,
Keep steaming

Every hour.
I'll give him
Antibiotics."
Not that they
Are going to do any good.
They had stopped the Theodor
In hospital
But she said,
"Give him his Theodor."
"Well," I said,
"The hospital doctor
wanted to stop it."
She said,
"He can't do without it.
Give him his Theodor."
And that was it.
I mean
I felt that he was at
A much higher risk
Having this flu
And pneumonia
And whatever
But I was just
Left to it
I mean that was it
For three weeks.

But I couldn't get him
Out of bed.
There was no way
I could get him
Out of bed.
I felt that somebody
In your position
We should have had a wee bit
More back up.

I did say
To the hospital doctor
About it
When we were in
The last time
And they don't comment
But she said
"Yours is one of
The better health centres."

I said
I was a bit disappointed
In the lack
Of support
And even the nurse
Agreed with me
When she came in
For his blood.

I said,
"I feel
I've just been left
With it
And what would have happened
If I had
Been taken ill?"
Because my daughter was ill
With the flu
My son was ill
With the flu,
I was totally
On my own.

So I mean
It took three weeks really
To get him back
On his feet
And this is the problem
Now
With his feet.
The nurse has been in
Because the diabetes
And his skin
Is so thin now
And the heels
I think
With him being in bed
So long as well
He's developed
These cracks
And there's
In each heel
Underneath
There is one
Very deep one

Which we can't
Get them healed.

It's just hard
To get these sort of things
Healed
And they are in
Such a bad bit now
He's just sort of
Shuffling around
Just now.
He's finding it
Difficult
And it's making him
A bit unsteady
As well.

I just don't know
What we're going to do
With them really.
Do you have a gun
In your bag?
He probably needs
A gun!

The nurses
Are coming in now
And, as I say,
I've been making sure
They Dettol everything
Because I know
You have got to be
So careful
With infection.

But I know
He is not
Much on his feet
Because they can't
Seem to get them
Healed
At all.

He has been on steroids
For so long as well

And his circulation
Of course
Isn't good
And that
Doesn't help.

In fact
If you were a horse
They would shoot you.
They would do you
A kindness.

Narrative as poetry

Why transcribe as poetry?

Careful study of the interview transcripts, and discussion of different ways of considering them, led the research team to think again about transcription itself, and its place in our interpretative practice. The transition from interview interaction to words and noises on a tape, to text on a page, is a difficult and complex one, yet one of vital importance for the later stages of any project. All researchers have to make many choices about transcription, each one having implications for analysis and reporting.[17,18] Research is always and inevitably selective, and researchers need to be aware of what and why they are selecting in, or excluding from, the analysis. Consequently, decisions about transcription are never merely technical ones. Just as language itself is not a transparent medium, so too the transcribing of it is never a transparent, or atheoretical process. Rather, the choices made embody the epistemological assumptions underlying the study and form part of our interpretative practice.

As part of the process of decision making at this stage of the study, we came to think the stories might be best represented as poems. We had read James Gee's work on the stanza as an example of a universal unit of human thought, which considers the implications for analysis of transcribing into stanzas.[19] Moving away from the tendency to assume that everyone speaks in prose, we experimented with the assumption that, at difficult times, people may launch into narrative poems. The common metres of English poetry echo and reflect natural breathing patterns. By listening carefully to the stresses and breaks in the accounts of heart failure we have presented above, we came to hear them falling into the rhythms and cadences of natural poetry and, once sensitised to this, we found ourselves responding to the interviews differently and writing them up differently.

This chapter gives only two full examples of the kinds of stories that arose in the interviews. In practice all but two of the participants regularly gave their responses in story form, particularly when trying to describe the daily experience of living with heart failure (two brief extracts are presented in the Box at the end of the chapter). When we listened again to parts of the interviews, we heard classic narrative markers, such as "Well, what happened was ..." or "You see, it all began when ..." We found that the accounts fell naturally into stanzas built around individual events, or people, linked by a recurring refrain. These usually carried the key message of the story, and built to a conclusion, often also marked by certain words or phrases, such as: "But I knew ...".

What can we learn from these two specific poems?

In both the stories presented above, patients and carers poorly understood and struggled with "the swelling". Mr HH's diuretic caused gout, which only increased the number of tablets he struggled to balance. He voiced the daily frustrations and uncertainties of progressive chronic illness: "You just keep wondering what's going to happen next," and "It's another step backwards ... I'm just an old crock really."

Mr N and his wife felt between a rock and a hard place due to his perceived dangerous treatment for asthma which made his heart "go crazy"; but they decided he would rather die with his heart stopping than die gasping for breath. They did not feel involved in decision making or empowered to work in partnership with professionals: "Then they just changed their minds again." Mrs N was disappointed at the lack of community support: "I felt I've just been left with it," "I was totally on my own," and the conflict between hospital and general practice advice about medication. Mrs N cried for help: "Do you have a gun in your bag, he probably needs a gun." As another patient [Mrs P] said: "I'm ready for the knacker's yard."

What can we learn from them in poetic form?

When comparing these tales with those from people with lung cancer, who were also interviewed for the study, it was clear that narratives of heart failure are not easy tales to tell. First, unlike cancer, there are few cultural narratives available for people to draw upon when fashioning their own accounts, although there are cultural tales of ageing and of disability that people do make use of. Secondly, the experience does not fit easily within the models usually employed for illness stories, the favourite one of which is the "restitution narrative", which tells of getting better,[4] for there is no clearly defined trajectory of major events (diagnosis, prognosis, treatment calendars, tests and checks, remission, recurrence), as with many other illnesses.

Rather there can be several years when very little seems to happen, and people describe an experience of endlessly circling round, rather than a linear progression. Even within most other chronic illness accounts there are key events, such as diagnosis, or epiphanic experiences, which give rise to biographical disruption, which can form the focal point of illness narratives in these conditions.[20]

Attempts to access, interpret and report on other people's experiences are always difficult, since they involve engaging with ontological and epistemological questions, regarding the nature of social reality and how we can be said to "know" it. Indeed whether or not it is possible to understand the experiences of others, and if so, what such understanding involves, forms the basic question underlying the philosophy of social scientific research.[21] However, looking at patient accounts in this poetic form did seem to provide new insights into the illness experience and sensitised us to aspects of it, such as its rhythms and emotional costs, and the ways in which individual illnesses and problems interact within each person's life to form a whole experience greater than the sum of its parts, that we might otherwise have missed, or misunderstood.

It is, however, a time-consuming approach, and so it may not be possible, given research constraints, to employ it across the whole data set. Consequently, we used this approach alongside more traditional analytic strategies, such as coding. Using both approaches set up a valuable dialogue between them, allowing us to transfer the insights gained from each.

The in-depth study of several poems gave us access to the broader interpretative frameworks which these participants were employing at the time of the interviews, and served as a counter-balance to the fragmentation and decontextualising that may beset qualitative research of this kind. Equally, having access to the coded sections from the larger data set allowed us to read and interpret the narratives in a broader local context. These narratives could also be read against other sets of counter, or parallel, narratives.

This approach is controversial and some practitioners and researchers feel uncomfortable with it. As we experimented with disseminating the project in this poetic form, we met both strong approval and excitement, and some cynicism. However one commentator wrote that, for him, the poems "echo the poetry of the prophets."[22] On various occasions, when we have used the poems as teaching aids with medical and nursing students, and other health professionals, many found them invaluable in bringing patient experiences to life, and in sensitising them in future consultations to the complexities, nuances, cadences, and emotional toll of patients' and carers' experiences of living with heart failure. When we shared the poems with the participants, they were delighted with them, feeling them to be a strong, and accurate depiction of their experience. "Yes, that's how it was all right," Mrs MM.

Social scientists, increasingly concerned by the debates engendered by the linguistic turn in social research, have been turning to experimental forms of writing. Part of this debate has centred on the role of the poetic voice in qualitative research[17,23,24] and the desire for "an aesthetic social science".[25] It is, however, a debate that has more often been focused on report writing than on transcription and the ways in which it can alter analysis and re-presentation. However, all acknowledge the special role and power of poetry: "poetry, as a special language, is particularly suited for those special, strange, even mysterious moments, when bits and pieces suddenly coalesce"[25] as they do in the participants' illness narratives.

Clearly, and despite all attempts to suppress them, patients and carers need to tell their illness stories. Consequently, we believe that healthcare professionals need to develop their narrative competence in order to learn how to hear, and work with, these stories in their daily practice.

In this study we have relied heavily upon people's words in research interviews to try to understand their experiences of living with life-limiting illnesses. However, words are slippery and often hard to understand, and the form and the meaning of words are inextricably linked. The meaning of any story is embodied in that story; that story is the only way to say what the narrator wants to say. Consequently, if we mistake the form in which research participants speak to us, we may also miss-take their meanings.

In what sense could these heart failure stories be described as poetry?

If poetry comes not as naturally as the leaves to the tree, it had better not come at all.

(John Keats)

Poetry is the spontaneous overflow of powerful feelings: it takes its origin from emotion recollected in tranquillity.

(William Wordsworth)

These accounts have to be understood as natural, spoken poetry, as opposed to formalised and stylised poetry which we are accustomed to see written down: an earlier, oral poetry. Good poetry concerns authentic experience and the ability to recreate that experience for the poet and others. Poetry can help us to find a voice of feeling, a voice to explore not only what happened but how and why, and what it meant to us as emotional beings.[26] WH Auden once defined poetry as "memorable speech" and there was an abundance of that in the interviews for this study. Germaine Greer, in "The name and nature of poetry", claimed that "Poetry is closer to speech than prose ... Only lecturers speak prose; otherwise prose is literary, a written form. We speak a kind of poetry."[27]

We found that by transcribing and presenting the stories as poetry, doctors, nurses, and researchers responded differently to them: for we are conditioned to respond differently to poetry than to prose. In thus changing the dynamics of the reading process we can elicit different responses[25] and in the process change ourselves and our own stories. We live in a world full of text, where patient accounts are presented (if at all) as a large block of text, which may be ignored or only skim-read; whereas, if presented as poems, they can be approached more slowly, and heard in the head with attention being given to their patterns of sound, image, and ideas, making for more emotional engagement with what is being said. As Robert Frost observed:

Poetry is the shortest emotional distance between two points: the writer and the reader.

For the researchers, transcribing into poetry opened up different processes of interpretative thinking, and issues of re-presentation and voice in the research process.

Research has consistently shown that patients value doctors, who, despite being busy, take time to listen to, and learn from, their experiences. For doctors to hear and conceptualise the "history of the presenting complaint" as an epic narrative poem may help them gain another perspective, and aid them in formulating holistic diagnoses and treatment plans.

The chapter ends with two brief extracts from accounts illustrating the experience of living with heart failure. The first, by Mr E, illustrates social isolation and the daily grind of hopelessness:

I just feel
some days
I'm better than others,
you know.
I'm getting I'm loath
to get up
in the mornings,
I've to force myself
because I'm getting
to think
What's in front of me
today?
Just the same
as it was
yesterday.

The second, by Mr GG, expresses problems with physical symptoms:

As I had been sleeping,
I had been
Slipping down
The bed,
And as I
Slipped down
The bed
My God!
Oh what panic attacks
I got!

And I had to sit up
In the bed
Like that
Oh, my God!
To get my breath
I couldn't
Get my breath
I felt
So scared.
You can't really
Actually tell people
What it's like.

Endnote

i   Severe heart failure has a 50% annual mortality rate and a high risk of sudden death; a worse prognosis than many cancers. Compared with other chronic conditions, heart failure patients report some of the worst physical and social problems.[7] A large, retrospective study of bereaved carers in the UK found that many such patients experienced uncontrolled symptoms, low mood, poor quality of life and had little understanding of their illness and its prognosis.[8] Until recently, much of the focus for research and service development in heart failure has been on medication to reduce mortality, and interventions to prevent frequent hospitalisation. But patients and carers seem to want a more holistic approach to care, one which enables service providers to take account of psychological, social, spiritual, and family needs as well as physical problems and medication.[9] Qualitative research in heart failure has revealed that patients tend to attribute symptoms to advancing age and that they feel unable to ask questions of their doctors, although they would like a frank discussion.[10,11] A study of elderly housebound patients, however, described a world view of living a day at a time, preferring not to consider such problems.[12] Collusion in doctor–patient communication emerged as a theme in an ethnographic study of cancer patients,[13] and maybe prevalent in people with heart disease, too.

References

1 Kleinman A. *The illness narratives: suffering, healing and the human condition.* New York: Basic Books, 1988.

2 Polkinghorne D. *Narrative knowing and the human sciences.* Albany, NY: State University Press, 1998.

3 Maines D. Narrative's moment and sociology's phenomena: towards a narrative sociology. *Sociol Q* 1993;**34**(1):17–18.

4 Frank A. *The wounded storyteller: body, illness and ethics.* Chicago: University of Chicago Press, 1995.

5 Kelly M, Dickinson J. The narrative self in autobiographical accounts of illness. *Sociol Rev* 45 1997;**2**:254–78.

6 Murray SA, Boyd K, Kendall M, Worth A, Benton TF. Dying of lung cancer or cardiac failure; prospective qualitative interview study of patients and their carers in the community. *BMJ* 2002;**325**:929–32.

7 Stewart AL, Greenfield S, Hays RD. Functional status and well-being of patients with chronic conditions. Results from the Medical Outcomes Study. *JAMA* 1989;**262**:907–13.

8 McCarthy M, Lay M, Addington-Hall J. Dying from heart disease. *J R Coll Phys Lond* 1996;**30**:325–8.

9 Gibbs JSR, McCoy ASM, Gibbs LME, Rogers AE, Addington-Hall J. Living with and dying from heart failure: the role of palliative care. *Heart* 2002;**88** (Suppl II): ii36–9.

10 Rogers AE, Addington-Hall JM, Abery AJ *et al.* Knowledge and communication difficulties for patients with chronic heart failure: qualitative study. *BMJ* 2000;**321**:605–7.

11 Higginson I, Addington-Hall JM. *Palliative care for non-cancer patients.* Oxford: Oxford University Press, 2001.

12 Carrese JA, Mullaney JL, Faden RR, Finucane TE. Planning for death but not serious future illness: qualitative study of housebound elderly patients. *BMJ* 2002;**325**:125–7.

13 The A-M, Hak T, Koeter G, Wal Gvd. Collusion in doctor–patient communication about imminent death: an ethnographic study. *BMJ* 2000;**321**:1376–81.

14 Riessman C. *Narrative analysis.* London: Sage, 1993.

15 Greenberg G. If self is a narrative: social constructionism in the clinic. *J Narrative Life Hist* 1995;**5**(3):269–83.

16 Mattingly C. *Healing dramas and clinical plots: the narrative structure of experience.* Cambridge: Cambridge University Press, 1998.

17 Glesne C. That rare feeling: re-presenting research through poetic transcription. *Qualitative Inquiry* 1997;**3**(2):202–21.

18 Lapadat J, Lindsay A. Transcription in research and practice: from standardization of technique to interpretive positionings. *Qualitative Inquiry* 1999;**5**(1):64–86.

19 Gee J. A linguistic approach to narrative. *J Narrative Life Hist* 1991;**1**:15–39.

20 Bury M. Chronic illness as biographical disruption. *Sociol Health Illness* 1982;**4**:167–182.

21 Fay B. *Contemporary philosophy of social science.* Oxford: Blackwell, 1996.

22 Launer J. *Rhythms of life. Q J Med* 2002;**95**:555–6.

23 Hones DF. The transformational power of narrative inquiry. *Qualitative Inquiry* 1998;**4**(2):225–48.

24 Poindexter C. Research as poetry: a couple experiences HIV. *Qualitative Inquiry* 2002;**8**(6):707–14.

25 Richardson L. The consequences of poetic representations: writing the other, rewriting the self. In: Ellis C, Flaherty M, eds. *Investigating subjectivity: research on lived experience.* London: Sage, 1992, pp 125–37.

26 Sansom P. *Writing poems.* Bloodaxe Poetry Handbooks, 1994.

27 Greer G. The name and nature of poetry. *Guardian Review* 2003:4–6.

4: Performance narratives in the clinical world

CHERYL MATTINGLY

Serious chronic illness and disability, bodily conditions for which there is no biomedical cure, expose our human vulnerability, a vulnerability we often try to elude or deny. When illness is protracted, when there is no chance of return to the person one once was, or when there is no hope of being "normal", a person's very sense of self is lived in a special way through the body. Personal identity becomes intimately tied to the pain, uncertainty, and stigma that come with an afflicted body. What might it mean to be healed when a cure is only a distant possibility or no possibility at all? The limitation of standard biomedical responses to this question has a great deal to do with why narrative is so irresistible. One common act, in the face of supreme uncertainty and suffering, is to tell a story. Even when the pain is beyond words, when no story can be adequately told about it, a person may find that she draws upon narrative to remember and recreate a self, reaching backward and forward in time in search of possible worlds, possible lives.

In this paper, I explore narrative and healing in this vulnerable space. I ask what work narrative allows us to do, how it helps or hinders living in this fearful place. And I look at narrative in an expanded sense, not only as something told but also as something that can be acted in the form of healing dramas. The call to narrative within medicine has been a call to humanise the practice of clinicians, and even society as a whole, by looking beyond the disease or the narrowly construed clinical case to see the "patient as person", one who experiences the disease and inhabits complex social worlds. Recently, narrative has been called upon as a vehicle for social change – including transforming how clinicians work, how the public perceives disease or disability, or how politicians and policymakers allocate healthcare resources. The role of narrative in an ethical critique of medicine also links to broader critiques of technical and scientific rationality that have served as underpinnings of medical practices. This chapter speaks to these critiques and concerns by exploring an important but nearly invisible aspect of health care, the enactment of what I will call "performance narratives" or "healing dramas" in the clinical encounter.

Performance narratives and the narrative nature of human time

Although most of the work on narrative and its place in medicine focuses upon *storytelling*, I consider narrative in a rather different way. Put simply, my claim is that narratives may be acted rather than told, and these performed narratives can play a powerful role in clinical care. Performed narratives are not retrospective accounts of past events but involve the active shaping of present moments. They are living narratives. As with any good stories, healing dramas reveal life in the breach, in this case a breach that suggests healing possibilities. In these dramatic moments, time itself takes on narrative shape, is imbued with those qualities we take to be the markers of a good story: suspense, riskiness, trouble, enemies, desire, transformation, and plot. By plot, I mean an emergent temporal configuring in which particular actions become meaningful as part of a larger, unfolding drama (cf. Ricoeur's extensive treatment of plot and its relationship to historicity.[1,2,3,4]) There are times when even an ordinary clinical encounter shifts into this dramatic form, offering the patient images of a possible future worth living.

In examining narrative in relation to clinical time, I will argue that healing itself can depend upon the narrative shaping of clinical time. Healing dramas are so important because of what they portend. They signify future stories – lives and events that will unfold in hopeful directions. Performed narratives that have healing potential are ones that engender hope. They can offer the capacity for healing, even in the face of a grim clinical prognosis. They involve the social creation of significant experiences, the transformation of routine (clinical) time into dramatic time. As Oliver Sacks[5] has said, "recovery is events … advents, which are births and rebirths" (p 154). When clinicians engender "births and rebirths", they do so not in mere words, but through embodied actions. Words, of course, are likely to play a key part of the action, as they do in any drama, but it is primarily the complex, embodied acts that carry the meaning. The significance of these dramas especially lies in the place they occupy as significant episodes, even key turning points, in a patient's (or family's) life story.

The language of narrativity I draw upon here comes primarily from philosophical considerations of the connection between narrative and the human experience of temporality. Most fundamentally, narrative gives us a form through which to apprehend the world, whether or not we put it into words. It places temporality at the centre of meaning. It is the intimate connection between human time and narrative, rather than its textual nature, that I emphasise here. We can observe and recount history (tell stories) because we are first of all historical beings, because we live in history. Time, as experienced, is by no means linear. It is, above all, practical. Heidegger[6] gives us a conception of human temporality that underscores the relationship between the experience of time and our practical orientation in the world. Human time, he says, is defined by Care. We encounter the world around us as "preoccupied" beings. Our sense of time depends on the things we care about, especially our commitments, what we want to come to pass, even who we want to become.

For Heidegger, existence is defined by potentiality. Becoming is basic to human existence. Who we most are is "not yet something"[6] (p 234). We are always, from a Heideggerian perspective, incomplete because we are always "ahead of ourselves". Our lives are "in suspense," and this time of preoccupation is one of waiting, planning, calculating, wishing, dreading. The present is always saturated with the future. Our life is not a simple succession of "nows" because our experience of the past and our anticipations of the future shape our experience of the present. We see ourselves as actors in particular kinds of unfolding stories. We enter a situation and ask what sort of story am I in here? As agents, we do more than passively interpret the scene – we also try very hard to influence it. We try to shape the stories we find ourselves in while we wonder, in suspense, how things will turn out. This is not to say that our life has the coherence of a well-told tale. We not only live in suspense, unable to control or even foretell the future, we also live out more than one possible plot at the same time. Thus the narrative quality of lived experience is wedded to possibilities rather than certainties.

The narrativity of life experience is not merely shot through with shadowy possibilities. It is uneven. Some moments are "more narrative" than others. We find ourselves in an unexpected place, presented with a possibility we hadn't known existed, at least not for us, surprised by joy, or terror, sensing that we are in a situation where something is very much at stake, where attention is required. Healing dramas are precisely these "more narrative" moments, ones in which we would say we are having "an experience" as opposed to those times we describe as merely routine or where, as we typically remark, "not much happened." Clinical moments that qualify as healing dramas are not only experienced (at least by one of the participants) as highly eventful, they are eventful or significant episodes in an unfolding healing narrative. They take their place in larger life dramas of recovery. Sometimes they are significant moments in re-envisioning what recovery or healing might mean, particularly when cure is not an option. Healing is not, it must be restated, synonymous with curing. Healing can even accompany dying, as I will try to show in this chapter.

Anthropology's classic investigation of non-Western healing rituals has a great deal to contribute to the consideration of healing as drama, as significant, and experientially potent event. Ethnographies drawing upon Victor Turner's social dramas as well as phenomenological investigations of the healing process are of particular relevance here. The sheer eventfulness of recovery, so often suppressed in biomedicine, is highlighted in a variety of non-biomedical healing practices. Because anthropology has such a long and important history of analysing healing from dramatistic perspectives, this tradition can illuminate healing as a locally situated, socially complex, and embodied narrative act.[i]

Healing rituals across a wide array of cultures have been noted for features that also characterise many clinical healing dramas. I list the key characteristics below.

1. There is a heightened attention to the moment, an "existential immediacy", which gives an authority and legitimacy to the activity.[10,11,12,13]
2. A multiplicity of sensory channels carry the meaning, sight, touch, sound, smell, creating a "fusion of experience".[14,15]
3. Aesthetic, sensuous, and extralinguistic qualities of the interaction are accentuated.[16,17,18,19,20]
4. The intensification of experience is socially shared, and it emerges through mutual bodily engagement with others.[21,22,23,24,25]
5. Healing actions are symbolically dense, creating images that refer both backward and forward in time – the patient is located symbolically in history.[26]
6. Efficacy is linked to potential transformations of the "patient" and sometimes a larger social community.[26,27,28,29,30]

Biomedicine seems an unlikely spot to discover healing dramas, but they are everywhere in the clinical world. Through the past 15 years of research in North American clinical settings, I have come to discover the complexity of what "recovery" can mean for those living in bodies relentlessly, perilously present as well as those that have grown largely "silent", to call upon Robert Murphy's eloquent image. I have grown to respect and even to wonder at the power of small moments, recovery located in a walk to the bathroom, putting on one's own shoes, a successful trip to the hospital gift shop in the new wheelchair.[31,32,33,34,35]

In a case I describe in this chapter, I will explore the ways that a 15 minute "routine" clinical visit by an oncologist becomes a performed narrative, embued with the aesthetic and dramatic qualities that anthropologists commonly attribute to non-Western healing rituals. It seems quite clear, however, the oncologist in this case is largely unaware of the power and profoundness of the actions he takes which shift the clinic from a purely "medical" encounter into a healing drama. And in fact, healing dramas are often well hidden from view.

Sometimes only the patients or family members notice them. Professionals are often quick to describe dramatic moments in the language of biomedicine so that they appear to be doing professional clinical work, not "playing" or "wasting time," "just being friends" with their patients or, perhaps most dangerous, going "outside their turf" by directing attention to matters that are supposed to be the province of psychological specialists like social workers, psychiatrists or clinical psychologists. Sometimes, health practitioners seem themselves to be unaware when they have helped to create a powerful healing moment, one that speaks to the patient or family in a deeply personal way. Sometimes practitioners seem embarrassed by their own good work. Rehabilitation therapists, for example, speak reluctantly about how they tailor their interventions to draw in a patient, sometimes defending themselves (in case they are perceived as not sufficiently scientific or objective) by saying that they need to "motivate" patients to get them to participate in treatment. Certainly the espoused theories of biomedical treatment do not advocate the creation of powerful dramatic moments as necessary to healing.[33,35]

Healing dramas, life stories, and family plots

To further consider clinical moments as powerful healing dramas and as short stories within unfolding and changing lives, I now turn to research I have been carrying out for several years in American hospitals in Chicago and Los Angeles. I, along with a group of colleagues, have been conducting ethnographic studies of African American families who have children with severe illnesses and disabilities, and the health professionals who treat them. This has involved accompanying families to clinical visits, videotaping those encounters, where possible, and separately interviewing the clinicians, family members and, occasionally, children. As part of the interview, we ask participants to "tell us what happened" in the encounters. We also observe and videotape children and families at home, at key family events, at school and in the community. This extensive participant observation has allowed us a way to understand how clinical events function as key short stories in the unfolding lives of families and children.

Over the past seven years, we have followed a cohort of 30 families. This longitudinal design has revealed a great deal about clinical encounters as events in family lives, about multiple perspectives between families and clinicians concerning the "same event" which has also been recorded on video or audiotape, and about how healing itself comes to be re-imagined and redefined through the course of an illness or a child's life. Even shifts in a parent's or family's life influence an ongoing interpretation of what healing can mean for a child who will probably not be "cured". Certain clinical events take on the qualities of performed narratives as they speak to larger personal and family stories that are in the midst of unfolding, ones where narrative endings are uncertain.

This research brings home the social nature of illness and healing. I am repeatedly reminded that illness (or disability) is also a social affair. It is particularly shared with parenting kin. Anthropologist Myra Bluebond-Langner offers an excellent account of the way a child's illness is shared by entire families.[36] In her ethnography of families caring for children with cystic fibrosis, she notes that family life is intimately related to "pivotal experiences or events" in the ill child's own illness trajectory. She describes what she calls a "natural history of the illness", by which she means "a series of events from diagnosis to death, which mark critical changes in the social and emotional life of the family as well as in the clinical status of the child" (p 13).

Healing, too, is something shared, and something that changes as the patient's body and life possibilities and limitations change. Even the possibility of recovery is a family matter. The parents see themselves as well as their children as sufferers, for it is tremendously difficult and often despairing work to watch over and care for one's very ill or severely disabled child.[35,37,38,39]

I now turn to a particular case, a family I have known for more than six years. I met mother Aliyah and child Keisha in October 1997, just a month after Keisha, four and a half at the time, was diagnosed with cancer.

Performance narratives and healing in the face of death

What if your life became a dream? A nightmare in fact? What if your little girl, your toddling three year old, were to fall mysteriously ill, vomiting so violently she seemed possessed by a devil, and you had to carry her in your arms, to beg and plead for the doctors to look at her, and they told you nothing, nothing at all? What if you had to carry her home in your arms while she lay listless and dull eyed? And what if this went on for an entire year, visit after visit to countless emergency rooms, until one day a doctor finally noticed something and you were told your child had cancer? This was the dream Aliyah woke up to, a dream that she still lives, almost six years later. Faced with news of a malignant brain tumour, which, by the time of diagnosis, was "the size of an egg", the prognosis was not good. Sixty per cent chance of survival, the doctors tell Aliyah. How can she create hope, and how can she see health care as a source of hope? And hope, I must underline, is not something discovered or wished. It is painfully created; it is performed. Healing is intimately connected to hope.

As treatment begins, Keisha sees numerous therapists, nurses, aides, and physicians. She has surgery, receives chemotherapy, radiation, and physical, speech and occupational therapy. The hospital becomes an integral part of life for Keisha and her mother over the next 18 months. Some of these clinical encounters take the shape of performance narratives, providing dramatic moments that generate significant and hopeful experiences for mother and child. Because of the dire prognosis, a hopeful narrative moment is not necessarily one that promises cure. Rather, healing and hope become linked to another aspect of clinical work, helping Aliyah and Keisha live a good life, the best life possible, despite Keisha's fragile medical state. This "good life" is bound up with Keisha receiving the best clinical care Aliyah can locate, clinical care in which Keisha is not just another "cancer kid", or worse, another "little black cancer kid", but someone understood and even cherished by the health professionals upon whom her life now depends. And, further, for Aliyah, healing and hope are also tied to the way professionals view her as mother, not dismissively, not even pityingly, but with respect. What she wants to cultivate and looks for is partnership in the hard work of trying to keep her child alive and as healthy and happy as possible.

In the following exchange, it becomes clear that Keisha's oncologist, Dr Hansen, helps to create a healing drama that communicates personal concern and care for Keisha, as a special and valuable little girl. This occurs not so much in what he says to Keisha but in the game he initiates, transforming a fearful moment into a playful one, even an affectionate and loving one, a temporary moment that more closely resembles a "good father" scene than a "good doctor" one. It is only after this brief "good father" drama that Dr Hansen begins his discussion of the latest MRI results and his examination of Keisha. Here, he moves into doctor mode but at the end of the visit, he pauses for a brief and neighbourly chat with Aliyah about the recent holidays they have both had. Clinical time, comprised of a quick physical examination of Keisha and a discussion of the latest MRI results – the activities recorded in the clinical chart – is thus couched within a family-like time that begins and ends this doctor's visit. The entire clinical encounter is no more than 15 minutes, but these are 15 very important minutes. In what follows, I draw from fieldnotes to recount not only this 15 minute exchange but to explore how this clinical time is shaped by doctor, mother, and child into a healing drama, and why dramas like this have the healing power they do.

The "yes I can" game and the MRI news

Aliyah and Keisha are taken into one of the treatment rooms. There is the usual exam table covered with a white sheet and two or three chairs. Keisha hops up on the table with her mother's help while Aliyah sits in one of the chairs. Keisha, as usual, pulls the otoscope and ophthalmoscope off the wall and begins playing with them while she and Aliyah wait for Dr Hansen. Aliyah is tense because she will hear about the results of the latest MRI. She waits, painfully, while trying to be calm for her daughter, fearing what he will tell them. Has the tumour spread? Or, she hardly dares to hope, has it shrunk or even disappeared altogether since the last bout of chemotherapy?

Finally, Dr Hansen enters. He smiles a greeting to Aliyah but goes immediately to sit beside Keisha. She instinctively puts her hand over her chest where her port is, fearing that he will give her a shot. She says nothing. He notices her protective move and smiles, "No, no, I don't do shots. That's those other guys down the hall. I'm just going to check you out a little, use my stethoscope. You remember this, don't you?" Keisha visibly relaxes, letting her hand drop to her side.

"Hey," Dr Hansen jokes, noticing the instruments still clutched in her right hand, "You can't have those! Give them back!" He playfully moves to take them from Keisha. She snatches her hand away, grinning. "No! I can have them!" she shouts. "No, you can't!" he says, raising his voice. "Yes I can!" she repeats, even more loudly, laughing now. "OK," he sighs in mock defeat. "I guess I'll just have to listen to your chest." Keisha hugs him and he puts his arm around her.

She leans against him and he strokes her head and back absently while talking to Aliyah about the results from the MRI taken a few days earlier. A moment later he jumps down, telling Keisha that he wants to show her mother the x-ray films. He holds them up to the light, as Aliyah walks over to him. Together they look as he points out just where the tumour is and he compares it to the last scan. "It's holding stable," he says. "It's not shrinking, but at least it's not growing. This chemo might yet work." Aliyah sits down again, relieved of her worst fears.

Dr Hansen returns to Keisha's side, telling her he is just going to check out a few things. He gently prods her, which she now submits to without protest. The room is silent.

A few minutes later, he looks up and asks of Keisha and then Aliyah, "How was your Thanksgiving?" Aliyah replies, "Okay, just my daughter and grandson came over this year. Very small." "Yeah," he says laughing ruefully. "My wife and I planned this big family dinner and then at the last minute, first my parents couldn't come and then my brother and his family couldn't make it. Then two kids cancelled out. So it was just us and a huge table of food. We're still eatin' that turkey!" Aliyah and Dr Hansen laugh at this familiar post-Thanksgiving problem as he turns his attention back to Keisha for a goodbye hug. Shortly after, he leaves the room.

In what sense is this a healing drama with properties noted earlier, ones that commonly characterise healing rituals in non-Western healing practices – a heightened attention to the moment, a multiplicity of sensory channels creating a "fusion of experience", an accentuation of sensuous and aesthetic qualities, a socially shared intensification of experience, symbolic density, and efficacy defined to potential transformations of patient and perhaps even a broader social community? And how is it a performed narrative, with the qualities we associate with a compelling story – drama, suspense, desire, a plot with a beginning, middle, and end?

In considering the dramatic qualities of this doctor's visit, the important place to begin is to note that, for this mother and child, every trip to the oncologist is, itself, an event. It may be routine for him, but it is portentous for Aliyah and Keisha. There will likely be some news, especially on visits after major tests have been done. The oncologist is privy to secrets about Keisha's body, thanks to exotic tools like MRIs, secrets that Aliyah, who knows her child so intimately, cannot guess. This privileged knowledge is not trivial; it concerns life and death. For Keisha too, as for many children, though she may not know exactly what is at stake, doctors are frightening people. The hospital has been a source of great pain for her, a place she generally dreads, especially on days when she receives chemotherapy. It is not a casual place. It demands vigilance. She instinctively places her hand over her port to ward off potential shots when Dr Hansen arrives.

Aliyah's heightened attention is not simply directed to Dr Hansen's words, but to the whole exchange among the three of them. The non-verbal communication is as important as what he tells Aliyah. For she too is vigilant; and her vigilance concerns more than the medical news. She simultaneously attends to an equally subtle text, a text she reads in his body and in what clinicians might consider the "informal" or "non-clinical" aspects of his communication. She is assessing whether Dr Hansen is doing all he can medically for her child. Race and class play a key role in the unstated text of their exchange. In our research (and this is widely corroborated by other studies) African American parents, especially those on public aid, watch to see if their children are receiving the latest and best clinical drugs and treatment protocols. They also watch to see if their children are being experimented upon. Will their child, though black and poor, or the child of a single mother, be given good care? Will the doctors try hard to keep her alive? Families try to ascertain this through a number of common means: by trying to get second opinions, by "surfing the Net" to see what they can find out, by talking to other patients and families to see what they can learn from others' experiences at a particular hospital or with a particular physician. Although they rely upon all these avenues to assess quality of care, one of the most important is the interaction itself. Does the doctor treat the parents with respect? Does he go beyond being a "mere professional," a distant scientist, to engage with them in a personal way? Does he know and like their child? Does he indicate that it would matter to him if a child died or was not cured? Medical encounters are not places in which such conversations take place in any explicit manner. These are not questions that families can put to clinicians and get answers to. Rather, their questioning must be indirect, a reading of signs in the clinical encounter itself.

And so, Aliyah reads the signs of Dr Hansen's actions. The power of these messages came through in an interview I did with Aliyah three years after Keisha's death. In looking back to how Dr Hansen had treated them, she mentioned that she had heard some negative gossip about him, but she didn't believe it. Others have said they thought Dr Hansen was prejudiced against blacks. "I don't know if it's true but I don't care," she told me, "he was good to me. He was good to Keisha. He really took care of her. He liked her. And not just like a doctor to a patient. But like a person, like a, like a," and here Aliyah hesitated at her choice of words, "almost like a father to a child."

How was this message communicated to Aliyah, that she and her daughter were in good hands, that he would not withhold treatment because of prejudice? This was not communicated in words. There is probably nothing Dr Hansen could have directly said to assuage this fear. Rather, he spoke through his playful manner with Keisha, his fatherly warmth, his relaxed confessional storytelling about a Thanksgiving fiasco. Such small exchanges held important meaning. For Aliyah, they take on the symbolic density characteristic of non-Western healing rituals – they speak to the possibility of hope and healing. They do so because they seem to indicate a very real sense of partnership with Aliyah – we are in this together, his actions seem to say. And his genuine and affectionate concern for her daughter are also evidence that they together hold Keisha's life dear.

Of all that he does, what Aliyah remembers best, and what ultimately helps her to believe that he has done his best, is his capacity to play with Keisha. For this is not just any play. His playful ritual with Keisha reveals that he has come to know her well enough to participate in an intimate family game, though he may be quite unaware that he is connecting at such a deep level. The "yes I can/no you can't" scenario is a familiar routine between Dr Hansen and Keisha nearly every visit in some fashion or another. It is an echo, in fact, of a game played commonly between this mother and child. Aliyah often gets Keisha to do things she does not necessarily want to do by telling her that she can't do them. She uses this tactic particularly when she wants her to do therapy exercises or a challenging task that Keisha shies away from. Aliyah, like a good therapist, will incorporate these exercises into play at home, but it is the "no you can't/yes I can" game that so often motivates Keisha to take on difficult activities. "You can't do that!" Aliyah will exclaim, having asked her to climb some stairs or perform some other task grown difficult for a child who has undergone surgery, radiation, and heavy doses of chemotherapy. "What?" Keisha will respond indignantly, but with a playfulness that indicates she recognises this as a pretend insult. "Yes, I can!" "Oh no you can't," Aliyah will reply. "Oh yes I can," Keisha will continue to protest. By this time they are both laughing. And so it will go as Keisha, giggling and mock defiant, climbs the stairs, swings on the swings, or throws the ball to her cousin.

Dr Hansen has mysteriously acquired knowledge of the "no you can't/yes I can" game and uses it for his own purposes, to put this frightened child at ease, a child who cries and pleads every week when she realises that her mother is taking her to the hospital again. He teasingly gets her to laugh with him, not by invoking just any joking routine, but one that connects their play to an intimate, familial child/adult play, one that characterises some of the best moments with her mother. The apparent carelessness of this play between doctor and child belies its utter seriousness in terms of what it communicates to this mother. It is fondly remembered by Aliyah years later. For her, it offers some of the strongest evidence she has that she found a doctor who has come to care for her daughter as a "little girl, not just another cancer kid," as she put it.

The level of connection is deep in another way. For in this hospital setting where a frightened little girl has no power but must surrender her body, week after week, for poking and prodding, he plays a game not only as an equal but, in fact, inverts their power relation. Not only does she do something that would ordinarily be forbidden – after all, otoscopes and ophthalmoscopes are not the toys of a child and Keisha clearly knows this. But when he (in pretend sternness) forbids it and she tells him no, he concedes. Her no, unlike the many nos Keisha voices futilely upon her trips to the hospital, wins the day. In fact, she can say no over and over and over with increasing delight. And, in the end, she keeps her stash of clinical tools clutched tightly in her hands while he moves into his examination or into conversations with her mother. Thus, in the middle of the grimmest scene, comes the possibility of play, of humour, a momentary forgetting of the terrible reasons that bring these three together. Ritual moments are famous for being "times out of time", for moving into emotional and social spaces that transgress ordinary social rules and social expectations. This small bit of play, lasting no more than two or three minutes, exactly fits these characteristics.

Dr Hansen would very likely say that he is just "being pleasant" to Keisha and her mother, or that he is "calming Keisha down", or some other small and modest assessment of his friendly and respectful attitude to mother and child. In interviews, he spoke of the clinical situation with Keisha, which concerned him greatly, but he would never think to recount something so "trivial" as his little "yes I can" games with her or his "chit chat" with Aliyah about Thanksgiving dinner. And yet, it is precisely the embedding of the strictly clinical within a kind of family drama, the three of them together, that carries such weight. He orchestrates an interaction where he and Keisha play while Aliyah laughs as appreciative audience. This creates a healing drama, a moment that holds promise even when the medical news is not especially good.

The sensuous, embodied messages communicated by the play between doctor and child are also reinforced through his storytelling. Dr Hansen points toward a kind of family scene and crosses professional/patient boundaries when he recounts Thanksgiving mishaps at his house. He and Aliyah jokingly exchange knowing glances about the family dramas that are so likely to accompany traditional holidays. Even more important, by referring to a common holiday, one celebrated across gender, race, class, and ethnic barriers, one quintessentially American, he also initiates a common identification. We are not just on opposite sides of every divide, this story says, we all share Thanksgiving moments. This storytelling, so far from biomedical talk, carries the implicit message that we are all people together here. Notably, he has told a confessional Thanksgiving story. He does not triumph in his little tale, but is the unwitting victim of more powerful family members who fail to show up to dinner as promised. As doctor, he may be the expert, but as family member who cooks too much turkey and has a hard time with his relatives, he and Aliyah seem to share a similar space. Here again, the prevailing power structure of the clinic is quietly and fleetingly overturned. A level playing field, even a homely space, momentarily appears.

For Aliyah, this small exchange takes its place, and gains its symbolic weight, as an episode in an unfolding story that centres upon the drama of cancer itself. Has the tumour grown and spread? Has it shrunk or disappeared altogether? Is it the same? It is this, the few sentences the oncologist utters while they look together at the x-ray films, gesturing with his hand to offer Aliyah a visual image of what he is saying, that comprises the life and death heart of this clinical visit. Here too, in a moment so unlike his play with Keisha, there is a ritual density that arises from the multiple sensual channels in which messages are communicated. Dr Hansen speaks as they gaze at the shadows on the films. This is "an experience" for Aliyah, and one where, at this moment at least, while both look attentively at the x-ray films, there is a shared moment of intensity. It is another episode in which she feels that the three of them are taking a journey together, one in which they all hope that Keisha will be able to live. The doctor is guide and messenger. He can travel to the very inner recesses of Keisha's body and bring back secret messages that he then deciphers and delivers to Aliyah. How important it is to trust a messenger who journeys to such hidden places and who has the power to decode the mysterious texts he returns with.

This clinical encounter is a significant episode in a contradictory, unfolding illness story, one where the ending is very much in suspense. On the one hand, it is an episode in a story in which Keisha is given back her life, is being gradually cured so that she can grow up like any other little girl. While a stable tumour is not the best news, compared to all the time when the tumour grew unchecked, even its arrest is a sign of life. But this encounter is also a potential moment, a next significant episode, in a tragically foreshortened life, one where the meaning of this play or this test result has to do with living as well as possible, fighting as hard as possible, with all the days one has left. The same encounter furthers both plots simultaneously.

In living out the story of her daughter's illness, this small moment, a single routine visit between an oncologist and his patient, takes on its profound meaning as part of a complex healing drama. This drama began long before Dr Hansen was on the scene, in the year of Keisha's increasing illness and her fruitless attempts to get an accurate diagnosis from doctors. Then, suddenly, everything changed with the delivery of a diagnosis more horrifying than Aliyah had imagined possible and the plunging of Keisha and her mother into an intense and uncertain journey through the medical world as her daughter received painful but necessary treatments and prognoses changed from month to month. In this terrible place, Aliyah felt she had come upon a doctor she could trust. Finding a good doctor is a measure of her own goodness and worth as a parent. The guilt she still bears for somehow not managing to get her child diagnosed earlier is palpable. Why did she listen to all those other doctors, she still asks herself? Should I have fought harder? Why was I so compliant when doctors diagnosed Keisha with flues, or allergies, and recommended changing her diet?

Her own sense that she had done everything possible for her daughter, had given her the best possible life despite illness, hinges, in an important way, on her relationship with Dr Hansen. For if she felt she had allowed her daughter to be treated by someone who would not do everything, who was prejudiced or incompetent, and who therefore denied or was ignorant of experimental medical trials or the latest treatment techniques, how could she live with herself? A best possible life for Keisha is one in which Aliyah is assured that she, and those she has allowed to treat her daughter, have done everything they could, have acted not only as professionals, but with a kind of personal commitment that will transcend the obstacles of race and class. Even if Dr Hansen is prejudiced, as she later hears, she does not waver in her opinion that she did the best for her daughter. She prides herself and her daughter for their capacity to break through colour barriers, to pull this doctor into a common humanity. The little "yes I can" games, the casual exchange of Thanksgiving stories, serve as indicators Aliyah uses to assure herself that she and her daughter have forged a relationship she can trust. She does not, in other words, simply trust this doctor. Trust is something created, developed. She trusts her own skills, and those of her affectionate daughter, to forge bonds of compassion. His playfulness, the gentleness of his hand on Keisha's back as he talks to Aliyah, are the signs she reads to assess her own ability to bring this doctor into a genuine connection with her and her child.

As in healing rituals in which efficacy is connected to personal and social transformation, so it is here. Though Aliyah hopes for a cure, ultimately healing comes to mean something very different. It means, instead, that Aliyah comes to change as she cares for a child who eventually dies at home in her arms. She is transformed from a distraught mother who, upon hearing the news that her child has a cancerous brain tumour, believes she will kill herself if her child dies, to a mother who now serves as a volunteer at this same hospital, working with other parents whose children are critically ill. She has become a guide who helps other parents through this terrible journey and the transformations that will be required of them and their children to stay the course.

How the story ended

Healing comes, ultimately, not from the medical community but from her religious beliefs and her own work to face death, that allow her to become a certain sort of healer herself, bringing comfort to parents afflicted with the same pain she has endured. What does this kind of efficacy have to do with biomedicine or with the work Dr Hansen does? Perhaps Aliyah's own words, uttered at Keisha's funeral, speak best to this:

I want to thank everybody, everybody who was a part of my daughter's life. And I am so grateful that my daughter, I'm, I'm gonna miss her. Oh, God knows I'm gonna miss her. But, she's never gonna leave me. [Audience: Amen] That little girl, she, she fought so hard for so long, you know. She had an excellent doctor, Dr Hansen. He told me everything, you know. I mean everything fell into place ... He was honest with me about everything. And — Hospital, they did a, they did a lovely job. Just wasn't their call. It was God's call. And I'm so grateful that my baby's in heaven, 'cause I know she's there right now. [Audience: Amen] I have no regrets. You know, 'cause she did everything she needed to do, and everything she wanted to do in her whole lifetime.

Aliyah's poignant funeral speech announces that healing is not only related to what God can offer, but what she, and the health professionals, could offer. Healing meant that each of them, in their own way, gave whatever they could to help Keisha stay alive, and be as happy and fulfilled as possible while she lived. For Aliyah, it meant that she could say "I have no regrets", because her daughter "did everything she needed to do, and everything she wanted to do, in her whole lifetime", even if that short lifetime was just a week shy of her sixth birthday. That included getting the best medical care she could for her daughter and finding an "excellent doctor", one who "told me everything" and who made sure that "everything fell into place". As things turned out, healing took place in another space, and by other hands, for Keisha was "healed in heaven".

Aliyah herself was transformed in this journey. Instead of thinking, as she did when Keisha was first diagnosed, that she would commit suicide if her daughter died, she came to a point where she could not only face this death but go on, as she continues to do, to help other parents whose children are critically ill. Healing gradually comes to take on a new meaning for her. Through this hard journey with her daughter, she came to grips with the difficult recognition that healing might not be the same as curing. Her funeral speech might indicate that Aliyah believes the role of the doctor and the hospital are over once they can offer no more by way of a medical cure. Quite the contrary. She expected that health professionals, especially her oncologist – who traffic in death every day – would make the same journey she did, shifting from a view of healing as curing to one in which they accepted that despite all they tried, it was "God's call". She did not expect them to share her religious beliefs. But she did come to think that she and Dr Hansen were partners in this terrible voyage and that, as partners, he would be there for the entire trip, even as she put it, "through the death part".

Being there might have taken several forms. At best, Dr Hansen might have come to this funeral. But Aliyah was not asking for this. At the least, it would have meant that he was the one to bring her the terrible news, namely that there was nothing more he or the hospital could do to keep Keisha alive. Instead, he delegated this task to the case nurse. In an interview about a year after Keisha's death, she talked frankly about how difficult his sudden disappearance was, exiting at the most difficult time of all. Aliyah reports, in vivid detail, the fateful conversation she had with the nurse case manager about her child's impending death.

Cheryl: Was it Dr Hansen who finally told you that the tumour had spread?

Aliyah: No, it was Cara, the case manager. It was right before Christmas and they didn't know if we wanted to stay there or go home and be hospice. Because she [the nurse case manager], at that time she said, "Well, there's nothing they could do now. Um, she's not gonna make it." I asked her, "Well, how long?" She said, "Maybe three, six months." You know. And she lasted exactly three.

Aliyah explains why this conversation with the nurse, one she thought she should have had with Dr Hansen, felt like such a betrayal. She moves beyond her own experience, speaking as part of a collective, for other parents who have had this same experience of doctors who "disappear" at the end.

Aliyah: That's what they [the doctors] do. That's bad. Because that's when the parent really wants to talk to the doctor. Because the doctor's been following their child, and they feel that only the doctor could be the one to tell them what's going on. They don't wanna see someone else come to bring bad news. They want their doctor to be there so they can even [she pauses] maybe cry to their doctor. And tell their doctor how they feel, you know? I mean, I enjoyed Cara while I was there with her, you know, as the case manager, but I wanted Dr Hansen to tell me. I didn't want somebody else. 'Cause I felt like he was running. I felt like he didn't wanna come to me and tell me, which I felt he was the only one that I would believe. I felt he should've been the one.

Cheryl: Sure.

Aliyah: I said, "Where is he?" That's the first thing I asked. She [the nurse manager] said, "He's on vacation." And I didn't want nobody else to tell me nothing.

Cheryl: Yeah.

Aliyah: So I think the doctors run away, or say that they're away. And when someone else told me that that happened to them, I said, "Oh, so it's just a routine."

Aliyah tried in other ways to have some final conversation with Dr. Hansen. She wrote to him and telephoned as well. But she never heard back.

Aliyah: I sent Dr Hansen a card, you know ... I just sent him a card, you know, thanking him for being, you know, doing what he could do for Keisha and everything. I left him a message, but I didn't hear from him any more.

She tried to puzzle out why he would not have contacted her. She is stunned by what she perceives as a "heartless" end to their partnership. She wonders if there is some institutional policy that dictates against it, a kind of institutional cold-heartedness. The message she receives from this is that they are saying "forget you!"

Aliyah: I don't know, maybe they're not supposed to speak with any of the parents. But, you know, it sure would make the parents feel better. And I've heard that from a couple of other parents, you know, they just feel like when your daughter, you know your son, whoever, is gone, it's like they say, forget you! And the part, the worst part is, it makes the parents feel so bad when you know um, when you feel like nobody cares, you know? It's heartless.

Cheryl: Yeah.

Aliyah: It's a cold-hearted feeling when the parents, you know, after they spend so much time there, you know, you would think that they would have some kind of feelings.

She continues to mull over this unexpected and abrupt withdrawal of the doctor. She offers another hypothesis. Perhaps it isn't a cold-hearted hospital policy but an understandable vulnerability in the doctors themselves.

Aliyah: Maybe, you know, it could be that they need therapy, too. ... It's like um, guys in the war, you know. After seein' so many dead people, they need therapy because they have flashbacks. I don't know. Maybe the doctors could need therapy, too.

The disappearance of Dr Hansen disturbs Aliyah partly because of its failure to fit the healing narrative she believed she was sharing with him, that they were living out together. This was one created from episodes like the clinical visit I described earlier in the paper. Such a visit was, from her perspective, a powerful short story in which the doctor was both a medical professional, a practising scientist, and a healer of a different sort, one who could join with her in delighting in Keisha's love of play, her joy in defiance, her affectionate nature. This was a doctor, the only kind one should trust, who saw Keisha as a little girl, not just a "cancer kid". Their trading of family stories and his ability to participate in a family game revealed a level of attachment that Aliyah associated with good care. She was not simply gauging a "compassion" factor. This was an important indicator of what kind of medical care her daughter was receiving, whether good treatments were being withheld because she was on public aid or because her daughter was African American and therefore, perceived as being less valuable.

Dr Hansen's failure to see things through to the end, or even to deliver the bad news, completely disrupts the healing narrative Aliyah thought she was living in. His actions violate the ending she anticipated, even what she thought would be the worst possible ending, the one where her child would die. In this narrative violation, a new and terrible fear emerges. Has she misjudged him all along? If he deserted her at this point, and does not even contact her long after the funeral when she tries to reach him, did he ever really care for her daughter? And if he did not, did Aliyah do all she could to get her child good care? Can she still hold to the healing story she told at the funeral, the one where her daughter had everything she needed in her short life? Aliyah is forced into a retrospective mistrust that she will likely struggle with the rest of her life. She is not alone in her way of assessing the quality of medical care. In this study, and in other studies of paediatric care, my colleagues and I have found that one of the most important criteria families use to judge the quality of the health professional is whether or not the professional likes their child.[40]

Conclusion

Narratives can play an enormously important role in health care. In this chapter, I have looked to stories that are acted rather than told, examining how the clinical encounter itself can sometimes take the shape of an unfolding narrative. These "performance narratives" or "healing dramas," as I have labelled them, are common but neglected elements of clinical care. Healing in Western biomedicine does its work, in part, not only through the biomedical treatments we associate with Western healthcare, but also through its ability to create healing dramas that point toward hope and possibility. Performed narratives, like any compelling tales, involve desire, drama, riskiness, the sense that something is at stake, and suspense. They provide heightened moments in which messages are embodied and symbolically dense. The power of a healing drama does not merely depend upon what happens during the encounter itself but on how that encounter functions as an episode in a larger narrative, a story of illness and healing that encompasses not only a patient's life, but very often, the lives of family members as well. Even in clinically desperate situations like the one I have described with Aliyah and Keisha, hope and healing are an important part of what clinical care has to offer.

Why should professional healers pay attention to this? Why should they try to understand and connect their moments with clients and kin to life plots and narrative horizons that extend far beyond their province as clinical specialists? Why especially, should they try to understand and contribute to the reconfiguring of healing in situations when they cannot cure, when, in fact, their patients die despite everything they do? In short, because they have been so important to the journey. Neglecting to understand the healing dramas they set in motion with patients and families and their place within larger illness and healing stories can deprive professionals of a sense of their own significant work.

Put most radically, the claim of this chapter is that in attending to the kind of performed narratives I have described, an expanded sense of both clinical care and of healing is required. Treatment efficacy cannot be confined to the measurable outcomes of particular protocols and their effect on curing patients or even ameliorating the course of disease or disability. All of this is a critical part of health care, but it is not the whole of it. Focusing on treating the body and the disease, but missing the healing drama, can mean neglecting the most critical elements of good care.

Acknowledgements

This paper is based upon research carried out with a long-time colleague, Mary Lawlor, and a team comprised of anthropologists and occupational therapists, including Lanita Jacobs-Huey, Ann Neville-Jan, Nancy Bagatelle, Jeannie Gaines, and Jeanine Blanchard. It is supported by a grant from the National Institutes of Health (HD3 8878). I want to give special thanks to Beverly, who has taught me so much about hope and vulnerability, and whose life has been a special inspiration for this chapter.

Endnote

i   The performative aspects of healing have been explored in some very interesting ways in anthropology, ways that have helped to introduce certain streams of phenomenology to anthropology. But, in an effort to distance themselves from earlier structuralist treatments of ritual, many scholars elaborating a phenomenological approach to the study of healing distinguish their approach from a narrative one. They frequently view narrative as offering only a disembodied semiotics of healing. This is unfortunate. What is needed is not a sharp distinction between a structuralist, narrative approach to healing, on the one hand, and a phenomenologically sensitive reading of the healing process, on the other. Rather, as in hermeneutic phenomenology,[1,2,7,8,9] narrative ways of knowing and doing need to be connected to embodied, extra-linguistic modes of experience. This link cannot be made without reformulating narrative itself as a construct such that it can be seen as connected, in complex ways, to the very shaping of embodied experience.

References

1   Ricoeur P. *Time and Narrative*, vol 1 (trans K McLaughlin, D Pellauer). Chicago: University of Chicago Press, 1984.
2   Ricoeur P. *Time and Narrative*, vol 2 (trans K McLaughlin, D Pellauer). Chicago: University of Chicago Press, 1985.
3   Ricoeur P. *Time and Narrative*, vol 3 (trans K Blamey, D Pellauer). Chicago: University of Chicago Press, 1987.
4   Ricoeur P. *Oneself as Another*. Chicago: University of Chicago Press, 1982.
5   Sacks O. *The Man Who Mistook His Wife for a Hat and Other Clinical Tales*. New York: Perennial Library, 1987.
6   Heidegger M. *Being and Time* (trans E Robinson, J Macquarrie). New York: Harper and Row, 1962.
7   Dilthey W. Introduction to the Human Sciences. In: *Selected Works*, vol 1 (RA Makkreel, F Rodi, eds). Princeton, NJ: Princeton University Press, 1989.
8   Gadamer, H-G. *Truth and Method*. New York: Seabury Press, 1975.
9   Carr D. *Time, Narrative, and History*. Bloomington, IN: Indiana University Press, 1986.
10 Csordas T. *Embodiment and Experience: The Existential Ground of Culture and Self*. Cambridge, MA: Harvard University Press, 1994.
11 Csordas T. Imaginal performance and memory in ritual healing. In: Laderman C, Roseman M, eds. *The Performance of Healing*. London: Routledge, 1996, pp 91–113.
12 Desjarlais R. Presence. In: Laderman C, Roseman M, eds. *The Performance of Healing*. London: Routledge, 1996, pp 143–64.
13 Schieffelin E. On failure and performance: throwing the medium out of the séance. In: Laderman C, Roseman M, eds. *The Performance of Healing*. London: Routledge, 1996, pp 59–89.
14 Briggs C, ed. *Disorderly Discourse: Narrative, Conflict and Inequality*. New York: Oxford University Press, 1997.
15 Tambiah S. *Culture, Thought, and Social Action: An Anthropological Perspective*. Cambridge: Cambridge University Press, 1985.
16 Stoller P. *The Taste of Ethnographic Things: The Senses of Anthropology*. Philadelphia: University of Pennsylvania Press, 1989.
17 Stoller P. Sounds and things: pulsations of power in Songhay. In: Laderman C, Roseman M, eds. *The Performance of Healing*. London: Routledge, 1996.
18 Stoller P. *Sensuous Scholarship*. Philadelphia: University of Pennsylvania Press, 1997.
19 Jackson M. *Paths toward a Clearing: Radical Empiricism and Ethnographic Inquiry*. Bloomington, IN: Indiana University Press, 1989.
20 Laderman C. Poetics of Healing in Malay Shamanistic Performances. In: Laderman C, Roseman M, eds. *The Performance of Healing*. London: Routledge, 1996, pp 115–41.
21 Danforth L. *Firewalking and Religious Healing: The Ana Stenari of Greece and the American Firewalking Movement*. Princeton, NJ: Princeton University Press, 1989.
22 Hughes-Freeland F. Introduction. In: Hughes-Freeland F, ed. *Ritual, Performance, Media*. New York: Routledge, 1998, pp 1–28.
23 Kapferer B. *A Celebration of Demons: Exorcism and the Aesthetics of Healing in Sri Lanka*. Bloomington, IN: Indiana University Press, 1983.
24 Kapferer B. Performance and the structure of meaning and experience. In: Turner V, Bruner E, eds. *The Anthropology of Experience*. Urbana, IL: University of Illinois Press, 1986, pp 188–202.
25 Schechner R. *The Future of Ritual: Writings on Culture and Performance*. New York: Routledge, 1993.
26 Kendall L. Initiating performance: The story of Chini, a Korean Shaman. In: Laderman C, Roseman M, eds. *The Performance of Healing*. London: Routledge, 1996, pp 17–58.
27 Turner V. *The Ritual Process: Structure and Anti-Structure*. Chicago: Aldine, 1969.
28 Turner V. *The Anthropology of Performance*. New York: PAJ Publications, 1986.
29 Turner V. Dewey, Dilthey, and drama: An essay in the anthropology of experience. In: Turner V, Bruner J, eds. *The Anthropology of Experience*. Chicago: University of Illinois Press, 1986.
30 Turner E. *Experiencing Ritual: A New Interpretation of African Healing*. Philadelphia: University of Pennsylvania Press, 1992.

31 Mattingly C. The narrative nature of clinical reasoning. *Am J Occup Ther* 1991;**45**: 998–1005.

32 Mattingly C. The concept of therapeutic emplotment. *Soc Sci Med* 1994;**38**(6): 811–22.

33 Mattingly C. *Healing Dramas and Clinical Plots: The Narrative Structure of Experience.* Cambridge: Cambridge University Press, 1998.

34 Mattingly C. Emergent narratives. In: Mattingly C, Garro L, eds. *Narrative and the Cultural Construction of Illness and Healing.* Berkeley, CA: University of California Press, 2000, pp 181–211.

35 Mattingly C, Lawlor M. The fragility of healing. *Ethos* 2001;**29**(1):30–57.

36 Bluebond-Langner M. *In the Shadow of Illness: Parents and Siblings of the Chronically Ill Child.* Princeton, NJ: Princeton University Press, 1996.

37 Mattingly C, Lawlor M. Learning from stories: narrative interviewing in cross-cultural research. *Scand J Occup Ther* 2000;**7**:4–14.

38 Mattingly C, Lawlor M. Disability experience from a family perspective. In: Crepeau E, Cohn E, Schell B, eds. *Willard and Spackman's Occupational Therapy*, 10th edn. Philadelphia: Lippincott, Williams, and Wilkins, 2003.

39 Mattingly C, Lawlor M, Jacobs-Huey L. Narrating September 11: race, gender and the play of cultural identities. *Am Anthropol* 2002;**104**(3):743–53.

40 Lawlor M, Mattingly C, Lewis G. *A Failure of Treatment.* New York: Oxford University Press, 2000.

Further reading

Becker G. *Disrupted Lives: How People Create Meaning in a Chaotic World.* Berkeley, CA: University of California Press, 1997.

Bruner J. *Making Stories: Law, Literature and Life.* New York: Farrar, Straus, and Giroux, 2002.

Cain C. Personal stories: identity acquisition and self-understanding in Alcoholics Anonymous. *Ethos* 1991;**19**:210–53.

Capps L, Ochs E. *Constructing Panic: The Discourse of Agoraphobia.* Cambridge, MA: Harvard University Press, 1995.

Charon R, Montello M, eds. *Stories Matter: The Role of Narrative in Medical Ethics.* London: Taylor and Francis, 2002.

Comaroff J. Medicine: symbol and ideology. In: Wright P, Treacher A, eds. *The Problem of Medical Knowledge: Examining the Social Construction of Medicine.* Edinburgh: Edinburgh University Press, 1982.

DelVecchio Good MJ. *American Medicine: The Quest for Competence.* Berkeley, CA: University of California Press, 1995.

Estroff S. *Making it Crazy: An Ethnography of Psychiatric Clients in an American Community.* Berkeley, CA: University of California Press, 1981.

Frank A. *The Wounded Storyteller: Body, Illness, and Ethics.* Chicago: University of Chicago Press, 1995.

Frankenberg R. Sickness as cultural performance: drama, trajectory, and pilgrimage: root metaphors and the making social of disease. *Int J Health Serv* 1986;**16**(4):603–26.

Gadamer HG. *The Enigma of Health: The Art of Healing in a Scientific Age.* Stanford, CA: Stanford University Press, 1996.

Garro L. Chronic illness and the construction of narratives. In: DelVecchio Good MJ, *et al*, eds. *Pain as Human Experience.* Berkeley, CA: University of California Press, 1992, pp 100–37.

Garro L. Narrative representations of chronic illness experience: cultural models of illness, mind, and body in stories concerning the temporomandibular joint (TMJ). *Soc Sci Med* 1994;**38**(6):775–88.

Garro L. Cultural knowledge as resource in illness narratives: remembering through accounts of illness. In: Mattingly C, Garro L, eds. *Narrative and the Cultural Construction of Illness and Healing.* Berkeley, CA: University of California Press, 2000, pp 70–87.

Good B. *Medicine, Rationality, and Experience: An Anthropological Perspective.* New York: Cambridge University Press, 1994.

Good B, DelVecchio Good MJ. In the subjunctive mode: epilepsy narratives in Turkey. *Soc Sci Med* 1994;**36**(6):835–42.

Good B. "Fiction" and "historicity" in doctors' stories: social and narrative dimensions of learning medicine. In: Mattingly C, Garro L, eds. *Narrative and the Cultural Construction of Illness and Healing*. Berkeley, CA: University of California Press, 2000, pp 50–69.

Greenhalgh T, Hurwitz B. *Narrative Based Medicine: Dialogue and Discourse in Clinical Practice*. Chicago: Login Brothers Book Company, 1998.

Holland D, Lachicotte W, Skinner D, Cain C. *Identity and Agency in Cultural Worlds*. Cambridge, MA: Harvard University Press, 1998.

Kirmayer L. Broken narratives: clinical encounters and the poetics of illness experience. In: Mattingly C, Garro L, eds. *Narrative and the Cultural Construction of Illness and Healing*. C Mattingly, L Garro, eds. Berkeley: University of California Press, 2000, pp 153–80.

Kleinman A. *The Illness Narratives: Suffering, Healing, and the Human Condition*. New York: Basic Books, 1988.

Kleinman A, Kleinman J. The appeal of experience: the dismay of images: cultural appropriations of suffering in our times. *Daedalus* 1996;**125**(1):1–24.

Komesaroff P. Introduction: postmodern medical ethics? In: Komesaroff P, ed. *Troubled Bodies: Critical Perspectives on Postmodernism, Medical Ethics, and the Body*. Durham, NC: Duke University Press, 1995, pp 1–19.

Mathews H, Lannin DR, Mitchell JP. Coming to terms with advanced breast cancer: black women's narratives from Eastern North Carolina. *Soc Sci Med* 1994;**38**:789–800.

Mattingly C. In search of the good: narrative reasoning in clinical practice. *Med Anthropol Q* 1998;**12**(3):273–97.

Mishler E. *Research Interviewing: Context and Narratives*. Cambridge, MA: Harvard University Press, 1986.

Monks J. Talk as social suffering: narratives of talk in medical settings. *Anthropol Med* 2000;**7**(1):15–38.

Montgomery Hunter K. *Doctor's Stories: The Narrative Structure of Medical Knowledge*. Princeton, NJ: Princeton University Press, 1991.

Morris D. *Illness and Culture in the Postmodern Age*. Berkeley, CA: University of California Press, 1998.

Murphy R. *The Body Silent*. New York: Henry Holt and Company, 1987.

Nelson HL. *Stories and Their Limits: Narrative Approaches to Bioethics*. London: Routledge, 1997.

Price L. Ecuadorian illness stories: cultural knowledge in natural discourse. In: Holland D, Quinn N, eds. *Cultural Models in Language and Thought*. Cambridge: Cambridge University Press, 1987, pp 313–42.

Redding P. Science, medicine, and illness: rediscovering the patient as person. In: Komesaroff P, ed. *Troubled Bodies: Critical Perspectives on Postmodernism, Medical Ethics, and the Body*. Durham, NC: Duke University Press, 1995, pp 87–102.

Wikan U. With life in one's lap: the story of an eye/I (or two). In: Mattingly C, Garro L, eds. *Narrative and the Cultural Construction of Illness and Healing*. Berkeley, CA: University of California Press, 2000, pp 212–36.

Young A. *The Harmony of Illness*. Princeton, NJ: Princeton University Press, 1995.

5: "I cut because it helps": narratives of self-injury in teenage girls

PETRA M BOYNTON, ANNABELLE AUERBACH

The story of this research

This chapter is based on qualitative research of teenagers' descriptions of self-injury. It is necessary to explain how this work began, since it did not follow the traditional format of research. Petra is a psychologist with an interest in teenage health. Annie is the editor of an online teenage magazine, *mykindaplace* (MKP). In 2002 Petra was invited by Annie to become the "agony aunt" for the website. Readers of the site sent in problems in the form of "Dear Petra" letters, which were answered by Petra and placed on the site by Annie on a fortnightly basis. A space was provided by each problem and reply for readers to add their ideas about how the writer might cope. This meant that the person who had written in with a problem received advice both from the "agony aunt" and also from their peers (see http://www.mykindaplace.com/agony).

Annie was already aware of the references to self-injury made by readers within the chat rooms on the site, where they frequently talked about "cutting" or "chicken scratching". What surprised us both was the number of references to self-injury that were made within each letter sent to Petra. We estimated that for every 15 letters received, around 10 would have some reference to self-injury. Typically, a letter might read something like "I am being bullied at school", "I have been sexually abused", "I am worried about my exams", or "I think I may have an eating disorder", all followed by "... and I cut myself". We realised that whilst readers needed specific advice about the various initial problems they had raised, the common issue of self-injury (which was almost always presented as a *response* to a problem rather than as a problem in its own right) also had to be tackled. This took up space within the replies, and it also meant that self-injury was becoming a recurring theme in Petra's answers. It almost felt like we were condoning the practice in some way. We decided to write a short piece about self-injury for the site, in which we outlined what we felt were the reasons why people self-injured; alternatives to harming; coping strategies; and links to related help groups (see http://www.mykindaplace.com/agony/cutting.asp).

At this stage we had no intention of conducting research. We were simply trying to explain self-injury in a way that avoided having to answer it in each reply. Usually when we posted a specific feature on the site, around 30 or so readers replied. But when we ran the self-injury feature, over 260 readers responded, with reactions ranging from a few lines to several paragraphs. Although the users of the site are not representative of all teenagers, the descriptions of self-injury and their views about it did appear to fill in some of the gaps within existing research, and in particular, they illustrated the experiences and perspectives of young women most of whom were (we presumed) not in psychiatric care (or indeed, any form of ongoing medical care), and hence were a much milder sample than those generally used for research studies on self-injury. The site had provided a space for young women to talk, and showed how they were able (or not) to manage self-injury.

The numerous detailed and candid postings, which illuminated this common and distressing problem, presented us with an ethical dilemma. We had a rich source of information that could help with research and care, but we had not set out to collect "data". We sought the advice of the local research ethics committee, who stated that since the quotes on the site were a public document (akin to a magazine), it was ethically acceptable to undertake an analysis of them.[1,2] We remained somewhat uneasy and therefore also approached the site users to see whether they would mind our analysing the quotes and using them to educate others about self-injury. Responses to this question were unanimously positive about the idea of a research study. We therefore undertook a thematic content analysis of the quotes posted on the site, which forms the basis of this chapter.

The quotes used in this chapter, and our interpretation of their meaning, were fed back to the site users, and we created an advice sheet based on the main themes and ideas from our analysis. This is included as an Appendix at the end of the chapter and may be reproduced with acknowledgement of University College London and Mykindaplace. We felt that it was important to create some form of summary of our findings that could be used by parents, teachers, healthcare staff, and teenagers. We kept the postings on the website in the context of education around self-injury and as an encouragement for others to seek help. We are aware that some sites (for example around anorexia) can be used to condone or facilitate further self-harm,[3] and we tried to reduce this risk by keeping references to self-injury linked with our advice space within the site.

Responses to the MKP website strongly supported our interpretation and encouraged us to publish the findings widely.

Please note that those affected by accounts of self-injury may find some of the following quotes act as a trigger. This may be worth considering if all or part of this chapter is to be used for any form of education or training with teenagers and/or current or former self-harmers.

Analysis of postings

As described above, our sample was 262 postings by girls aged 11 to 21 who were members of the teen website MKP. Participants' details were anonymised for the analysis, and indeed, many respondents had already created fictional identities for the purpose of posting on the site. In this chapter, respondents have been referred to by a number, but it is worth noting many used names on the site that reflect feelings of unhappiness around self-injury, such as *depressed, useless, alone, ashamed, frustrated fear*, and *It's AlWaYs ToO lAtE wHeN yOu GoT NoThInG*. We have deliberately avoided editing the quotes for spelling or grammar, choosing instead to let them appear as written by respondents.

We used standard qualitative research methodology to undertake a thematic content analysis of respondents' free text accounts.[4] One of us (Petra) initially read through each posting and noted the issues raised in it. From this we established a coding schedule of 38 categories (themes) (see Table 5.1). Each quote was then co-rated by Annie and the occurrences of each theme were recorded in a database (using SPSS).

The accounts revealed that 61 respondents (23%) had self-injured in the past, and 100 (38%) were current self-injurers. Fifty-four respondents (21%) were writing about someone who self-injured (most commonly it was a friend or boyfriend). Only 20 (8%) asserted they did not self-injure. The remaining respondents (10%) discussed self-injury but did not state whether they engaged in such activities themselves. Although the sampling frame for this research (those who choose to post on a website about self-injury) is of course highly selective, we were still surprised at the high proportion who had actually engaged in the activity personally. These figures suggest (though they do not prove) that the current estimate of prevalence of self-injury (around 13%) may be an under-estimate.[4,5]

Self-injury: the story fragments

Most postings were only a few lines long, and few contained a coherent, linear sequence of events that fitted the conventional

Table 5.1   Main themes identified in postings

General category	Themes
Knowledge/experience of harming	Friend/boyfriend/family member self-injures; I used to self-injure; I currently self-injure; I don't self-injure
Why do it?	Family problems/bereavement, cope with stress; to release feelings; because I can't stop; I like how it feels when I self-injure (and I like how it looks during and after); I don't know why do it; I feel depressed and/or angry (I hate myself); being bullied; low self image (eating disorders); people copy each other; attempted suicide; sexual/physical/emotional abuse
Where I self-injury	Locations on body; venues where harm (for example, at home, or at school)
"Management" of self-harm	What I use to self-injure; how I hide scars; how long I've been doing it for; I don't do it all the time; I don't do it very deeply
How I feel	Ashamed or secretive; wish I'd never started; I don't feel anything before or during harming ("numbness"); distressed/take comfort from scarring
What helps	Alternative forms of coping; friends; telling someone; schools should offer more help
What doesn't help	Teachers and counsellors dealing with SI "inappropriately"; thinking it's attention seeking; thinking it's "just" youth culture; people's ignorance about the issue
Talking to each other via the messageboard	Replies/advice to other postings on the board; Please can you help me? (asking site); Don't do it (telling others to stop/not start)

narrative form. Nevertheless, many accounts appeared as "story fragments" (two or more actions and events loosely and implicitly linked in time). The main events linked to self-injury in this way were family problems (including divorce and bereavement), stressors such as schoolwork, or friendship difficulties. Less commonly, bullying, physical abuse or sexual abuse was mentioned. These experiences led to teenagers feeling angry, depressed or frustrated, and self-injury became a way of releasing the frustration and/or restoring control:

> ... you know that feeling when everythings going wrong and you just want to curl up in bed and vanish till its all back to normal thats what most people do or wish, but selfharmers try to make it better they make themselves feel bad or in pain to make the thing that seemed bad not so bad any more compared to what they just did to themselves (cutting, scratching) (respondent 22).

Some respondents did not link the self-injury to a particular event or experience. Rather, the story began with simply "feeling stressed" or "in a bad mood". Implicitly, the nature of the events leading up to the emotional state were not particularly critical – self-injury was a response to the state itself.

I also self-harm, hiding the scars aint easy but its the only way. i told a few of my mates some reacted better than others, the same question was asked why, why and why,?, and i had 2 admit i didnt know i just liked the feeling, when i was stressed, angry, upset, 2 me its almost like crying, a release of your feelings, but i h8 crying i feel weak, stupid and vunrable, no 1 really understands (respondent 11).

Several respondents identified "being in a bad mood *with myself*", and couched the self-injury act in terms of punishment.

... it's very tempting when im in a really bad mood or hurt and angry to take it out on myself because i feel things are always my fault (respondent 15);

i do it because i hate myself and i think i deserve pain (respondent 101).

Interestingly, a number of girls reported they initially harmed themselves by accident, and, finding that it led to relief or pleasure, then repeated this behaviour during a later stressful situation.

i was ironing my school uniform 4 the next day wen i suddenly looked at the iron without thinkin about it i leant it against my arm (respondent 97);

Then one day I was cutting some veg and my dad made me jump and i cut my arm with the knife and it didn't hurt, it felt good like a release (respondent 171);

For me its a spur of the moment thing, I tell myself not to do it and then all of a sudden I realise I've done it again (respondent 188).

A few respondents gave very precise explanations for the reasons behind self-injury, and also showed keen awareness of the ambiguities of self-harming as a form of self-healing:

The scientific part is your body lets out these sensations where the cut is to help the body deal with pain that's why some people feel better when they cut/burn/scratch themselves. The truth of the matter is that you cut yourself because you're unhappy soon it could become your unhappy because you cut yourself (respondent 55).

The act of self-injury: strategies of how and where

Seventy-one respondents (21%) described their self-injury strategies. Most commonly, respondents cut themselves with scissors, knives, and razors. Others made reference to using compasses, pins and keys, or to scratching their skin or picking at scars. Some burned themselves using an iron or matches, and a minority harmed themselves by hitting or biting themselves or pulling their own hair. Sixty-four (24%) revealed where they harmed themselves. The most common sites chosen were the arms, tops of legs and stomach, although wrists, hips, thumbs, and hands were also mentioned. The main locations for harming were the home (mainly their own home in their own room), but a minority admitted harming themselves at school too. Thirteen respondents (4%) were keen to point out they did not do it "all the time", and seven (3%) emphasised that when they did cut, they did not do it very deeply – as though emphasising either that self-injury was only used as a last resort or that the amount of release needed was less than the maximum possible:

> *i have started to cut my arms, not very deeply but enuff so it bleeds. i dont do it often, just when things get to much for me (respondent 93).*

Many respondents (23%) enjoyed the sight and feeling of self-injury and described a sensation of pleasure in feeling pain or seeing blood appear:

> *ive just started cuttin myself i like the way the blood dripz outta me n runs down my arm it makez me feel betta afterwardz (respondent 80);*

> *it helped so much to see my blood coz of how much it hurt me (respondent 146);*

> *"I sit alone at night with a knife in my hand, thinking of all the times when life was good, thinking should i or should i not?, I press the knife down hard on my arm, i see blood comeing from my arm, it feels so good (respondent 233).*

It appeared from many postings that the ritual of self-injury, especially the release of blood, served as a physical metaphor for release from emotional distress.[6] But despite the clear impression that self-injurers gain pleasure from the act, none of the postings specifically suggested attention seeking as a motive or pleasure gained from the response of others to the self-harming behaviour. On the contrary, many told stories of efforts to conceal scars or other evidence from parents or teachers.

Many respondents were concerned about hiding their scars, discussing how they used long sleeves, bracelets or bands to hide them. Some said they blamed their scars on their pet cat, whilst others went on to explain that hiding wasn't always necessary, for example:

I hav scars all over me and the only ppl who notice r ppl who look for them, and not many ppl do. Honestly. If the cuts r new and its obvious that they werent an accident, do try and hide them till they arent as obvious, but afta that no-one notices. When they're at the stage where you can pick them, shave over the top of them so there's nothing to pick, it stops them being as obvious and it doesnt even hurt. (respondent 44);

alot of people think that people who self-harm do it for attention but this is not true as we normally dont like anybody seeing the scaring and try and make it as discreet as possible (respondent 56);

it's not a trend or fashion statement it's about people who need help (respondent 16).

In contrast to these findings, it is widely believed that self-injuring is a learned "attention seeking" behaviour acquired by copying peers or media role models. The postings we analysed suggested that youth culture, attention seeking, or copying is not as big an issue as might be expected.

Other players on the stage: professionals, parents, and peers

Respondents stated that they found schools and counsellors for the most part to be unhelpful, although 45 (17%) felt that you should tell someone if you were harming. Teachers, they said, tended to either downplay or ignore the issue, or threatened the girls with telling their parents. This seemed to add to the stress associated with self-injury:

My friend used to cut herself and it took a long time for anyone to help. We all knew but she asked us not to tell so we didn't. When our tutor found out SHE didn't tell anyone either and I thought that that was out of order. When our assistent head found out she told her mum and dad who threatened to have her taken away to boarding school, which made her even more depressed (respondent 42);

I found that there is never, the support, awareness, or info, when you need it and it creates isolation, when you want somebody to realize, and nobody does. i found it hard to stop, i wanted somebody to help me but didnt want to tell anyone (respondent 69);

i cut ma self at the moment but things hav been really hard 4 me bcoz one of the teachers at school has found out and it's terrifiyin coz she always luks at my arm! so i've decided 2 do it sumwhere else now where she wnt expect! (respondent 26);

i fink that skools r partly 2 blame 4 the ppl all self-harming, becoz they put so much pressure on us and its just to hard to keep up and keep on top of things! (respondent 55).

The perception that professionals just wanted the behaviour to stop was common, and several respondents commented that this ignored the pervasive and compulsive nature of the problem, which was frequently compared to smoking and drug taking and described in the language of addiction:

A lot of people don't realise that cutting is hard to give up, like smoking or drinking, and you won't give up unless you make the descion to do so (respondent 125);

I have been cutting myself for about 9 months now. I am apparently depressed, but I went to see a therapist and couldn't stand talking to her so I lied to her. It is shameful. I mean you cut because you feel it will make you better and then you feel bad because you cut, so you cut again. Then you have to hide and lie about cat scractches. You MKP people say talk to some one about it. How can you when it is such an embaressing thing to do? It is like an addiction you can't stop. I did it once and I now do it every day some times more than once a day. Its a load of crap and I wish I had never started, but I can't stop now (respondent 30).

For those girls whose families were in crisis, the thought of a teacher telling them about self-injury led to a fear of punishment or ridicule. And for those girls who felt they had a "happy" family, they worried their parents would be upset or feel let down if they knew their daughter deliberately hurt herself. Some also worried they would add to their parent's problems:

i said i would tell my mum but i never did, but if it starts again i woudlnt know how to tell her, she already has her hands full with my sister let alone me (respondent 37);

These are supposed to be the best years of my life but i just feel trapped angry and sad. I cant tell my mum because I'm keeping her together she can't know and i cant see a GP without her knowing (respondent 82).

Fifty respondents (19%) noted that they resented other people's attempts to prevent them from harming, most commonly because they had not worked out any alternative strategies:

sometimes i dont want help, because ... What would i do instead of doing that, its the only thing I've ever done (respondent 6).

A minority of respondents recounted positive stories of getting help from counsellors and GPs, or from parents. These accounts were characterised by three themes: the respondent had felt listened to, had felt that she was not being judged, and had been offered practical coping solutions:

I've also told my mum and she helps by letting me turn my music up full blast when i get mad or she buys me flowers and chocolate to make me fell better and loved when i get down so i'm less likly to cut myself (respondent 40);

i went to one of my school teachers and told her about everything and she took me to the school nurse–they both told my mum because i was really worried about what she'd say to me. but luckily she was o.k about it and she supported me brilliantly. i got some councelling from my doctor and now i feel fine (respondent 67).

Despite these positive postings, the main source of help identified by the respondents who currently self-injured was overwhelmingly friends and peers, who were mentioned by 44 (16%):

friends can really help you overcome this problem so i think anyone who is a friend of a victim of self-injury should talk to them about it. its helped me and made me realise that friends are so important to u and if it upsets them then its not worth it! (respondent 168).

Respondents who wrote about friends who were self-harming worried about how they could best help them, implying a strong sense of responsibility for supporting a fellow teenager with a serious problem that could not be safely shared with professionals. The high proportion of positive recommendations to confide in friends, and the apparent willingness of friends to help, suggests that it may be appropriate to offer peer support or training to young people so they can assist those at risk of self-injury. However, this places a great deal of responsibility on a young person in a very emotive area. One posting on the board illustrated how hard it was to deal with a person who "comes out" as a self-injurer:

My boyfriend recently told me that he had cut himself about a year ago. At the time he was having a lot of trouble at home because his parents were splitting up. He told me he was so angry that he didn't feel any pain. What he told me has scared me. I keep thinking he's mad. If he can get into such a temper he turns a knife on himself, what might he do to other people? I suddenly have found I don't want to be near him any more (respondent 4).

Several other contributors picked up on this posting, accusing the respondent of being unfeeling and implying a moral responsibility to get involved (implicitly because professional sources of help would be no use). Clearly, there are both practical and ethical ambiguities to address before peer intervention can be used in the prevention of self-injury.

How will my story end? – concerns about the future

Amongst those who were currently self-injuring, the main fear expressed for the future was that they would be unable to stop, and that their self-harming behaviour would become more destructive and frequent:

I used 2 cut myself alot and now do it sum times. it is really hard 2 stop. Cutting urself is just a way of expressing frustrarion and anger without havin 2 explain 2 people (respondent 109).

Some respondents did not want to stop:

i have SH, i do it quite deeply and often. i have dun it so many time that i have dont have much space left to do it. i havnt told ne 1, not because im asshamed but because im worried about wot they will say or do. but personally i dont think that there is ne fing rong wit doin it. i do want to stop in a way just so i dont hav da scars ne more, but if i didnt hav SH then wot would i have!! (respondent 71).

This response suggests that although respondents were not attracted to harming *per se*, they felt it was the best strategy for relieving the emotional pain they were feeling.

Thirty-two respondents (12%) explicitly mentioned contemplating or attempting suicide. Respondents who had self-injured in the past but were not currently engaging in such acts said that their main fear was that the temptation of self-injury was very great and they could not rule out returning to it when life became upsetting.

Thirty-two respondents (12%) offered an alternative to self-injury, including poetry-writing, music, sport, religious rituals, physical expressions of anger, or keeping a "happy box" or diary:

Now when I want to cut myself I go for a long run, I just keep running and running and that helps (respondent 24);

when i get angry or upset now i write everything down even if it doesnt make sense, i feel better then keeping it inside or cutting myself (respondent 23);

When I get really upset, I write in my diary. I'm glad to have it, especially as it locks up, so all my thoughts are kept private. When I get angry, I kick or push the wall, imagining the commotion and mess it would make if it fell down (respondent 154);

There r plenty of other ways of dealin with depression: Go 4 a run, and pretend ur squashin ur problems with every step u take. Cry, long and hard and dont feel ashamed 4 it. As sum1 has already sed, make a happy box full of things that make u feel better like a photo of a loved one. Listen 2 music, scream, shout and generally b a nuisance 2 the neighbourhood (hey, ur folks mite not enjoy it, but im sure theyd prefer u 2 do that than harming urself!) Write all ur feelings down, then rip up the piece of paper, burn it, screw it up, throwin all ur problems away. JUST PLEASE DONT SELF-HARM!. (respondent 197)

It was noteworthy that those who were not currently self-injuring were more likely to suggest alternatives, whereas those currently self-injuring generally focused on the act of injury as a means of releasing emotions.

A commonly expressed fear about the future was that if they disclosed their self-injuring activities to a teacher or healthcare professional, that person would in turn inform their parents and all would act to "medicalise" the problem and take steps to prevent them from self-injuring:

I cud never tell my parents or a teacher or doctor cuz im scared of what wud happen (respondent 165).

In the eyes of the respondents, parents, teachers, and healthcare staff should be educated to look at the causes of self-injury and work around those, rather than simply attempting to stop the behaviour. There was also implicit resentment that the support from peers was not acknowledged or valued by the various adults involved:

if you know anyone whos doing this stand by them because all the medical stuff just doesnt help it just makes it harder for them. Dont send selfharmers to councillors make them talk to their friends and family their normally more help than you think (respondent 21).

Self-injury – a review of previous literature

Narratives of self-injury are common in our language, as metaphorical expressions rather than depictions of real actions, with frustration expressed in phrases like "I'm tearing my hair out" or "I feel like I'm banging my head against a brick wall". Self-injuring is traditionally viewed by psychiatrists as an external response to internal distress.[4] Some religions have incorporated either actual self-injury into mourning rituals,[7] or symbolic gestures of tearing at clothing (for example, the act of Kriah in the Jewish faith). The deliberate infliction of injury by doctors to "release" the unhealthy build-up of harmful agents (as in the act of bloodletting, or, in more extreme cases, lobotomy) used to be standard medical practice.

However, there is a marked difference between these cultural and historical activities and the more taboo issue of deliberate and sustained self-injury. Whilst self-injury is discussed within health care, it tends to be in the language of case reports and numbers – quantitative surveys that tell us how many people harm themselves, as opposed to explanations of why they do it. Part of the reason for this silence, is that self-injurers are secretive in nature,[8] and because Western society appears to want to ignore the upsetting notion that people, particularly young people, want to mutilate their bodies to secure some form of psychological relief. Reactions from the medical profession have ranged from appreciating that self-injury is a somatic language of distress[9] that needs to be understood and treated appropriately, to self-injury being a form of parasuicide requiring intervention,[4] or misunderstood as "attention seeking" or erroneously linked with body piercing or tattooing. Within these different responses it is also recognised that there is an increase in self-injury amongst young people, particularly teenage girls,[4,5] although information is lacking about the reasons why they choose to hurt themselves. Therefore healthcare staff, parents, teachers, and teenagers remain uncertain about what self-injury is, and what to do about it.[10,11]

Part of this problem is linked to the way self-injury has been researched and managed. Where evidence exists it tends to be based on older adults, those at risk of suicide,[4,12,13] who are being treated for mental health problems, frequently in secure units. Self-injury has been addressed in terms of a symptom of mental illness, rather than an act within itself, and treatment has tended to be around dealing with the mental health problem, or stopping attempts at self-injury, rather than trying to understand why and how people choose to injure themselves.[14] As a result, the needs and experiences of teenagers and others without any recognisable mental health problems have not been adequately addressed. Given the number of young people currently harming in the UK and elsewhere, it is necessary to understand the reasons why they are opting to self-injure.

The qualitative research that exists on self-injury is equally limited, given its location in case histories of psychiatric patients, accounts from children who are looked after in care,[14] or descriptions from adults recalling self-injury practices of their childhood.[6] Although these descriptions are useful in telling us about self-injury, they are limited to a particular population. As a consequence, self-injury is seen as a mental health problem, rather than a coping strategy, and certainly not a strategy that affects teenagers more than older adults, girls more than boys.[4,5,15]

Gender issues

It has been suggested that girls are twice as likely to injure than boys,[5] because of the way most cultures raise them.[15] Whilst boys are encouraged towards active sports and expression, girls are less likely to be directed in this way,[16,17,18] although attempts are being made to change this with charities like UNICEF or YWCA working to improve the lives of young women. And whilst boys are not necessarily encouraged to be verbally and physically aggressive, girls are more likely to be penalised for such behaviours.[16] Furthermore, particularly in Western cultures, but increasingly in other parts of the world, younger women are encouraged to monitor and criticise their bodies.[19,20] Girls are more likely to be victims of sexual abuse and eating disorders.[21,22] Boys do attempt to harm themselves, and have specific problems around coping with masculinity[23,24] that means they are more likely to be harmed through violence, and more likely to attempt, and succeed, at suicide.[24,25] Girls are encouraged to be quieter, stiller, to not make a fuss, to disappear, often physically through dieting. It is therefore not surprising that girls adopt the route of self-injury, since their voices are not and cannot be heard elsewhere. This research focuses on teenage girls, who are most at risk from self-injury, but we acknowledge the pressures of masculinity placed on young men, and encourage others to address the specific risks posed to boys.

Contagion, enjoyment, and media effects

Some of the silences around self-injury are linked to a fear that talking about it may increase it. There is some evidence of "contagion", where young women who are aware of other's self-injury may copy.[4] Yet our research shows that whilst this does occur, many people are unaware of self-injury, believing they are the "only one" who does it. Although it is understandable that parents, teachers, and healthcare providers may be concerned that in voicing the issue of self-injury they may perpetuate it, not discussing it may also mean self-injury continues untreated. This paper offers some ways to tackle the issue of harm that may be useful to readers. Linked with contagion is the belief that the media is responsible for an increase in self-injury. It is true that more people appear to be self-injuring, and there has been discussion of the practice in the press, including features in newspapers, magazines, television chat shows, and soap operas (for example, the UK soap *Hollyoaks* featured the character Lisa, who self-injured. See helplines at the end of this paper for more information). It is hard to say whether increased media coverage is exacerbating self-injury. It may be that in being open about the problem more people feel empowered to out themselves as a current or ex-harmer. When more charities began to acknowledge and address child abuse at the end of the twentieth century, it appeared that there was an increase in child abuse, but what was actually seen was a clearer picture of the prevalence of harm towards young people. It is likely that rather than the media causing self-injury, the media is reflecting the way young people are coping with stress.[26]

An even more unpalatable issue is that many people who self-injure report enjoying the behaviour.[6,27,28,29] This may range from pleasure in preparing to injure, or fantasising about how it may be achieved; to the act of self-injury, followed by the treatment of wounds or scars inflicted during the episode.[6] To some extent, our findings confirmed these concerns. It is, of course, hard to talk about or educate around self-injury if such a dangerous practice appears to give such relief and sometimes overt pleasure.

Why do people self-injure?

Although research on self-injury is limited, there is some evidence about the prevalence of self-injury, with estimates suggesting around 13% of young people deliberately self-injure.[4,5] Less is known about the causes and events that lead people to harm themselves, or about the way self-injurers feel about their bodies or their lives. Where information exists, reasons given for harming are: to feel more in control of one's life, as a stress reliever or a means of dealing with internal rage, grief or anger; or conversely to make a person actually feel something (if they feel emotionally numb generally). Some people have talked about the pleasure gained from feeling pain, witnessing the act of harming, or caring for their injuries.[6,27,28,29] Yet most of these accounts come from adults reflecting on harming in the past, or those in psychiatric care. The voices of the girls themselves are largely absent, and our own study is thus an important addition to the existing literature.

The underlying reasons for self-injury are, of course, critical for understanding and treating the problem, particularly since a wide range of healthcare staff will have to treat those who have attempted self-injury.[10,11,12] Currently, health professionals may only be aware of severe cases, and may not be fully aware of the experience of or reasons for self-injury. Our own study provides an important insight into the world of self-injury in less "medicalised" cases, and offers some ideas from the teenagers themselves about how treatment options may be approached.

Conclusions and recommendations

A number of reports and papers have already called for more awareness, training, and services around self-injury.[4,14,30,31,32,33] Most of these have suggested support for those at risk from self-injury as well as those who care for them. We applaud these recommendations, and add our own from the basis of our research.

This paper is an insight into self-injury. More needs to be done around awareness, education and support – particularly for parents and healthcare providers.

We need to understand the reasons why teenagers self-injure, as much as we need to know how many are at risk.

A high level of awareness of self-injury is needed when dealing with all teenagers, not just those in looked after or psychiatric care (although the latter groups are more at risk).

Self-injury needs to be tackled systematically in schools. A possible option for prevention and treatment is teaching communication and life skills to enable boys to lessen the risk of violence to themselves and others, and to assist girls in becoming more assertive and less likely to direct their feelings inwardly via self-injury.

Links with bullying, physical/emotional/sexual/substance abuse, and eating disorders need to be tackled alongside self-injury.

We need to understand that self-injury is a form of language in itself, a language of distress[9]; but we should not allow our anxieties about self-injury to silence us. We do not believe that in discussing self-injury we will cause it to spread, but our silences around it may cause it to grow. As one contributor to the site stated:

No-one takes teen problems serious enough ... its time we did something about it (respondent 17)

Acknowledgements

We would like to thank all the members of MKP who contributed to this research, and Jo Surnam for her help.

References

1 Denzin M, Lincoln P. *Handbook of Qualitative Research*. London: Sage, 1994.
2 Sharf B. Beyond Netiquette: the ethics of doing naturalistic discourse research on the internet. In: Jones S, ed. *Doing Internet Research: Critical Issues and Methods for Examining the Net*. Thousand Oaks, CA, London and New Delhi: Sage, 1999.
3 Pollack D. Pro-eating disorder websites: what should be the feminist response? *Feminism Psychol* 2003;**13**(2):46–51.
4 Hawton K, Rodham K, Evans E, Weatherall R. Deliberate self harm in adolescents: self report survey in schools in England. *BMJ* 2002;**325**:1207–11.
5 Ross S, Heath N. A study of the frequency of self-mutilation in a community sample of adolescents. *J Youth Adolesc* 2002;**31**(1):67–77.
6 Lutzenberger J. Cutting, craving and the self I was saving. In: Johnson ML, ed. *Jane sexes it up: true confessions of feminist desire*. New York and London: Walls Eight Windows, 2002.
7 Overview of World Religions http://philtar.ucsm.ac.uk/encyclopedia/index.html.
8 Rubenstein JL, Halton A, Kasten L, Rubin C, Stechler G. Suicidal behavior in adolescents: stress and protection in different family contexts. *Am J Orthopsychiatry* 1998;**68**(2):274–84.
9 Clark, A. Language of self-harm is somatic and needs to be learnt. *BMJ* 2002;**324**:788.
10 Reid S, Henry JA. Deliberate Self-Harm. *Primary Care Psychiatry* 2002;**8**(1):1–7.
11 McAllister M, Creedy D, Moyle W, Farrugia, C. Nurses attitudes towards clients who self-harm. *J Adv Nurs* 2002;**40**(5):578–86.
12 Runeson BS. Suicide after parasuicide. *BMJ* 2002;**325**:1125–6.
13 Bennewith O, Stocks N, Gunnell D, Peters TJ, Sharp DJ. General practice based intervention to prevent repeat episodes of deliberate self-harm: cluster randomised controlled trial. *BMJ* 2002;**324**:1254–66.
14 Bywaters P, Rolfe A. Look beyond the scars: understanding and responding to self-injury and self-harm. NCH (National Children's Home) http://www.nchafc.org.uk/page.asp?auto=336.
15 Shaw SN. Shifting conversations on girls' and womens' self-injury: an analysis of the clinical literature in historical context. *Feminism Psychol* 2002;**12**(2):191–219.
16 Hyde JS. *Half the human experience: the psychology of women*, 5th edn. Lexington, MA and Toronto: DC Heath, 1996.
17 Renzetti CM, Curran DJ. *Women, Men and Society*, 3rd edn. Boston, MA: Allyn and Bacon Worldwide, 1995.
18 Burton, Nelson M. *The stronger women get the more men love football: sexism and the culture of sport*. London: Virago, 1994.
19 Moore S, Rosenthal D. *Sexuality in adolescence*. London and New York: Routledge, 1993.
20 Doyal L. Abusing women. *What makes women sick: gender and the political economy of health*. Basingstoke: Macmillan, 1995.
21 Dohm FA, Striegel-Moore RH, Wilfley DE, Pike KM, Hook J, Fairburn CG. Self-harm and substance use in a community sample of black and white women with binge eating disorder or bulimia nervosa. *Int J Eating Dis* 2002;**32**(4):389–400.
22 Santa Mina EE, Gallop RM. Childhood sexual and physical abuse and adult self harm and suicidal behaviour: a literature review. *Can J Psychiatry* 1998;**43**(8):793–800.
23 Connell RW. *Masculinities*. Cambridge: Polity Press, 1995.
24 Men's Health Forum. *Soldier It! Young Men and Suicide: an audit of local service provision and young men's uptake of services*. MHF, 2002.
25 Kimmell MS. Masculinities as homophobia: fear, shame and silence in the construction of gender identity. In: Whitehead SM, Barrett FJ, eds. *The Masculinities Reader*. Cambridge: Polity, 2001.
26 Gunnell D. Reporting suicide: the effect of media coverage on patterns of self-harm. *BMJ* 1994;**308**:1446–7.
27 Favazza A. *Bodies Under Siege: Self-Mutilation in Culture and Psychiatry*. Baltimore, MD: Johns Hopkins University Press, 1987.
28 Hyman JW. *Women Living With Self-Injury*. Philadelphia: Temple University Press, 1999.

29   Strong M. *A bright red scream*. New York: Viking, 1998.
30   Royal College of Psychiatrists. *Managing deliberate self-harm in young people*. Council Report CR64. London: RCP, 1998.
31   Australasian College for Emergency Medicine. *Guidelines for the management of deliberate self harm in young people*. The Royal Australian and New Zealand College of Psychiatrists, 2000.
32   Auditor General Western Australia. *Life Matters: Management of Deliberate Self Harm in Young People*. Report No.11, 2001.
33   NHS Centre for Reviews and Dissemination. *Effective Health Care* – Deliberate Self Harm. December 1998;**4**(6):1–12.

Appendix 1: Self-injury – what to look out for

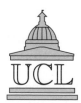
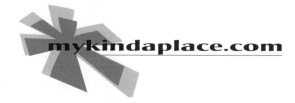

People who self-injure are, usually, both secretive and ashamed about what they are doing. This means self-injuring can continue for some time before it is detected – if it is detected at all. Here are some ways in which people could be hiding harming behaviour, and what to do about it.

Advice for friends

Self-injurers report they are most likely to tell a friend if they need help, and also find friends the most supportive place to go for advice. Before this happens, you might notice the following:

- Your mate might become more withdrawn or unhappy than usual.
- They may not want to do activities that involve undressing (e.g. sport – particularly swimming).
- They may wear increasingly baggy clothes, or clothes that cover the body (such as tops with long sleeves).
- They may be reluctant to undress in front of you.
- They may seem snappy or irritable.
- Places where they have cut or bruised themselves can hurt – they may flinch away from you if you touch them.
- They may talk about things like "cutting" or "scratching".
- You may notice they're wearing bandages or plasters on a regular basis.
- They may also have problems with their body image, or their attitude towards food.
- They may talk negatively about how they feel about themselves.

If you notice these, don't force them to tell you what is going on. Ask your friend if they are okay. If they admit they are self-injuring, try and find out why – are they angry, afraid, being bullied, or feeling depressed? Try and get help for those issues as they will be what drives harming behaviour. And don't forget to get help or support for yourself whilst this is going on.

What parents may hear or notice ...

As above, plus

- An unwillingness to share feelings and thoughts as much as usual.
- Increasing requests for privacy.
- Being quiet or withdrawn.
- Blaming cuts or scratches on other things, e.g. "the cat scratched me".

Young people who harm are often afraid their parents will be angry with them or feel disappointed. These worries can stop them confiding in you. Again, don't force them to tell, and if they do admit to harming do not shout at them or accuse them of being silly – this could make them worse. Also, don't feel you have failed as a parent or there is something wrong with your child. If they are harming it is because they are unhappy and you can help them feel better about this.

What teachers may hear or notice ...

As above, plus

- Conversations about cutting.
- Excuses not to take part in certain lessons or activities – particularly drama or physical education.
- Homework being missed, late, or not handed in.
- Bullying – many self-injury after being bullied.

Many young people do not trust teachers, they worry you'll go straight to their parents about this – which makes them more frightened and less likely to tell. If someone reveals they are injuring themselves, give them time to talk, don't threaten with telling the family, act dismissive or ignore the problem. This can make them feel more rejected.

What to do if you suspect self-injury is happening

- Don't get angry, shout or make accusations.
- Don't be dismissive, or think it's just "showing off".

- Make sure you talk to the person; make them aware they can confide in you.
- Offer support or referrals to other services (e.g. GP or school counsellor).
- Deal with problems that arise (e.g. low self esteem, or fear of bullies).
- Keep checking the harmer is okay.
- Offer solutions to help them deal with stress or anger.

It seems many young girls and some young boys are self-injuring in a response to stress, unhappiness or coping with "teenage problems". Rather than it being a sign of them having a mental health problem, for many it is a way of getting through life. However, this does not mean their behaviour should be ignored. You can find out more at http://www.mykindaplace.com/agony/cutting.asp.

Appendix 2: Support groups and useful resources

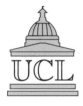 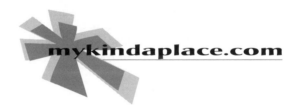

Channel 4 Television – Self-injury, as displayed by character Lisa on *Hollyoaks*
http://www.channel4.com/life/microsites/H/helplines/phone_h_selfharm.html
Childline (support for children who are victims of abuse)
http://www.childline.org.uk; Tel: 0800 11 11
Deliberate Self-injury in Young People – Advice sheet for parents and teachers from Royal College of Psychiatrists
http://www.rcpsych.ac.uk/info/mhgu/newmhgu30.htm
Eating Disorders Association
http://www.edauk.com/young_home.htm
Info Injection – resources for primary care workers about self-injury and suicide
http://www.le.ac.uk/li/clinical/outreach/infoinjection/suicide.pdf
National Children's Bureaux – includes a database of self-injury initiatives
http://www.selfharm.org.uk
National Self-injury Network
http://www.helen.ukpet.com

Read the signs – advice on mental health (including eating disorders and SH)
http://www.readthesigns.org/index.asp
SIARI (Self-injury and Related Issues) – support for self-injurers and those close to them
http://www.siari.co.uk
Self-injury Alliance – support group for self-injurers
http://www.selfharmalliance.org
Self-injury Advice – support for SH and advice on causes and treatment
http://www.palace.net/~llama/psych/injury.html
Self-injury Resources
http://www.selfinjury.freeserve.co.uk
Self-injury Resources and Biography
http://www.users.zetnet.co.uk/BCSW/pdfleafs/resources.pdf
Success Unlimited – anti-bullying site
http://www.successunlimited.co.uk
Unicef's Go Girls! Campaign
http://www.unicef.org/noteworthy/girlseducation/index.html
Young Minds – Children's Mental Health Charity
http://www.youngminds.org.uk
YWCA UK – *Hurting Inside Out.* Report can be ordered from
http://www.ywca-gb.org.uk/pcpublications.asp

6: The DIPEx project: collecting personal experiences of illness and health care

ANDREW HERXHEIMER, SUE ZIEBLAND

How DIPEx came about

The Database of Personal Experiences of Health and Illness (DIPEx) launched its website in July 2001 (http://www.dipex.org)[i]. This chapter describes how and why it came about, what it covers, and the many issues the project has raised about the methodology of collecting patients' narratives.

Andrew Herxheimer (a clinical pharmacologist) and Ann McPherson (a GP in Oxford) had the original idea of setting up a database of people's accounts of their experience of hospital treatments. The database was intended to complement the Cochrane Library (which reports on the best evidence from medical treatment trials) and help people facing treatment decisions to

---

Box 6.1 Poem written two weeks after a total knee replacement

Renewal

After *70 years the knee was tired, weak, rebellious,*
though still a friend and part of me.
They replaced grating bone with plastic and steel,
fixed to the old bones, bound by faithful muscle and skin,
new parts of me on probation.

I bend them to my will to make them a full member of the team:
a happy and confident knee, setting off only a few alarms.
Ends need means, said the foot to the hand.
Read our lips said the hips, gritting their teeth.

(Andrew Herxheimer, 1996)

decide what to do. The idea for the database resulted from Ann and Andrew's own "illness experiences" – Ann was treated for breast cancer in 1995 and Andrew had a knee replacement in 1996. Ann had written a personal view in the *BMJ*[1] and Andrew, a poem about his new knee (Box 6.1). These experiences sharpened their awareness of the value of hearing from others what it has been like to be ill and be treated.

In 1996 Andrew asked the Consumers' Association, with which he had worked for many years, for a small grant of £1000 to help develop the idea of a Database of Patients Experiences (DIPEx). Local research ethics committee approval was obtained for distributing a self-completion questionnaire. GPs and hospital consultants were asked to give this to people who were undergoing hospital treatments. Rachel Miller (a health researcher) joined the group to help with the survey and Barbara Sackett (temporarily in Oxford from Canada) provided administrative support. A poster introducing the DIPEx idea and results from the survey was presented at the Cochrane Colloquium in Amsterdam in October 1997.

In many ways the questionnaire responses were disappointing. Doctors forgot to ask patients to complete them. People who did fill them in wrote little about their experience and feelings about illness – tending to treat the questionnaires as patient satisfaction surveys ("the food was horrible and the nurses were lovely"). The group therefore decided that different methods were needed and asked Sue Ziebland (a medical sociologist working in Oxford) for advice about undertaking interviews with patients. Sue recommended using qualitative research methods to conduct systematic and rigorous studies of each condition or disease included in DIPEx. This would require using purposive (or maximum variation) sampling methods to ensure that the broadest possible range of experiences was included. Rachel had used similar methods before and we started to plan DIPEx as a set of good, publishable research studies that would also make a website resource for patients. We all read Arthur Kleinman's *The Illness Narratives*.[2] Andrew and Sue went on a Wellcome History of Medicine oral history course in the summer of 1998 which further influenced us to use a very unstructured "oral history" approach to collect people's narratives. We also learned from the methods of consent and copyright that oral historians use to deposit interviews at the British Sound Archive at the British Library. These formed the basis of our later multicentre research ethics committee approval.

At this stage DIPEx meetings were very informal and conducted around Ann's kitchen table. Andrew and Rachel were both based in London and drove over for meetings every 4–6 weeks. Sasha Shepperd (a health researcher then based at Imperial College, London) joined the group to advise on the health information side of the site. Sasha had recently developed a tool entitled DISCERN for evaluating the content of consumer health information and we were keen to ensure that information included in DIPEx met these standards. During this time Ann and Andrew (in particular) went to many meetings to promote the DIPEx idea to try to get funding. Almost every time we met to discuss the project we (or others) thought of another potential use for the resource: for carers as well as patients; to improve scientists' understanding of the public as well as public understanding of science; to help balance the relationship between patients and health professionals; in teaching medical students; illustrating medical text books; contributing to shared decision making; for health issues (for example, screening and smoking cessation) as well as illnesses; as a resource for patients' representatives on committees; and many more.

DIPEx: what it is and what it does

DIPEx is now a registered charity with a research group based in the University of Oxford Department of Primary Health Care. Its primary aim is to describe the widest practicable range of peoples' individual experiences of health and disease, and to provide a rich information resource for people affected by diseases and for those who look after them. The steering group, responsible for strategic planning and policy, comprises the co-founders (AH and Ann McPherson, also medical director), the research director (SZ), a medical consultant (Rachel Miller), a senior member of the research team (Alison Chapple), the director of the DIPEx charity and a patient/user representative (Gill Needham). The research team of nine are all senior qualitative researchers with backgrounds in medical sociology, anthropology, history or policy research, and each is responsible for collecting the data and analysing one module. Each researcher is supported by another DIPEx qualitative researcher and one of our medical team, as well as by members of their project advisory panel. Many of the researchers have said how much they enjoy being part of a project that has a product of such tangible benefit to the patient group they have become involved with in the study. (This benefit is sometimes contrasted with some of the more nebulous outputs of academic research).

Box 6.2 A story from the DIPEx breast cancer database

Okay last August one Sunday evening I was reaching over on my desk to get a pen and felt a dreadful pain inside my right breast. Prior to that I had had some itching, my nipple was itching very, very intensely and er I didn't think about it, itchy nipple to me didn't mean anything suspicious. But when I felt

(Continued)

Box 6.2 (Continued)

the pain and the lump er I immediately was struck with fear and foreboding and didn't know what to do. My family were away visiting the in-laws and I had a dreadful night, but I had an appointment at the doctor's for the next day for something else, something totally unrelated. When I saw the doctor that day, the next day after finding the lump er, when we'd finished about the prior consultation I mentioned that I'd found a lump in my breast and I was terribly afraid. He sent me in to see the nurse, the practice nurse, and er she basically dismissed it as being hormonal, my age, "80% of breast lumps are nothing, don't worry, go home, keep a diary."

I went home feeling still very anxious and very worried and er kept a diary. That was on the Monday, on the Thursday I hadn't slept for 2 nights, I felt dreadful and er so I phoned the nurse again and told her. And she said "We need an appointment with me and the doctor so can you come in on Tuesday?" That was 8 days after the original appointment, which I agreed to. I went to the surgery that day and sat in the nurse's room for 22 minutes, half naked, feeling absolutely ghastly. She came into the room and said that the doctor was too busy to see me. That was like somebody stabbing a knife in me. Er she took my blood telling me that this was all hormonal and I had nothing to worry about, go home. I went home, I went outside of the practice and broke my heart in the car. It still hurts to talk about this bit of my treatment because I felt as if I wasn't worthy of even seeing a doctor at that point. To be told that the doctor is too busy to see you when you have an appointment, when you're very worried and you've got a breast that won't even fit in your biggest bra was dreadful.

Anyway I went home and my sister who was a mammographer of all things was away on holiday. She came back on the Saturday and I confided in her. It was at this point that my life was turned around. She made me promise her that I would go to the doctors and demand an examination. That I did on the Tuesday. I had the appointment for the results of my blood test and I walked into the doctors, put my diary on the table and said "I demand an examination." The doctor said he had examined me and I told him he had not and he said "Okay let's examine you now, I'll go and get the nurse." Prior to this the nurse had told me she wasn't qualified to examine breasts, but that appointment she did examine my breast with the doctor there. Again I felt as if I wasn't worthy of the doctor's attention, that the doctor was shunning me again but at least he did the right thing and he sent me straight to hospital.

The first two DIPEx collections ("modules") dealt with hypertension and prostate cancer. Now, in April 2004, eight more modules have been added, on cancer of the breast, bowel, lung, testis and cervix, epilepsy, heart failure, and children with congenital heart disease. Work on 12 further modules is progressing (see Table 6.1). We have a list of 100 conditions that we would like to cover in the next five years, but which we will actually do depending on funding. There are some issues (for example, experiences of medically unexplained symptoms) that, though important, are not associated with a particular voluntary group

Table 6.1 DIPEx programme (April 2004)

Module name	Completion expected	Funded by
Rheumatoid arthritis	Autumn 2004	Arthritis and Rheumatism Council
End of life	Summer 2004	Gatsby Charitable Fund
Sexual health of young people	Summer 2004	Department of Health
Chronic pain	June 2004	The Health Foundation
Breast screening	Autumn 2004	National Screening Committee
People with dementia and their carers	Autumn 2004	Alzheimer's Society (part)
Depression	August 2004	Department of Health
Antenatal screening	October 2004	National Screening Committee
Ovarian cancer	Spring 2005	Cancer Research UK
Antenatal care	Spring 2005	National Screening Committee
Terminations for fetal abnormality	2005	National Screening Committee
Teenage cancers	Summer 2005	Wooden Spoon

or area of Department of Health funding, whereas the cancer modules have attracted funding from several sources (see Table 6.1).

Several other UK research groups see the website as a means of public dissemination and added value for their own research on health and illness and therefore collect interviews that are compatible and copyrighted for DIPEx. We are keen to encourage such collaborations. We also promote the use of DIPEx resources in teaching clinical communication and qualitative research methods as well as for secondary analysis by researchers.

DIPEx enquiries use the qualitative method of in-depth interviews. Participants are encouraged to talk without interruption about all aspects of their experiences that have mattered to them. This type of "illness narrative" provides raw data and has long been used in social science analyses. In the 25th Anniversary edition of the journal *Sociology of Health and Illness* (2003), Julia Lawton[3] reviews how in-depth interviews have been widely used by medical sociologists, often to "champion patients' perspectives, by putting them centre stage" (p 25). However, sociologists do not simply record peoples' views and perspectives and present them without comment. Research informed by medical sociology typically examines the contexts in which illness and health behaviours take place, and seeks to understand how society, self, and physical bodies, shape experience of illness. Important explanatory notions which have arisen from this sociological approach include the careful analyses that led to Charmaz's perspective of "loss of self",[4] Bury's concept of "biographical disruption",[5] and Williams' notion of "narrative reconstruction".[6] These concepts have helped to build understanding of experience of illness, and have inspired research into many different conditions.

The rich qualitative data behind every DIPEx module have convinced us that building a website is not enough to alert a diverse audience to the significance of our findings. Papers, announcements, and chapters reporting our findings could help all who communicate and deal with patients, as well as some research communities, and time for writing these is built into the DIPEx programme.

We want DIPEx research to contribute to qualitative social science as well as to clinical practice. We therefore aim to publish our results in journals with differing readerships, covering self-help groups, GPs, nurses, various clinical specialists, researchers, medical sociologists, and managers.

Examples of findings from DIPEx narratives

The DIPEx researchers have undertaken, analysed, collated, and indexed over 750 narrative interviews so far. We list below some examples of findings that we believe have widespread implications for the management of patients and the design and delivery of health services.

Getting the right information

Many people still do not know how to find information they need when facing a diagnosis or dilemma. This applies to those with common diseases, such as breast and prostate cancer, which are frequently written and talked about and for which information resources and self-help groups are well established. Health professionals are not good at guiding people at an early stage of their disease to sources relating to personal needs and preferences.

In our evaluation, based on focus groups with breast and prostate cancer patients, respondents reported that information provided by health professionals had been "patchy, inconsistent, contradictory, and haphazard". As one man with prostate cancer reported: *"The information is there but it's not generally and freely put to you unless you go and drag it out of the system."*[7] Most participants regarded health professionals as a reliable source of general medical information, but several pointed out that it could be difficult to get unbiased information about treatments from consultants, who often appeared, perhaps not unreasonably, to favour the particular treatment they advocate and offer. People we interviewed distinguished between medical advice, which they said they would not accept from the unqualified, and the practical and experiential information and support they could receive from other patients. They valued DIPEx because it offers access to the experiences of others without the emotional demand involved in personal interaction. Some people are happy to join a support group, but others hesitate to expose themselves to perceived additional emotional demands. Private access to personal information through Internet resources can help those who are shy, uncertain, or simply unconvinced that they could benefit from a support group.

Follow-up – quality and frequency

Specialist cancer services in the UK are under considerable pressure, sharpening attention on the need for appropriate and cost effective follow-up after hospital treatment. When there is little evidence to support specialist follow-up, an individual patient's preference is particularly important. We have explored the follow-up needs and preferences expressed in DIPEx bowel cancer interviews, and have also surveyed follow-up practices in UK hospitals within colorectal cancer collaborative services.[8] We discovered a wide variation in follow-up patterns, involving different tests, time periods, and personnel, yet very few (3/35 (< 10%)) policies that we were referred to stated that patients should be given a choice about the type and pattern of follow-up. Analysis of DIPEx interviews indicates that not all patients welcome specialist follow-up. Some had little faith in tests offered by specialists, were made anxious by hospital visits, or thought bowel cancer patients should be given better information about symptoms and should be encouraged to report any problems to their GP or specialist nurse. Patients' needs were rarely judged resource-intensive: generally, those interviewed wanted a responsive and interested GP, guidance about where to find information and support from the voluntary sector, and clear consistent advice about diet.

Understanding the meaning of "screening"

Interviews with men with prostate cancer revealed that many had had the Prostate-Specific Antigen (PSA) test, often as part of routine private health screening, without being fully informed of the implications of the test results. The UK National Screening Committee does not recommend a national screening programme because there is insufficient evidence, as yet, about the effects of screening, or treatment, on longer term morbidity and mortality. However, we found that men with prostate cancer felt strongly that healthy men should be screened with the PSA test, even if they knew that the test lacks accuracy and that earlier diagnosis has not been shown conclusively to lead to more effective treatment. DIPEx informants believed that early diagnosis *would* reduce mortality, improve quality of life *and* save the NHS money. They argued that testing should be available because (a) symptoms can be ambiguous, (b) screening is seen as responsible health behaviour and would encourage men to look after their health, and (c) there is equivalent screening for women's cancers.[9] These perspectives explain why prostate cancer support groups campaign to establish a PSA screening programme.[10] Our sampling methods require that we include the broadest range of views, but the research team had to make considerable efforts to find men to interview who were not in favour of PSA screening.

Our study also included interviews with men who much regretted having been PSA tested, because the test result came to dominate their thoughts and, in some cases, led to invasive treatment with unpleasant complications. Once a raised PSA has been found, and has therefore to be followed by regular repeat measurements, the man and his family often worry and feel that "something must be done". Such pressure can be hard to resist, but we hope that the careful balance of views expressed in the DIPEx prostate cancer module, may help men to make a more informed decision about whether to have a PSA test, or not.

[Un]informed treatment choices

People's accounts of what treatments they were offered revealed that some potentially appropriate choices were frequently not mentioned. Sometimes such choices were considered only when the patient had obtained independent information (often from the Internet). For new treatments this is understandable, but a man with prostate cancer expressed a frustration that other men also felt, when he complained that it was hard to get an unbiased assessment of the pros and cons of treatments, because surgeons tend to favour surgery and radiotherapists tend to recommend radiotherapy:

> *The problem with the options was that it was very, very much compartmentalised. When I went to see the surgeon I think his idea was that radical prostatectomy is the thing. And that's what I've heard from everybody else, because all urologists are basically surgeons and they say to a hammer everything looks like a nail, and I think that's very much the way it is. And so you know, if I went to him he could only give me information about surgery. I was put onto somebody who was involved in radiotherapy and he gave me a lot of information about external beam radiation. (Testimony of a 51-year-old man who chose to have brachytherapy in 2000)*

An example from the cervical cancer study is a woman who was offered hysterectomy, but learned through her husband – who was a doctor – about a new operation, trachelectomy, which would leave her uterus intact and so not preclude future pregnancy. The patient consulted the surgeon who happened to be introducing this procedure in another hospital, and she was happy to become the first patient in the UK to undergo the procedure.

In two striking scenarios, it seemed quite common for patients not to be offered a well-established treatment option. The first was where "watchful waiting" (also known as "active monitoring") for men with prostate cancer was judged appropriate as an alternative to surgery or radiotherapy, each of which has potentially serious drawbacks.[11] The second example concerned the management of testicular cancer. Testicular prostheses have been available since the 1970s, and men should be informed, in advance, about the possibility of inserting a prosthesis at the time of orchidectomy. However, a number of men reported that they were not told that prostheses were available, and some of those who were told were given no time to decide what to do.[12]

What people say about their medicines

In ordinary practice doctors focus on specific questions, for example, whether the patient is taking the medicine, whether particular effects have occurred. DIPEx interviews differ from such conversations in that the participants have no clinical relationship with the social scientists who interviewed them, they were interviewed at home and may have felt less inhibited, when talking about their perceptions about a medicine and how they use it, than if interviewed in a healthcare setting. People's beliefs, understandings, and routines often become clear only when they feel free to talk about the medicines and anything else that is important to them, *without interruption* and *for as long as they want*. Box 6.3 summarises perceived benefits and concerns about hypertension medication, and the following quotes from the hypertension study illustrate some of these key issues.

Box 6.3 Perceptions of taking anti-hypertension medication

Benefits
Feeling protected against stroke
Migraines stopped
Perceived symptoms reduced

Concerns
Side effects, now and in the future
Dislike of taking any drugs
Questioning the necessity of taking any drugs
Not being able to forget about the hypertension

A 61-year-old doctor interviewed for the hypertension module explained why he did not want to take beta blockers, although the impotence that he feared is not, statistically, a notable problem with the medicine:

I never wanted to take beta blockers because they were the main thing that seemed to cause impotence. Those were the ones where impotence was high profile. And therefore I thought I would cut out that worry … I think I am quite suggestible and once you'd read that the beta blockers might make you impotent … I said "Oh to hell with that. I'd rather try something that was less up-front about it."

A professional woman aged 60 described how she disliked taking beta blockers and how her perspective on the effects of the medicine differed from that of the trainee doctor she saw:

I saw a young GP, in fact I don't think he had yet passed his exams, who said "High blood pressure, no problem, we will put you on beta blockers." And immediately did this and took my blood pressure a week or so later and it was down to 120 over 80.

He said, "That's fine we have solved the problem."

And I said, "I feel awful, I feel much worse than when I wasn't taking anything and I don't think beta blockers suit me and can we try something else?" and he said "No, these work. What's your problem?"

And I got absolutely enraged with him because he was not listening to what I was saying which was that the quality of my life was wrecked by these things.

I felt physically exhausted, I could barely climb the stairs. It was quite a low dose, about 20 mg. I could barely climb the stairs without my legs aching so much I wanted to collapse and I felt depressed … That's what depression is like … I remember it very vividly. And this was directly related to that medication.

It is also quite possible to feel that medication protects against a condition, whilst voicing considerable concerns about side effects. However, some participants questioned whether they really needed to take the prescribed drugs, and suspected that they might have "white coat hypertension", which only manifests itself in a hospital clinic. Participants with home blood pressure monitors were able to reassure themselves that they really did have hypertension, which removed the concern about taking tablets unnecessarily. For this woman in her

50s, dislike of taking medication was serious enough to make her consider not taking any drugs:

And I am seriously thinking of not taking the tablets. I do feel ... I wake up in the morning and I actually feel quite good and then I take the pill and I seem to lose energy. I really ... I don't know if I am imagining it but I seem to not have that life force that I had before I took the pill and I don't know whether that's because I secretly don't like drugs – do you see what I mean? And obviously I'm not stupid and if I knew my risk was incredibly high I would just say "Well I'd rather be here than not be here, rather be here feeling a bit rough than not be here" and I would take them.

What emerges is more complicated and more interesting than "compliance" or "concordance" viewed mechanistically. For example, many people with hypertension, for various reasons, chose not to take their tablets at least part of the time. Some – among them a doctor – "forgot" to take the medication, because they did not want to be reminded there was something wrong. Others felt that the side effects of the medication were greater than could be justified by the risk that they would run if they did not take the medication. One man reasoned that since so many people with hypertension are not being treated, if he left off his tablets, he believed he would be no different from them.

How people seek information about their health, and why

DIPEx interviews contain many accounts of how, and why, people have sought information. Many of our respondents had used the Internet – either directly or via a friend or relation – to try to find out about their condition. Their experiences are interesting because little empirical research has so far examined the possible effects of health information on the Internet,[13] though there has been much speculation.

We have analysed the various ways in which people with cancer talk about using the Internet, and have identified not only a far broader range of purposes than has previously been noted, but have also looked at what accessing health information means for patients. People use the Internet to check the significance of symptoms, to find out about diagnostic tests, to check that they are being offered the best treatments, to learn how others may have told their children about their illness, to give and gain support, and to share information and campaign. They also describe considerable caution in interpreting the information they find on the Internet – checking it against several different sources and being very sceptical about information that is found on only one site. We conclude that this facility enables people to display – to family, friends, and health professionals as well as the researcher – their expertise; thereby they maintain their sense of "social fitness", which can be threatened by serious illness.[14] This positive aspect of Internet use has escaped many other commentators, who have often been more concerned with the dangers of inaccurate and misleading Internet information, or perceived threat to professional identities in medicine.[15,16]

Uncomfortable topics

Doctors recognise some aspects of diseases as important, but frequently find them too uncomfortable to discuss, among them, incontinence, stigmatisation, sex, and how to tell children when a parent is seriously ill. People who have had cancer describe how sexual difficulties were ducked, and how they struggled to maintain their previous persona. For example, although bowel cancer is often described as an "embarrassing" illness, our interviews suggest that the word is quite inadequate for the utter humiliation and loss of adult identity that many patients experience when they lose bowel control.[17] Professionals who do not understand this are in danger of sounding glib and out of touch when they give advice. Stories of how people had (or had not) told their children about their disease help others to decide what to do themselves. We would have found it hard to imagine how a mother could tell her four-year-old son that she had bowel cancer.

A major theme in the prostate cancer stories is that *"hormone drugs attack a man in every department where he feels he is a man"* – impotence, labile mood, lack of energy, inability to work. Patients may not be warned about these possible effects, and by the time they have had the treatment it is too late.[18] This contrasts with the experience of men with testicular cancer, who seldom reported feeling less masculine after treatment. Most could resume normal life, including sexual activity. An unexpected discovery, which may help in consultations, concerned the way they used jokes. Many who had lost a testicle initiated jokes to manage feelings, to hide embarrassment, to reduce tension, to share a sense of solidarity with others, and to encourage others to examine themselves. These men also described their reaction to jokes made by others, which was usually positive; jokes helped to dispel tension and reassure them that they were being treated as normal by their family and friends. Exceptions were men born with only one testicle who then developed cancer, those who had lost both testicles, and a man who could not ejaculate. These men were sometimes upset about jokes made by others, or by the idea of jokes being made, fearing humiliation, stigma, and prejudice.[19] Although the ability to "take a joke" is an important part of young male identity in the UK, these findings demonstrate the need for clinicians to be careful about using humour until they are confident of the patient's perspective.

Attitudes to the National Health Service

Positive accounts of experiences within the UK NHS were reassuring at a time when weaknesses in the delivery of health care were receiving widespread media coverage. For example, the parents of children with congenital heart disease expressed enthusiastic admiration for health services, and the way their predicament was handled, and seemed untarnished by the reports on events in Bristol and at Alder Hey Hospital in Liverpool. This was a welcome contrast to the stream of criticisms of the NHS at this time (2002–3), suggesting that it was dysfunctional and ready to collapse. In some cases, an abnormality had been detected during pregnancy, in others it had not been correctly predicted. Whatever the story, parents praised the sympathetic attention and explanation they had received; and when surgery had been needed, they were particularly appreciative of the support from the cardiac liaison nurse, who could be reached at any time. Parents said that they were never made to feel their request for advice was unnecessary, and that the response received was always prompt and appropriate. Intensive therapy units were also universally admired: mentions included the anticipatory visit which was always offered to the patients interviewed, the constant individual care (one nurse per patient), and the impressively advanced technology used. Open-heart surgery was being performed in tertiary hospitals, often quite far from the family's home, with the resulting potential for expense and domestic disruption. Thoughtfully, funds had been provided for journeys (in one instance visits to outpatients entailed a plane journey), and in some places accommodation was provided for parents and other children if required, with beepers so that relatives could quickly be called to their baby's bedside.

DIPEx participants with lung cancer were asked if their experiences had had any effect on their views of the NHS – a question phrased carefully and neutrally to prompt positive as well as negative responses. Either implicitly (by using phrases such as "I couldn't find any fault") or explicitly in their accounts, patients contrasted their own (usually good) experiences of care with their (usually poor) expectations of the NHS. Low expectations included: that it would take a long time to see the specialist, or that they would have to wait for treatment; and that doctors and nurses would be too busy to give explanations.

Methodological and theoretical issues

The DIPEx initiative has raised a number of methodological and theoretical issues around the collection, analysis, and publication of patients' stories. From the start, we were concerned that a long and detailed interview might upset some patients. Reliving unresolved problems and experiences can be painful; public exposure of private reflections might cause some harm. These possibilities cannot be entirely prevented, but the risk is lessened by employing only experienced qualitative researchers skilled in handling sensitive issues, and by the interview method.

At the start of each DIPEx interview the participant is asked to tell the story from the point when she or he first suspected that there was something wrong. The researcher provides an audience for this story, avoiding interruption, until the account has arrived in the present, the day of the interview. Some respondents are able to relate a coherent and lengthy story covering the many issues we would ideally like to hear, while others are evidently less confident in talking about what has happened to them. We describe this section of the interview as the oral history or "narrative" part, because the floor is very much handed over to the respondent to tell their story in whatever way they want. The researcher may then ask for clarification or expansion of some of the issues raised, before using a set of additional semi-structured questions and prompts to explore topics that we are always interested in (for example, ideas about causes, medications, and side effects, where information has been sought, views on the NHS and medical communication) as well as further issues particular to the condition concerned, identified from the review of the literature and earlier interviews.

Unlike many research studies that set out with a single, closely defined research question, this type of qualitative study aims to understand the different perspectives, priorities, and interpretations of the research participants.[20] Interviews have lasted between 1 and 6 hours and have sometimes involved more than one visit. They are a very rich form of data for many different types of analysis.

In a narrative interview the respondent controls its structure, length, and content, and intrusive questions are avoided. To guard against publication of material that might cause embarrassment on the website we are careful about our consent and copyright procedures. After detailed explanation about the nature of this research and the publication intention of the researchers, participants sign a consent form before the interview but they are not asked to sign a copyright form (which gives permission for the interview to be used in broadcasting, teaching, and research) until later. Participants receive a copy of the transcript and are free to withdraw the interview, limit the selections to anonymous written or audio clips, or to identify sections to be withheld. To date about 10% of participants have chosen to remove part of their interview, very few have withdrawn the full interview. Researchers are now categorising the removed sections (for example, personal detail about self or family; pejorative comment about health professional) to elucidate further what types of information people withdraw.

In contrast to most quantitative studies, such as surveys that are designed to answer a limited number of precise, pre-defined questions, the relatively unstructured nature of narrative interviews means that interviews for DIPEx projects can be used for many different qualitative analyses. An individual narrative interview can be the focus of an analysis (using, for example, sociolinguistic methods), or interviews can be looked at in their condition-specific collections of 30–50 interviews, or a particular theme can be analysed across several collections. Each of the DIPEx collections is selected as a maximum variation sample (chosen to include people whose experiences are likely to differ because of condition-specific factors as well as the usual age, gender, ethnicity and treatment choice), which is not intended to be numerically representative of the population from which it is drawn. Analyses based on the assumption of a statistically representative sample would therefore be misleading, even though relatively large numbers could be achieved by combining different collections.

Patients telling their story have a sense of altruism and solidarity with others, analogous to giving blood. We have been struck by how they feel more part of the wider community in sharing their story; some may even gain greater self-understanding and self-esteem. Many participants have become enthusiastic about DIPEx and feel a bond with it. We also feel a bond with those who have contributed, and want to maintain some contact with them. We have held launch parties for several of the modules, when interview participants are invited and many attend. Participants who had contributed to recent modules, and their guests, came to an event held at the House of Lords in March 2003. Many very much enjoyed meeting other DIPEx participants – some had never before talked to other people with their condition.

Conclusion

We believe that the DIPEx collections bring qualitative health research findings to medical audiences and the public, and in the process, *bridge* the different views, interests, and perspectives of these distinct audiences. There is considerable interest in promoting public understanding of science – we believe that a parallel enterprise should be to further science's understanding of the public. To this end we have encouraged the use of DIPEx interviews in undergraduate and postgraduate education of doctors and other health workers.

Patients' experiences are an important touchstone for the modern NHS, yet there is little agreement about how to incorporate and make use of them. Many committees now routinely have a patients' representative, but there are concerns that they are rarely "truly" representative of their identity group (a criticism that, it is only fair to point out, is rarely levelled at the sole GP, epidemiologist, pharmacologist or sociologist on the committee). The DIPEx collections are freely available to all and are a straightforward and powerful way for patients' representatives to enhance their understanding of the experiences of other patients – including those who would never be willing or able to take part in a committee. As more modules are published many different health service committees will be able to draw on DIPEx data to identify the patients' perspectives. The selection of national, maximum variation samples in all DIPEx collections is important for this purpose and should enhance the ability of patients' representatives to contribute to their committees.

We are also keen to persuade clinical scientists and their funders to include a patient-centred qualitative component in research.[21] We have made a start by proposing a link between individual Cochrane reviews and the corresponding DIPEx module.[22] For example, the review of chemotherapy for advanced colon cancer would be linked to the summary of what patients who had undergone such treatment had to say about it in DIPEx interviews.

To date, DIPEx collections have only included participants who are living in the UK – although people of minority ethnic groups have been included in all our studies. There is, however, considerable potential for international collaborations and we are keen to encourage groups to start collecting compatible narrative interviews of patients in their countries, using the local languages. That should eventually make it possible to compare illness experiences in different cultures and health systems. The first step in this direction has been to publish accounts of the project in other major languages – articles have now appeared in German, Italian, Japanese, Spanish, and Chinese[23].

Acknowledgement

We are grateful to all of the interview participants and to our colleagues for their help with this chapter.

End Note

i   The original name was "Database of Individual Experiences", but we found that 'individual' was a word that few people use, so substituted 'personal'. In 2004 we also finally realised that 'DIPEx' means nothing to people, and adopted an additional internet address www.personalexperiences.org which leads to the same site.

References

1 McPherson A. The quality of the b(r)east. *BMJ* 1995;**310**:1339.
2 Kleinman A. *The illness narratives: suffering, healing and the human condition.* New York: Basic Books, 1988.
3 Lawton J. Lay experiences of health and illness: past research and future agendas *Sociol Health Illness* 2003;**25**:23–40.
4 Charmaz K. Loss of self: a fundamental form of suffering in the chronically ill. *Sociol Health Illness* 1983;**5**:168–95.
5 Bury M. Chronic illness as biographical disruption. *Sociol Health Illness* 1982;**4**:167–82.
6 Williams G. The genesis of chronic illness: narrative reconstruction. *Sociol Health Illness* 1984;**6**:175–200.
7 Rozmovits L, Ziebland S. What do patients with prostate or breast cancer want from an internet site? A qualitative study of information needs. *Patient Educ Couns* 2004;**53**:57–64.
8 Rozmovits L, Rose P, Ziebland S. In the absence of evidence who chooses? A qualitative study of patients' needs after treatment for colorectal cancer. *J Health Serv Res Policy* (in press).
9 Chapple A, Ziebland S, Shepperd S, *et al.* Why men with prostate cancer want wider access to Prostate Specific Antigen (PSA) testing: qualitative study. *BMJ* 2002;**325**:737–9.
10 Rowlands D, Rowlands S, eds. *PSA Newsletter* 2000;**4**:2–6.
11 Chapple A, Ziebland S, Herxheimer A, McPherson A, Shepperd S, Miller R. Is "watchful waiting" a real choice for men with prostate cancer? A qualitative study. *BJU International* 2002;**90**:257–64.
12 Chapple A, McPherson A. The decision to have a prosthesis: a qualitative study of men with testicular cancer. *Psychooncology* (in press).
13 Eysenbach G, Powell J, Kuss O, Sa ER. Empirical studies assessing the quality of health information for consumers on the world wide web: A systematic review. *JAMA* 2002;**287**:2691–700.
14 Ziebland S, Chapple A, Domelow C, Evans J, Prinjha S, Rozmovits L. How the Internet affects patients' experience of cancer: a qualitative study. *BMJ* 2004;**328**:564–7.
15 Eng TR, Maxfield A, Patrick K, Deering MJ, Ratzan SC, Gustafson DH. Access to health information and support: a public highway or a private road? *JAMA* 1998;**280**:1371–5.
16 Coiera E. The internet's challenge to health care provision. *BMJ* 1996;**31**(2):3–4.
17 Rozmovits L, Ziebland S. Expressions of loss of adulthood in the narratives of colorectal cancer patients. *Qualitative Health Res* 2004;**14**:187–203.
18 Chapple A, Ziebland S. Prostate cancer: embodied experience and perceptions of masculinity. *Sociol Health Illness* 2002;**24**:820–41.
19 Chapple A, Ziebland S. The role of humour for men with testicular cancer. *Qualitative Health Res* (in press).
20 Popay J, Rogers A, Williams G. Rationale and standards for the systematic review of qualitative literature in health services research. *Qualitative Health Res* 1998;**8**:341–51.
21 Herxheimer A. Factoring in the patient – proposal for a third dimension in trial design. *CERES News* 2003;issue **33**:1–3.
22 Herxheimer A, Ziebland S. Illustrating Cochrane reviews with narrative clips describing patients' experiences of the interventions. *Cochrane Collaboration Methods Groups Newsletter* June 2003;**7**:5–6.
23 Successively updated translations of the original paper (*Lancet* 2000;**355**:1540–3) have appeared in: *Zeitschrift f Allgemeinmed* 2001;**77**:323–7, *Ricerca e Pratica* 2001;**17**:181–9, *The Informed Prescriber (Tokyo)* 2002, *Atención Primaria* 2003; **31**:386–8, *Chinese J Evidence Based Med* 2003.

7: Narratives of spirituality and religion in end-of-life care

ARTHUR W FRANK

To invoke spirituality or religion at any point in a life is to shape the experiences of that life to fit a particular narrative. In contemporary medical care, spiritual and religious narratives are most often invoked in end-of-life care. One great contribution of the hospice movement has been to make spirituality an explicit focus in end-of-life care. But to shape an experience one way is necessarily to neglect, avoid, or reject other narratives. This chapter is about what particular narratives see and what they ignore, and the clinical problem of recognising when clinicians and patients are not telling the same story.

Narrative is too expansive a concept to define, so in place of a definition, I will use a metaphor of narrative that I find especially helpful due to its simplicity. The literary critic Frank Kermode suggested that the basic form of a narrative is "tick … tock."[1] The "tick" creates an expectation that the "tock" resolves; narratives are built from embedded cycles of expectation and resolution. What is called genre describes particular types of ticks and the corresponding tocks that readers have a right to expect as proper resolutions. The tick of characters discovering a dead body at the beginning of a story leads readers to believe they are probably reading a murder mystery, and that they can expect the final tock will reveal who-done-it. One advantage of an established genre is to specify what counts as a proper tock that resolves a certain kind of tick, and what the story's listener or reader can expect on the way to that tock.

If we think of our lives as narratives, then dying is The Big Tock, in at least one sense. Throughout our lives the tock that ends one episode often does double duty as the tick that starts the next episode. Death is a unique kind of tock. Since humans cannot be sure that death is the start of anything else, the stakes on doing the ending right are often high; not always high, as I will suggest at the end of this chapter, but often high for dying persons, their families, and professional caregivers. And because life stories are often indeterminate as to which genre they fit into, the dying person and those around him or her are often unsure what a proper tock is supposed to sound like. Dying, like many stories, seeks its own proper ending; the story is about finding a good end to the story.

The clinical work of end-of-life care has at its core the alignment between the dying person's sense of the kind of life he or she has lived – the tick – and what seems a fitting end in the form of his or her death – the tock. Caregivers seek to honour the dying person's story, but they also have their own sense of the right kind of tock. Different narratives of spirituality and religion are central to people's tick/tock. These narratives express and determine the expectations that shape dying and what sort of resolution is considered "good". In end-of-life care, as throughout narrative-based medicine, the question is what makes a good story, because a good story is a good life.

Narrative constructions of death

The legal scholar Ronald Dworkin, writing about euthanasia requests, joins many commentators who argue that people self-consciously understand their lives as a particular story. Dworkin understands this narrative sense of life as raising the stakes on how people die, because death is taken to be the culmination of life's story.[2] He observes that some people believe the best ending to their lives is one that affirms the values exemplified throughout life. This best ending is often defined negatively. What counts is that dying should not diminish or contradict these values. These people may be willing to hasten death in order to avoid an ending that undoes their life's work of sustaining certain values.

A story about people who see their deaths this way is told by a Cuban-American social worker, Gladys Gonzalez-Ramos, writing about the death of her parents.[3] The story is tragic not because of how her parents understood what counted about how they lived and died, but because of what their circumstances demanded, in order for them to remain true to these values. Gonzalez-Ramos begins with her memories of leaving Cuba in 1960, when she was six. Her parents eventually settled in New Jersey, with extended family spread over the east coast and some remaining in Cuba. Her parents worked, as she puts it, day and night, achieved a reasonably middle-class level of comfort, and because they remained within a Spanish-speaking community, never mastered English sufficiently to be able to converse with the specialist physicians they needed when her father suffered a major heart attack and her mother developed Parkinson's disease.

The diseases are the tick that sets in motion the tightening web of desperation that becomes the story of her parents' lives. Each of their attempted responses to illness is frustrated. They cannot find specialists who speak Spanish so they endure what their daughter describes as the humiliation of being unable to negotiate their way in the healthcare system. The best nursing homes have no Spanish-speaking staff or residents; alienated there, they return home. But home care proves increasingly difficult; homecare aides who speak Spanish are unable to speak sufficient English to accompany the couple to medical appointments. Problems involve more than language. "There were different customs, different foods, different sayings," Ms Gonzalez-Ramos writes. "No matter what arrangements my father and I made, my mother's longing for privacy with her husband never stopped. They now slept in separate bedrooms, and the evening aide reported that my mother called out for my father endlessly until the morning hours. Inevitably, my father often heard my mother calling for him and went to her side, but the stress started giving him chest pains" (p 32).

Her father describes her mother's physical decline as "fading out just like a candle slowly dies" (p 29). He becomes increasingly depressed, but psychiatric care consists of a 20 minute appointment once a month to renew a prescription for Zoloft. Ms Gonzalez-Ramos writes that the psychiatrist "seemed to see his role as a psychopharmacologist, not as someone needing to attend to the sadness that Zoloft cannot repair" (p 32).

On 18 October 1999, Mr Gonzalez acted out what was apparently a well-considered plan, killing his wife and then using the same gun to shoot himself, having stood so that the blast would also knock him out of the window of their 11th-floor apartment. Ms Gonzalez-Ramos, basing her interpretation of what happened on her father's extensive letters, explains their choice of dying in terms that exemplify Dworkin's argument. "They had lived a long and happy life together. They had traveled and prospered, and they did not want to end their lives in slow deterioration. They wanted to die as they lived: side-by-side. They wanted to stop the interminable suffering" (p 32). Ms Gonzalez-Ramos is left with no doubt that her mother agreed completely with her father's decision.

I called this story tragic. It is a tragedy for society that satisfactory care – care that the family considered satisfactory to meet not only their medical needs, but also their needs for dignity and autonomy – was not available to help this family. Gonzalez-Ramos makes a convincing case that even with her parents' economic resources and with her expertise as a social worker, care was *not* available. But from the perspective suggested by Dworkin, I do not understand the Gonzalezes' deaths as a tragedy. They found the means to effect a death that, given the circumstances, fitted their view of the best possible tock to the tick of their lives. I finished reading the story feeling the real tragedy would have been for them to have lived in increasing despair. Others will understand this story differently, and those differences are consistent with a narrative-based approach. The intensity of disagreement about the necessity and the morality of what happened underscores how high the stakes are on affirming one type of narrative as appropriate to a good death.

This narrative which emphasises not undermining the values and dignity of accumulated past experience does not shape everyone's hopes and fears about dying. Dworkin describes an alternative narrative of death. Here the concern is not with avoiding an ending that seems headed toward contradicting the values of the life that has been lived. This view emphasises holding onto life in the hope that something more might yet happen that could give new meaning to what has been lived. An eloquent expression of this belief is found in the story of a hospice patient named Leonard Patterson, narrated by ethnographer Yanna Lambrinidou as part of a major research study of palliative care.[4]

At one point in Mr Patterson's care he is in pain, and for a complex of bureaucratic reasons his medical services are hopelessly inadequate to give him even the pain medication he needs. His physical pain is compounded by worry over the continuing care of his family after he dies. He asks his pastoral care worker, Steve, if there is a pill that could help him to die. Steve's description of his reaction to this request exemplifies the narrative in which something else may still happen that could give new meaning to the life that has been lived:

Inside myself I am thinking, "Holy shit! We are not going down that road." … What I have seen is that there are still miracles and blessings that can occur with people of faith in their understandings of who God wants to be for them, experiencing God in some very powerful ways that are awesomely reassuring and, of course, sharing their struggles with their family members. So I think euthanasia would be inappropriate because he was not clear at that point. He was still struggling and trying to negotiate that and come to some kind of resolution. (p 172)

I note a subtle inconsistency within Steve's story of his reaction. He starts off making a case that what matters is leaving time for changes in "understandings of who *God wants* to be for them" (emphases added). It's God who does the wanting, and I hear Steve saying that life should be sustained on the chance that God may act. The dying person's spiritual quest is to remain open to any last-minute intervention by God that might change the person's sense of "who God wants to be for them", as Steve says.

But Steve then qualifies the implications of this God-driven narrative, since in the last sentences God is no longer the active subject who wants. Instead it is the dying person who is or is not yet at some "point". So long as the person is "still struggling and trying to negotiate" some form of resolution, then that person should remain alive and in that process. The activity has shifted to the human side, seeking God. This shift from God as the active subject to the dying person as active is a subtle one, but I find it consequential for how Steve shapes Mr Patterson's experience into a narrative that has practical implications for care. In his first sentences Steve seems to close off any possible occasion for euthanasia since we must wait for God. In his last sentences Mr Patterson's movement in the spiritual dimension of the dying process matters most; he was not "at that point" yet, but he possibly could get to that point. Thus Steve starts off with an argument that seems to reject the Gonzalezes' way of dying, but he ends with an implication that some people reach a point where further waiting on God is no longer useful in their lives. In the telling of this story, as in many stories, distinctions that at first seem clear then blur.

Both these stories suggest how class bias can affect what is seen as the preferred narrative for dying people. The Gonzalezes have lived lives that a middle-class observer can readily suppose to have been good; they have "traveled and prospered" as their daughter writes. By contrast, the same middle-class observers, and I include myself, are tempted to see Mr Patterson's life as diminished. We then want something to elevate the ending of that life, and in the projection of our desire we miss what the story is about for him. On a visit home from the nursing home, Mr Patterson lies in his bedroom. "It was hot," Lambrinidou writes, "and the smell of the cat's urine was overwhelming. But Mr Patterson seemed blissful. Turning his head slowly, he looked around at his room and said to us, 'This is my life.' He paused for a second and continued: 'I'm proud of it'" (p 166). Particular care is required when we approach the narratives of lives that we ourselves might not be proud of.

Before turning to some different tick/tock issues, both the stories above – the Gonzalezes' deaths and Steve's response to Mr Patterson's euthanasia request – can be opposed to a medical intensive-care narrative, exemplified by a story narrated by physician Eric Cassell.[5] The story affects me because its details are so close to the death of my mother-in-law. Here is the story as Cassell shapes it:

A forty-nine-year-old woman developed recurrent breast cancer three years after a lumpectomy, radiation, and chemotherapy. It progressed very rapidly so that within a few weeks she had extensive spread of her cancer to the lungs, bones, and liver. The severity of her liver disease made adequate chemotherapy impossible, but her oncologist continued to talk of cure "once the liver is better." When she became sicker and deeply jaundiced, she was admitted to a major teaching hospital. Because of gross edema and abnormalities of electrolytes, a nephrologist was called who took over the problem of kidney function. Her liver function worsened, but the oncologist's stated optimism did not wane. The house staff were kind and attentive, but busied themselves with her abnormal liver function. She and her partner, supported by the physician, continued to make plans for her future and would not hear of the possibility that she might die. Reluctantly, she accepted the advice that her parents be told of her illness. She was discharged from the hospital but was readmitted in three days with a pathologic fracture of the hip. The hip was pinned, but postoperatively her liver function worsened and her blood pressure fell. She was transferred to an intensive care unit. The oncologist said that as soon as the problems with her liver and kidneys were straightened out, he could start treating her cancer. In a few days the nephrologist announced that her kidneys were now doing well. Her sickness deepened and she became confused. The orthopedist came and pronounced the wound healing well. He asked the nurses whether they could get her up and walking. She died the next morning.

This story can be read as the tragic complement to the Gonzalezes' story: their final tock had to be hastened; this woman's final tock is unexpected, with no time to connect it to the preceding tick of her life. Thus the tick of this woman's life seems to have been denied any culminating tock. Treatment kept on happening, and then to everyone's apparent surprise, she was dead. Yet that interpretation projects the tock I think I want onto the tock of this woman's death; the culminating-moment narrative may be mine, not necessarily hers. This death may have been just as she wanted. It remains unknown who – medical staff on one side, patient and spouse on the other – was responding to whose narrative desire.

But Cassell does leave us certain that no work was done with patient and staff to explore narrative options. What happened took place by default, so far as the medical centre was concerned. Default, however, is not chance. The ill woman and her spouse chose a treatment setting that could be predicted to treat them as this one did. Narrative enquiry has to be careful not to diminish any storyteller's agency; even this dying woman is enacting a story of her life.

Narrative conflict

If pressed to specify what is wrong – perhaps frightening or horrifying – in Gonzalez-Ramos' story or Cassell's story, many people would probably express a sense that something had been violated by people feeling forced to act this way or being treated this way. If asked what was violated, people would probably have recourse to words like soul and spirit. Steve reacts to Mr Patterson's euthanasia request in religious language not only because he is a pastoral care worker. No other language seems adequate to the gravity of the situation. The contemporary distinction between spirituality and religion is like the proverbial elephant and the blind men; the distinction is drawn differently by each academic and professional interest that grabs a particular part of it. This chapter seeks to depict spirituality and religion as different narrative shapings of experience. Each places different emphases on what counts as tick and as tock.

The narrative conflict between spiritual and religious narratives is found in another hospice story narrated by Lambrinidou (pp 212–32).[4] This story concerns a patient named Stanley Gray, who has the distinction of being the only patient who was still alive when the research study was completed. Mr Gray is dying of congestive heart failure and end-stage chronic obstructive pulmonary disease. He has lived a life he describes as sinful and apparently most people would agree. But recently he found God through the teaching of a television evangelist. Hospice staff, including the chaplain, alternate between their suspicions that Mr Gray's highly punitive religious beliefs compromise his health and their belief that God, or Mr Gray's belief in God, may be what forestalls a death that medical prediction declared inevitable years before.

Spiritual and religious narratives conflict in a scene when a hospice chaplain, Carl, guides Mr Gray through what Carl calls a spiritual exercise, which takes its inspiration from gestalt therapy techniques. The chaplain instructs Mr Gray to imagine Jesus sitting in an empty chair at the kitchen table and to tell him his worries. Then he is to listen to what Jesus tells him. After a period of silence Mr Gray does not hear anything, but Carl reports hearing how much Jesus loves Mr Gray. Carl then has Mr Gray place his troubles – including his guilt over his inability to stop smoking – into Jesus' hands.

Lambrinidou reports that the chaplain, Carl, was pleased with the exercise, but Mr Gray had reservations. "On the one hand," she writes, "he was relieved by the opportunity to unburden his worries, and on the other, he saw his interaction with Jesus as a convenient but immoral way of detaching himself from his responsibilities. He argued that God expected His followers to take charge of their own lives" (p 219). Mr Gray's objections to the spiritual exercise seem to reflect his desire to learn scripture "as it is supposed to be taught – as God wants it taught – verse by verse, book by book. Not trying to change it to suit man as he would like to have it" (p 222).

I respect the courage of Mr Gray's convictions even if I would probably disagree with much of their content. Mr Gray shapes his experiences according to a narrative that can be called religious; this shaping is particularly evident in his emphasis on not changing divine word to suit the contingent preferences of humans. Carl, at least in this scene, shapes experience as a spiritual narrative. As the story is told, Carl's emphasis seems to be on people constructing their own beliefs to fit their lives and situations. It is significant that the form of the "spiritual exercise" is taken from gestalt therapy: the spiritual narrative invokes goals that are psychotherapeutic. This spiritual narrative leads another chaplain who visits Mr Gray to object that the "closed system" of Mr Gray's evangelical beliefs "made people disinterested in new ideas, gave them a false sense of security, and prevented growth" (p 226). These objections amount to saying that Mr Gray is telling the wrong story, which in turn amounts to saying that he is living the wrong life. The staff considers Mr Gray's religion to be "rooted more in fear than in the love of God" (p 218). They worry that these beliefs are not conducive either to Mr Gray's spiritual growth or to the kind of death they want for him – a death that would be free from diffuse anxieties including fear of God's punishment. They are probably right, but being right depends on the story being a psychotherapeutic one. I question whether they recognise that Mr Gray is telling his story within a different narrative, with different values and goals. If what counts in care is the story that the patient tells about his or her life, the staff are missing Mr Gray's story.

Mr Gray shapes his story within a religious narrative when he affirms the importance of receiving divine word as God intended it and refuses to change its meaning to suit himself. Belief in the fixed interpretation of divine word will lead to the kind of "closed system" that the chaplain objects is antithetical to individual "growth". Again, the chaplain is right about growth, but wrong in failing to recognise what Mr Gray's story is about. Narratives are defined by what they presuppose about the nature of reality and the goals of life; stories told within particular narrative frameworks apply these concepts of reality and purpose to specific situations. Thus stories are both *defined* and *defining*. In the religious narrative, reality is that divine word which has a fixed interpretation, and the goal of life is to live according to this word. Mr Gray's story is a good example of how hospice philosophy's embrace of therapeutically driven spirituality can imply a complementary suspicion of religion – and why people who shape their lives within a religious narrative can be equally suspicious of what they describe as formless, all too convenient spirituality.

Restitution, chaos, and quest narratives

Spiritual and religious narratives are general frameworks into which particular life events can be placed. These narratives endow particular meanings, they suggest what counts more or less, and they make events recognisable to other people who live in a culture where stories like that are told regularly. In the early 1990s as I studied personal narratives of illness experience, I realised that these stories fit three basic narrative types, which are woven together with different emphases to form any person's story of illness.[6,7] The medically preferred type of narrative I call the *restitution* story. In Cassell's case history the orthopaedic specialist presupposes a restitution story when he asks the nurses when they are going to get his patient up and walking, since the hip surgery is healing well. Each medical professional – the orthopaedic specialist, the nephrologist, the oncologist – considers only the restitution of the body part that is the focus of their particular specialty. No narratives other than restitution have credibility; no other stories make sense to people. The patient follows this medical lead – which may also be her expectation of medicine – as she continues planning her life after treatment. Meanwhile, she dies.

Some people do not want to anticipate the final tock; they want to keep living a restitution story. No story is, in itself, wrong, but what can go wrong in care is the constraining of a storyteller's shaping of experience by what sort of narratives that potential listeners are prepared and willing to hear. If the dying woman had given up the restitution story, no other narrative would have been readily available to her, at least in communicating with those hospital workers. Many illness experiences do not fit a restitution narrative, and those experiences have no story.

When no narrative is available to express what is being experienced, what is expressed is *chaos* – words that never quite form stories, because there seems to be no narrative going anywhere, only accumulations of suffering. The Gonzalezes' story, as it is lived, is a chaos narrative: every way they try to improve their situation seems closed to them; the constant refrain of the story is: "but that won't work either". Disease turns to depression, and psychosis seems on the horizon. The narrative point of these psychiatric labels is not their diagnostic truth; rather they are tropes in a story of increasing desperation. The chaos narrative constricts its listener in a maze that has no exit, and then turns up the heat. The gun shots that end the story come as a kind of relief, allowing listeners to debate the morality of what the Gonzalezes did, rather than having to remain with them in the maze as the healthcare system closes off option after option. The Gonzalezes need to die for their story to become a coherent narrative.

What about ill people for whom the restitution story is either no longer available – their disease proves unresponsive to treatment – or they have decided that restitution is no longer morally satisfactory? What narrative is available when people no longer choose to have medically defined goals shape their life stories? They move to what I call, somewhat reluctantly, the *quest* story. My reluctance involves choosing a term that buys into a narrative owing a great deal to Joseph Campbell's work on myth.[8] What I admire is Campbell's insistence that the truly heroic quality of action is not overcoming an adversary but enduring suffering. Campbell's heroic model is more feminine than masculine, finding its earliest paradigm in the journey of Inanna to the underworld. Inanna undertakes the journey, suffers helplessly, is rescued by helpers from the world she has left, and returns to sort out matters with those who did not contribute to her rescue. She wields no weapons; her strength is her perseverance. This trope of heroism as perseverance is most useful to people who are ill and dying.

But I am troubled by what happens when Campbell's notion of the heroic is transformed into self-help prescriptions for a happy life; reconstructing the myth within a contemporary spiritual narrative loses the heroic. Though Inanna increases her power and divinity through her journey, she does not enter the underworld to have a personal growth experience. She goes because it is her fate to go. She is called to the underworld as preparation to become the goddess whom she can become only by making that journey and incurring such suffering. The cosmic order requires her becoming and thus her journey. Neither the journey nor its aftermath makes her happy by most human standards. Inanna does increase in wisdom and stature, but this "growth" is neither personal nor linked to pleasure.

The notion of fate that pervades Inanna's heroism seems increasingly intolerable to more individualistic notions of the person. When Campbell's idea of the hero is reinterpreted to fit ideals of a culture that privileges "lifestyle", strange and perhaps unfortunate ideas appear about spiritual quests. Thus I am in deepest agreement with the objections of a friend who emailed me from the bedside of her dying father after she saw the programme of a spirituality and medicine conference at which this chapter was originally presented:

> My father's dying has been a spiritual journey for me, but I'd be pissed as hell if someone suggested that it must be, or that it was inferior if it wasn't laced with spirituality. Don't know if that's where you're heading, but it's what I'm thinking these days. It's kind of a sneaky/ smug way to medicalise death via spirituality.

That's exactly where I'm heading, but the argument has to proceed carefully. I want to show the spirituality narrative to be what it is: a version of the quest narrative, one narrative possibility among a variety of possible narratives, and like all narratives, a potentially deaf spot to other narratives, especially those closest to its concerns. Knowing spirituality as a narrative should not undo the good work of the last several decades that has made spiritual care a component of all good medical care. I was in the audience in the early 1970s when Cicely Saunders came to New Haven, Connecticut and gave the lecture that marked the beginning of the first hospice in the United States. I heard Dame Cicely speak again during the time I was writing the paper that forms this chapter, and I found her faith even more evident as the foundation of her work. Hospice brought spirituality into the care of the dying, and the continuing need to generate more spiritual awareness within medical settings is illustrated by Cassell's story of the patient dying amid specialists' respective successes. Whether or not the dying woman herself wanted spiritual care, what is frightening in the story is the specialists' narrowness of focus. Whether or not the patient received spiritual care, it is the physicians who need such care.

One requirement of spiritual awareness is not being locked, unreflecting, within a single narrative, including a single spirituality narrative. Spiritual awareness seems to require the capacity to use different narratives flexibly and responsively. What is troubling in the care of Mr Gray is whether those around him are being responsive, or whether they are requiring Mr Gray to fit their agenda with a single-mindedness that rivals the physicians in Cassell's story. In Mr Gray's case, the ideal of "growth" risks becoming another form of restitution, at least for Mr Gray's caregivers.

Blurred narratives and voices-in-relation

In end-of-life care, spiritual and religious narratives seem to be more than arbitrary choices among a variety of narrative possibilities; these narratives seem to have some claim to priority, and at some point, the spirituality and religious narratives blur. For most people, throughout most of human history, looking squarely at death has required some spiritually informed sense of The Big Tock. That need has articulated powerful dialogues on dying. In 1974 Sam Keen, then a staff writer for *Psychology Today*, made overtures to interview the philosopher Ernest Becker, who had recently published *The Denial of Death*. He received word that Becker, then 49, was dying of cancer but wanted to proceed with the interview. Becker would receive the Pulitzer Prize posthumously for his book. He begins the interview by reflecting that his unexpected dying has put him in a situation to see if he can now practise the ideals he wrote about.[9]

Becker and Keen approach death by discussing the idea of heroism in contemporary life; the gender bias of their language is worth questioning but seems unrelated to the point that emerges. Becker first describes the hero most broadly in terms of leaving behind "something that heightens life and testifies to the worthwhileness of existence. Making a beautiful cabinet can be heroic. Or for the average man, I think being a provider is heroic enough" (p 183). Keen describes this conception as "the hero as self-sufficient man" (p 183) and Becker, perhaps hearing in that reply the limitation of what he has said, adds more. "But I don't think one can be a hero in any really elevating sense without some transcendental referent .... The most exalted type of heroism involves feelings that one has lived to some purpose that transcends one" (p 183).

Here the spiritual and religious narratives blur. Incongruous as it may seem, I hear echoes of Becker's heroism in Mr Gray's adherence to televangelism. Becker's desire for a transcendental referent is expressed in Mr Gray's insistence that God intends a specific meaning to scripture, and that humans are not free to adapt that meaning to suit themselves. Mr Gray wants an external, greater-than-human standard against which to be judged. Jesus is not some cosmic sponge to wipe away every human trouble so that people need not take responsibility. Mr Gray seeks not his own peace with himself – which is too often what "growth" means to the psychotherapeutic consciousness – but a sense that he has tried his best to act in accordance with a will beyond his own – something kin to Becker's transcendental referent. For Mr Gray, any "growth" can be assessed only with reference to a will outside himself, to which he must attend, and to which he can fail to attend sufficiently. That risk of failure is crucial to the religious ethic; without it one is simply creating beliefs to suit oneself. Mr Gray believes that it is not sufficient to say he's sorry and then feel better. He seeks to prove he *is* sorry by changing his actions and possibly – he can never be sure – earning forgiveness. Mr Gray has made little that is beautiful in his life; he has not even provided for his family. I respect him for not accepting forgiveness too easily.

Ernest Becker's interview with Sam Keen exemplifies self-reflection on the narrative that is shaping one's life. Becker uses the dialogue with Keen to craft a tock that is the culmination of, and clarifies, the values of the tick that has preceded it. Becker's good fortune (not exactly luck) is to have an interlocutor who does more than listen but who never imposes. Keen speaks Becker's language, he enters his narrative framework, and a story emerges that is greater than either's individual participation. They become voices-in-relation, achieving a kind of narrative synthesis.

How loud is the final tock?

Narrative inquiry is a perpetual regress: every story is embedded within some narrative, and every narrative is embedded in another narrative. The story I have told about dying is part of a narrative that takes dying seriously – the final tock is understood as a big deal. That too is a narrative shaping, and some people do not shape their experience that way. My friend's email about her father's death describes a different narrative possibility. Unlike Ernest Becker or Mr Gray, her father did not need to find any transcendental referent to make his life, and his death, meaningful. The work of making the final tock meaningful had already taken place during his life. My friend objected strongly to people "remarking on Dad's manner of dying and how fortunate we are to be able to 'say things we've always wanted to say'."

Huh? I wanted to scream, what the hell does that mean? Like I could script something relevant to the deathbed scenario that I never said in the dailiness of our friendship? Maybe I'm lucky, or an oddity, but I felt enormously loved by my father and I know he knew how much I loved and respected him. What else is there to say?

My friend is lucky. Many deathbed scenes are the last remaining occasion to say things that have been left unsaid and that need expressing: each person needs to tell the other what value their life has had to them; that the dying person has lived better because of those who are left behind, and that the bereaved will grieve but also will keep aspects of the dying person alive in their lives. These things often do not go without saying; affirmation is needed.

People die as they live: within narrative frameworks. No final story provides textbook guidance. Attention to multiple narratives complicates issues in order to sort out where differences and distinctions lie. One moment these narratives differ and conflict, and the next they blur. This chapter has tried to show that process, drawing distinctions and then blurring them. Life and clinical care are that complicated, but on another dimension, both are also simpler. As my friend writes so beautifully about her father, what matters most is that people be assured of each other's love. Perhaps the family of the woman who dies in Cassell's story was left feeling that in her unwavering commitment to staying alive, she expressed her love for them. Even a terrible death like that of the Gonzalezes is not quite a tragedy because their surviving daughter, who tells the tale, understands what happened as filled with love: love of the dying couple for each other, their love for their children, and their daughter's love for them. Their deaths show how terribly sad death can be, but also that the ending can be the least important part of a life. When the narrative understanding of life inflates the value of a proper ending, it can be profoundly misleading. The final tock may not matter that much.

References

1 Kermode F. *The Sense of an Ending*. Oxford: Oxford University Press, 2000, pp 44–6.
2 Dworkin R. *Life's Dominion: An Argument About Abortion, Euthanasia, and Individual Freedom*. New York: Knopf, 1993.
3 Gonzalez-Ramos G. The 18th of October 1999: In Memoriam. *The Hastings Center Report* 2000;**30**(4):28–33.
4 Barnard D, Towers A, Boston P, Lambrinidou Y. *Crossing Over: Narratives of Palliative Care*. New York: Oxford University Press, 2000.
5 Cassell EJ. The Principles of the Belmont Report Revisited: How Have Respect for Persons, Beneficence, and Justice Been Applied to Clinical Medicine? *The Hastings Center Report* 2000;**30**(4):12–21.
6 Frank AW. *The Wounded Storyteller: Body, Illness, and Ethics*. Chicago: University of Chicago Press, 1995.

7 Frank AW. "Just Listening": Narrative and Deep Illness. *Families, Systems and Health* 1998;**16**(3):197–212.
8 Campbell J. *The Hero With a Thousand Faces*. Princeton, NJ: Princeton University Press, 1949/1972.
9 Keen S. *Voices and Visions*. New York: Harper & Row, 1974, pp 175–98.

8: The death of the narrator

CATHERINE BELLING

Some of the challenges that face those who care for terminally ill patients emerge from an obvious but perhaps undervalued fact: such care is about endings. In a narrative sense, those who make or guide the patient's last healthcare decisions may significantly influence the end of a life story – and therefore its final meaning. I suggest here that the notion of narrative endings plays an active if submerged role in end-of-life care, and that articulating this notion might elucidate some of the apparent contradictions that can affect such care. While it is of course accepted that terminal illness concerns the end of life, the association between biological death and the cultural endings we construct in narratives is less widely accepted in medical spheres, though this appears to be changing.

A 1996 study found that hospice in-patients who had witnessed the deaths of other hospice patients were significantly less anxious and depressed than those who had not.[1] Protection from the grim details of actual dying appears not to shield patients from anxiety about their own deaths, whereas confronting death by observing the dying of another person may help to allay fear. A narrative approach, I will show, can make sense of this finding and suggest ways in which the experience and knowledge of dying can be clinically beneficial. In my discussion, I draw on published autobiographical accounts by writers with terminal illness in order to consider some implications of a narrative view of dying. I suggest ways in which such a view may be helpful in clinical decision making at the end of life, particularly in terms of a patient's sense of control over life's ending, as evinced in two occurrences: the request for assistance in committing suicide and the creation of advance directives.

Narrative and identity in the closing chapter

[T]he great crises and ends of human life do not stop time. And if we want them to serve our needs as we stand in the middest we must give them patterns.[2] (p 89)

A friend spoke of something his elderly mother said near the end of her life: "I can't die yet. If I do, I'll never know how it all turned out." Her words capture the contradiction that both fuels and challenges the human will to see our lives as stories. The world continues without us, when we are not here to look back on our lives complete and make sense of things. The endings of our lives, because we end with them, are finally – as far as we can tell from this side of death – obscure to us.

This fact, whether consciously registered or not, may contribute to the anxiety about dying which is almost universal in the face of a terminal prognosis. One helpful response may be to approach the last stages of a lethal illness as an opportunity for the patient to author the last chapter of his or her life narrative. This approach may provide a constructive way of thinking about some of the more intractable problems facing the dying and those who treat them.

We conceive ourselves in stories – or, as the philosopher Anthony Paul Kerby puts it,[3] "self-narration [is] fundamental to the emergence and reality of [the self]" (p 4). Whether or not one subscribes to the postmodern idea that identity is entirely a discursive construct, it is true that we tend to think of, or imagine (or construct) our sense of self as unified and constant over time, over the period of the life of the person who identifies with it.[4] "I", in other words, is always a biographically defined subject, whether or not one ever writes that (auto)biography down.

Stories, however, derive much of their meaning from the way they end. Much thought has been given to the significance of closure, of the ending that somehow ties up loose narrative threads, and how the possibility of a meaningful conclusion contributes to our sense of existential security. The literary critic Frank Kermode[5] describes the intolerability of the infinite: "tracts of time unpunctuated by meaning derived from the end are not to be borne" (p 162). The novelist Henry James considered it a fundamental task of narrative literature to give meaning to the endlessness of reality, saying "relations stop nowhere, and the exquisite problem of the artist [the novelist] is eternally to draw, by a geometry of his own, the circle in which they shall happily *appear* to do so" (emphasis in original).[5] Stories end, and by ending they allow us the illusion that events and lives can be looked on complete, summed up, and made sense of. This extends to our personal stories, as Kerby[3] points out: "[Self-]narrating generally seeks closure ... by framing the story within [the structure of] a beginning, middle, end ... Closure of this sort ... is not only a literary device but a fundamental way ... in which human events are understood" (p 6).

The philosopher Walter Benjamin (a doctor by training), linked the prospect of dying to the origins of human storytelling.[6] The dying person, he argues, has an authority bestowed on him by virtue of being situated at (I would say "near") the end of a life that can now be transformed into a complete biographical narrative: "a man's ... real life – and this is the stuff that stories are made of – first assumes transmissible form at the moment of his death" (p 94). For Benjamin, a historical decline in storytelling is linked to society's increasing denial of death, especially an increasing effort "to make it possible for people to avoid the sight of the dying" (p 93). The direct recognition of death as a reality is necessary to the construction of a coherent narrative about living. When we are protected from knowing death, we are also prevented from being able to draw clearly those "geometries" that according to Henry James enable us to make sense of our lives.

There is a fundamental problem with this, whether or not we avoid the sight of death, particularly when the lives and deaths we deal with are actual rather than fictional: how does a narrator apprehend and describe the moment of death itself? Narrative is inherently retrodictive, told (or thought), that is, in the past tense from a vantage point in the future, from which things can be looked back on, the patterns and connections identified. Autobiography and memoir rely on remembering what we have already known. We may look back on our lives so far, or on what happened a minute ago, but never – at least as far as we can tell – on our deaths. We begin by saying "I was born", but how do you say "I died"? My death is, to me, unnarratable. I cannot tell the end of my story because my ability to know it ends with me.

This problem is confronted directly when a patient diagnosed as being "terminal" decides to write the end of his or her life, to become its author. Writing about his final illness, Harold Brodkey[7] describes how being diagnosed with Aids disrupted the narrative experience of living: "In ... my mind," he says, "was an editorial sense that this was wrong, that this was an ill-judged element in the story of my life" (p 6). He explains this new element as a threat to his sense of self: "This inability to have an identity in the face of death – I don't believe I ever saw this written about in all the death scenes I have read .... It is curious ... how my memories no longer apply to the body in which my words are formed" (p 173). An identity based on a series of memories, a constructed autobiography told by the "I" as narrator, finds itself at odds with the physical and dying body of the author, Brodkey himself. Narrative reconstruction is needed in order to make sense of this radical discontinuity between author's body and narrator's voice.

Another writer, Barbara Rosenblum,[8] explains, on learning she has advanced breast cancer, that her "body no longer contains the old truths about the world" (p 165). She experiences what she calls a profound "crisis of knowledge, a sort of epistemological anxiety" about herself (p 179). To resist this, she decides to "live self-consciously (and perhaps die self-consciously) in an exemplary manner," and to do this she, like Brodkey, writes (p 13). But neither can keep writing and die at the same time.

In another account of breast cancer, Christina Middlebrook is explicit about the problem of narrating: "The dead cannot tell their story. We have so much more experience surviving the death of a loved one than we have of dying. When I was first diagnosed, I thought of death this way, from the aspect of the survivor, from the feelings of the person who attends the funeral."[9] We all, I think, wish we could emulate Tom Sawyer and attend our own funerals to hear how things turned out – but we cannot.[i] Middlebrook captures this difficult truth in the subtitle of her book: "A memoir of dying before I die".

For Anatole Broyard, dying of prostate cancer, self-consciousness is synonymous with life. Alluding to the words of the British psychoanalyst DW Winnicott, Broyard[11] says that he aspires to "be alive when I die" (p 30). Winnicott's fragmentary autobiography actually contains that impossible sentence "I died." This follows the prayer to which Broyard alludes: "Oh God! May I be alive when I die."[12] As quoted by Winnicott's wife, the autobiography itself begins:

I died.

It was not very nice, and it took quite a long time as it seemed (but it was only a moment in eternity).

There had been rehearsals ... When the time came I knew all about the lung heavy with water that the heart could not negotiate, so that not enough blood circulated in the alveoli, and there was oxygen starvation as well as drowning. But fair enough, I had had a good innings ... .

Let me see. What was happening when I died? My prayer had been answered. I was alive when I died. That was all I had asked and I had got it.[12] (p 4)

Winnicott writes as if he is in a position to look back on his death and describe it. We know, as does he, that the position is fictional, the writing speculative. Yet just as his earlier experiences of illness were "rehearsals" for death, so this writing is a way of practising, not for the physical experience of dyspnoea, but for the metaphysical ones of conclusion and closure and, most importantly, of consciously and actively recognising that closure, by "being alive" at the point of death.

Anatole Broyard's wife, Alexandra, recalls her husband's use of Winnicott's prayer. Writing the last lines of his book, she assures us that Broyard was indeed "alive" at his death. The two stories of dying have something else in common, then: in both cases, the surviving spouse is the one who must recount, or at least edit, the ending of her husband's life. Broyard's wife tells us how he was at the end, but this is the point: *she* has to tell us. She recounts his dying because he cannot. Though we can read what he wrote from the time of diagnosis to very near death, this is not enough. Oliver Sacks, in his foreword to

Broyard's book,[11] observes that the writer "takes his pen almost to the darkness. His final journal notes go to within a few days of his death" (p xii). Those few, crucial days, though, form the gap between the death of the narrator and that of the author, the story's protagonist who, deprived of the narrator's necessary lagtime, cannot say "I said my last word, took my last breath. I died. And this is what it meant".

In her account of approaching death, Barbara Rosenblum's writing has a counterpoint; the title is *Cancer in Two Voices*,[8] and the second voice is that of Rosenblum's partner, Sandra Butler. As a couple, their narratives alternating, the two construct the story of Rosenblum's dying, but it is, of course, only Butler who can present the death itself, saying in her lone voice, in the past tense, "Barbara died today" (p 204). Harold Brodkey[7] describes how this silencing begins. Once dying, he says, you are "no longer the hero of your own story, no longer even the narrator" (p 6).

This silencing of the narrator is not just a matter of the physical inability to write, of the effects of pain or even of necessary sedation or narcosis (and we are seldom alive, in Broyard's sense, by the time we die, and certainly we are hardly ever, in the law's sense, competent to give an account of ourselves). But even in the absence of these barriers, even if the author is, like Broyard, alive right to the end, it is not enough.

Broyard[11] describes his illness as "a kind of incoherence. I could only become coherent if I were to get well or if I were to die" (p 68). Writing, as the most concrete form of converting inchoate experience into coherent narrative, is effective in this effort to record and so pin down the self while it can still speak. Near the end such writing becomes almost "live" in the way live television is, without editing or perfecting, but even here actual simultaneity remains impossible.[ii] Narrating is an attempt to provide coherence, then, but only dying will actually achieve it. As the literary critic G Thomas Couser observes, "closure in autobiography is always fictive, arbitrary, *premature*".[14]

Authoring the end: suicide and advance directives

Your own death lies hidden from you.[2] (p 161)

This gap between the narrator's silencing and the patient's death may help explain one seemingly paradoxical response to the prospect of dying of an illness: an effort to hasten death. Many terminally ill patients consider or actually commit suicide.

A recent qualitative study of HIV-Aids patients' attitudes to assisted suicide casts light on connections between problems of narrative closure and the desire of terminally ill patients to end their own lives.

The study concludes that these patients did not view suicide simply as a way to escape predicted pain and suffering. Instead, the researchers conclude, suicide is understood as a "means of limiting loss of self".[15] In another study of assisted suicide, hospice nurses and social workers in Oregon were asked about the reasons patients gave for requesting help in ending their own lives. The conclusion was similar, though its terms were different: the majority of patients gave as the most important reason "the desire to control the circumstances of death".[16] In the gradual disintegration of coherence and the isolation that comes as dying begins, the narration that constructs the self begins to fail. A chosen, controlled death enacts the will of a self not yet lost.

Suicide may then be seen as a radical act of authoring, of making the story end at a time chosen by the author. To end one's life is to determine actively the coherence that dying diminishes but that the completeness of death promises to bestow. The implicit logic goes something like this: "if we can't wait around to see how it all turns out, at least we can try to force it all to turn out, now, while we're still here." The act tends not, of course, to work out this way, but the intention and ability to commit suicide may well help restore a temporary sense of narrative coherence. Brodkey[7] considers suicide in this way: in small acts of rebellion – "I haven't eaten or taken my pills," he says – he restores some self-determination in what he calls his "little suicide[s]" (p 164). This view of suicide may be useful both in apprehending the urge in the terminally ill actively to seek out death, and in finding alternatives to suicide, for there is another strategy for approaching the gap between the failure of narrative and death itself, and it is here, I suspect, that narrative competence in clinicians becomes fundamental to end-of-life care. I will call this strategy *proleptic narrating*.

Most narration is retrodictive, telling about events in the past tense from a vantage point in the present. This, as I have shown, is the reason it is impossible to narrate the experience of having died. I will not here include accounts of near-death experiences, although these are a fascinating and fertile area for thinking about apprehending death. Even in these cases, the gap between being "near" death and being dead exists. As the philosopher AJ Ayer pointed out when describing his own experience of cardiopulmonary arrest, to die "in this sense" is not the same as brain death.[17] He says of the things he saw while "dead" that they "have slightly weakened my conviction that my genuine death … will be the end of me," but even these insights, close as they may come to experiencing the end of life, are not "genuine death". Ayer does not know from his experience what his death will be like: not even narrators like Ayer are in fact returned from Hamlet's "undiscovered country". He was, however, in a far better position after his experience to *imagine* his death.

A significant role of literature is, arguably, to enable us to imagine the state of being dead as one from which to speak (we might even argue that a great many narrators, particularly the kind we call omniscient, speak from an implicitly posthumous place). We imagine ghosts (and the one in *Hamlet* certainly describes his own death by poisoning, though he is prohibited from describing his subsequent existence in purgatory), and sometimes we imagine tales told in the voices of the dead. A very successful recent novel, *The Lovely Bones* by Alice Sebold, is narrated entirely by a murdered adolescent girl.[18] These imaginative preconstructions are enormously valuable, but, like accounts of near-death experiences, do not quite solve the problem each individual faces, of being able to finish telling one's own life from beyond its ending. But these efforts do suggest ways in which the imagination might make it possible, though difficult, to narrate death as a future event, out of chronological order, as if it has already happened.

Many autobiographies or memoirs make use of *analepsis*, the flashback. The starting point, from which the narrator remembers, is a point later in time than what happens in the story being narrated. *Prolepsis* is its opposite, not recollection but the anticipation of events in advance of their occurrence. Prolepsis relies on a narrator who knows ahead of time how the story will proceed beyond the point of telling. The narratologist Gerard Genette discusses how an autobiographical narrator, looking back on life from a point near the end, is in an especially good position to describe events proleptically: "The 'first-person' narrative lends itself better than any other to anticipation, by the very fact of its avowedly retrospective character, which authorises the narrator to allude to the future and in particular to his present situation."[19] For Genette, this means primarily describing events already in the narrator's past, though they may happen later in time than any given point in the story, but there is also room for a less common form of prolepsis that follows a line of action to a conclusion beyond the point at which the narrator stops narrating. It is only by this means that an autobiographical narrative can encompass the death of its narrator.

Alexandra Broyard tells us that her husband was alive when he died. He is silent, she speaks. But remember whose words she uses. The intention to "be alive when I die" was his, told in advance and then presented by his wife, quite explicitly, as the words he himself chose. She is his surrogate narrator. In writing the epilogue to her husband's book, then, Alexandra Broyard fulfils what we might call his advance directive to her, to tell the end just as he would have – or, more precisely, in the way that, proleptically, he already has. A similar tactic may be used, given adequate communication among patient, family, and clinicians, in all foreseeable medical deaths.

The advance directive and the living will are verbal acts that can be narrative and are always proleptic. In making advance directives, we do more than speculate about our deaths: we determine, verbally, some of their conditions. If these usually rather reductive legal documents – listing undesired procedures or the name of a surrogate consenter to, or refuser of, treatment – were to be expanded, either in writing or by a sustained and recorded conversation with physician and family, then perhaps the "loss of self" that motivates the need for suicide might be diminished. I imagine a thick description of dying, one that includes place, people, lighting, issues to be addressed and those to be left unspoken, pain either fully treated or withstood for the sake of lucidity, last wishes and activities, and so on – a description producing the kind of control that tends to characterise carefully planned assisted suicide, perhaps. But in order to foretell the story of our deaths we need experience of dying, and the best source of this is concrete knowledge about the deaths of others.

The majority of patients still do not have advance directives. In a 1998 study in the *Archives of Family Medicine*, the most frequent reason given by those who did have one was "experience with the prolonged death of a friend or family member."[20] This may be not only because such an experience was so horrible that the patient fearfully did the paperwork needed to prevent it. It may also be because this experience was the only opportunity offered for the patient (or future patient) and family members actually to imagine what dying could be like. And prolepsis is impossible without a conception of the likely details of the future. The subject protected from the prospect of dying is denied the opportunity to foretell his own death.

In an intriguing editorial decision, Anatole Broyard's wife chose to end her husband's last book with an essay he had written years earlier about his father's death from cancer. It is as if she allows her husband's experience of the end of his father's life to stand in for that of his own, in a kind of doubled narrative agency by proxy. There are of course problems with this; as we have seen, the survivor's version is intractably other than that of the one who dies. But implicitly, in this book, Broyard's sharing of his father's death facilitated his own ability to write, as proleptically as possible, about his own.

The patient–author, then, cannot tell the end of life in isolation. One more verbal act is essential to establishing narrative closure. Told by the physician, this is the account that, along with diagnosis, begins the story of dying: prognostication. No memoir of terminal illness can be written without it. The author has to learn that it is time to begin the ending. Prognosis, as a kind of quantified uncertainty, may appear to be the antithesis of narrative, and numbers – months, years, probabilities – statistics, with their reductive and deceptive clarity, can be ambiguous or inaccurate. But if prognoses can be made in the context of dialogue – and a narrative – about dying, and revised, where needed, in ongoing conversations about expecting death, this may be a first step in protecting the self from incoherence.

The clinician understandably may desire to minimise the brute facts of narrative incapacity at the end of life in order to shield patient and family from suffering they may well have to experience all too soon. There is a tension, however, between such protection and the necessity of confronting the realities of dying, confronting them in order to know them. The study already mentioned showed how direct confrontation of the prospect of death, usually in the form of witnessing the death of another, tends to be more reassuring than traumatising for terminally ill patients.[21] Learning in advance what dying can be like makes it possible to imagine the facts of dying in the context of a story not yet finished. Such imagining is necessary to help keep the patient as narrator alive and telling, and then, when necessary, to allow him to pass the story on, almost told already, to the one who will add the last sentence: *you* died.

Endnotes

i "That was Tom's great secret – the scheme to return home with his brother pirates and attend their own funerals." [10]
ii Ross Chambers makes a similar point about the diaries written by Aids patients.[13]

References

1 Payne S, Hillier R, Langley-Evans A, Roberts T. Impact of witnessing death on hospice patients. *Soc Sci Med* 1996;**43**:1785–94.
2 Kermode F. *The Sense of an Ending: studies in the theory of fiction, with a new epilogue.* New York: Oxford University Press, 1966.
3 Kerby AP. *Narrative and the self.* Bloomington, IN: Indiana University Press, 1991, p 4.
4 Sprinker M. Fictions of the self: The end of autobiography. In: Olney J, ed. *Autobiography: essays theoretical and critical.* Princeton, NJ: Princeton University Press, 1980, pp 321–42.
5 James H. Preface to *Roderick Hudson.* Quoted in Kermode F, *The Sense of an ending.* New York, Oxford University Press, 1966.
6 Benjamin W. The storyteller. In: Arendt H, ed. (trans H Zohn) *Illuminations.* New York: Schocken Books, 1968, pp 83–109.
7 Brodkey H. *This wild darkness: The story of my death.* New York: Metropolitan Books, 1996, p 6.
8 Butler S, Rosenblum B. *Cancer in two voices* (expanded edition). Duluth, MN: Spinster Ink, 1991, p 165.
9 Middlebrook C. *Seeing the crab: a memoir of dying before I do.* New York: Harper Collins, 1996, p 204.
10 Twain M. *The Adventures of Tom Sawyer* (1876). In: Twain M. *Mississippi writings.* New York: Library of America, 1982, p 117.
11 Broyard A. *Intoxicated by my illness and other writing on life and death* (compiled and edited by Alexandra Broyard). New York: Clarkson Potter, 1992, p 30.
12 Winnicott C. D.W.W.: A reflection. In: Winnicott C, Shepherd R, Davis M, eds. *D.W. Winnicott: Psycho-analytic explorations.* Cambridge, MA: Harvard University Press, 1989, pp 1–18.
13 Chambers R. *Facing it: AIDS diaries and the death of the author.* Ann Arbor, MI: University of Michigan Press, 1998, p 8.

14 Couser GT. *Recovering Bodies: Illness, Disability, and Life Writing*. Madison, WI: University of Wisconsin Press, 1997, p 69.
15 Lavery JV, Boyle J, Dickens BM, Maclean H, Singer P. Origins of the desire for euthanasia and assisted suicide in people with HIV-1 or AIDS: a qualitative study. *Lancet* 2001;**358**:362–7.
16 Ganzini L, Harvath TA, Jackson A, Goy ER, Miller LL, Delorit MA. Experiences of Oregon nurses and social workers with hospice patients who requested assistance with suicide. *N Engl J Med* 2002;**347**:582–8.
17 Ayer AJ. What I saw when I was dead. *National Review* 1988;**40**:38–41.
18 Sebold A. *The lovely bones*. New York: Little Brown and Company, 2002.
19 Genette G. *Narrative discourse: an essay in method* (trans JE Lewin). Ithaca, NY: Cornell University Press, 1980, p 67.
20 Bradley EH, Wetle T, Horwitz SM. The Patient Self-Determination Act and advance directive completion in nursing homes. *Arch Family Med* 1998;**7**:417–23.
21 Yedidia MJ, MacGregor B. Confronting the prospect of dying. Reports of terminally ill patients. *J Pain Symptom Management* 2001;**22**:807–19.

9: Narrative, emotion, and understanding

PETER GOLDIE

It is a very natural thing to do, in discourse about our own past lives, to relate what happened in the form of a narrative. Moreover, it often takes considerable effort to talk about our own past lives in some other way than by relating a narrative. This, I think, is as true in formal encounters with doctors, nurses, psychiatrists, psychotherapists, counsellors, and so forth as it is in discourse with one's partner over dinner, with a friend over a drink, or in discourse between strangers who meet on a plane or a train.

There is, of course, a question whether autobiographical narrative *ought* to have a place in the sort of formal encounter that is involved in a clinical setting. Speaking as an occasional patient (not as a member of the medical profession, being a philosopher by trade), I should hope the answer is yes: if I may be forgiven the pun, the clinician ought to be someone to whom one can relate. But in this chapter I want to skirt around this question, and address myself to those who, unlike me, are members of the medical profession, and who, like me, also want the answer to the question to be yes, finding patients' autobiographical narratives to be of great utility in their practices. What I want to do is consider some concerns about narrative to which we yes-sayers have a duty to respond: concerns that autobiographical narrative cannot meet the standards of truth and objectivity that evidence-based medicine can achieve.

There are two concerns here. The first is that autobiographical narratives cannot realistically aspire to truth in the same way that scientific discourse can; autobiographical narratives, and factual narratives in general, should be assimilated to fictional narratives, "true to life", perhaps, but not true *period*. I shall try to allay this concern: factual narratives can be true *period*, and there is nothing about the nature of narrative that excludes this possibility.

The second concern follows on from the first. Even if autobiographical factual narratives can aspire to truth (to be true *period*), they cannot realistically aspire to objectivity. My response here is to distinguish. If being objective is contrasted with being perspectival, then I agree that narrative discourse is not objective, for it is essentially perspectival, involving the narrator's perspective on the related events. But being perspectival does not imply failure to be objective in another sense of that slippery term. A narrative can be objective in this sense: the narrator's perspective can be *appropriate*, involving an appropriate evaluation of, and emotional response to, what is related. So a narrative can be objective, albeit emotionally engaged and perspectival. Narrative discourse does not and should not aspire to be like scientific discourse, dispassionate and non-perspectival, and thus objective in the other sense of that term.

I hope that discussing these concerns in the way that I will do in this chapter will reveal an important truth: an act of narration is a kind of *action*, done for reasons, and an account of these reasons can explain why someone related *this* particular narrative at *this* particular time in *this* particular way (perhaps distortingly, perhaps passionately but without distortion). Because of this, an audience has a double interpretive task of considerable complexity in understanding an autobiographical narrative, as we all know from our own experience: one has to interpret the content of what is narrated; and one has, at the same time, to interpret the act of narration and the narrator's perspective on what happened. If the clinician can realise that there is this *double* interpretive task, then both patient and clinician can be empowered: the patient can have greater confidence that the clinician will be able to understand his or her reasons for relating this particular narrative at this particular time in this particular way; and the clinician will be, in this respect, someone to whom the patient can relate.

Narrative theory: emplotment

I want now to begin by drawing on narrative theory in order to see how narrative works. I will then illustrate the theory through an example that will be familiar to many readers of this book. It is drawn from Chapter 1 of the predecessor volume to this one, *Why Study Narrative?* by Trisha Greenhalgh and Brian Hurwitz.[1] It is Robert's story. Robert was a patient of Hurwitz, and he had related to Hurwitz a narrative of events that took place some 30 years earlier, involving awful mistakes in diagnosis by the medical profession during the onset of Robert's diabetes. The conversation between Robert and Hurwitz was recorded on tape and was reproduced by Greenhalgh and Hurwitz almost verbatim, with the patient's consent. Robert's story, as told by him, is now reproduced again in full in the Box. But first a bit of theory.[i] An autobiographical narrative emerges from a process of *emplotment*, an active process which is undertaken by the narrator. I will give three characteristic features of narrative that emerge from this process, and will then use the chosen text to illustrate them.

The first characteristic feature of narrative is *coherence*. Emplotment gives coherence to a narrative by taking the "raw material" – representations of

Robert's story

BH: *How long have you been diabetic for?*

RG: *Since September 1969.*

BH: *Tell me how you first found out that you were diabetic.*

RG: *Well my tongue started to get very, very dry and also I was drinking excessive amounts of liquid and also I had an upset stomach. So I went to my doctor and told him all this, and all he told me was that I had an "upset stomach" and I told him then that I think I am a diabetic and he told me that I was talking a load of rubbish.*

BH: *Why did your symptoms suggest diabetes to you?*

RG: *Because I had been with a diabetic before who has now died. I had known him since he was 9 years old, so the symptoms I had he described to me before and that is how I knew I thought I was a diabetic. So I went to another doctor and he told me the same thing, that I had an upset stomach. So I waited and waited and waited, then I decided to go back to my doctor, when my water was starting to crystallise and he told me that I had VD.*

BH: *What do you mean by "when my water started to crystallise"? How did you know your water was crystallising?*

RG: *When I was passing the water the end of my penis started getting all white and also some times when the water hit the pan it was starting to go clear white.*

BH: *What happened next?*

RG: *Well, I decided to go down to the VD clinic down in London and I went in there on the Friday night and I handed him the letter and he read it and he said to me "What do you think you have got" and I said "I think I have got diabetes" and he said "What F-ing B sent you here, he should have seen this before you were sent here". So he said to me "Look, I cannot do anything for you tonight, but please report down to the hospital the next morning (and that was the Saturday morning)." So I went back home and I came down the Saturday morning, but with me walking down on the Friday night and the Saturday morning, which normally takes me about 5 minutes, took me 35 minutes just to reach the bus stop.*

BH: *Why was that?*

RG: *Because I was so weak I could hardly move at all. So I went down, got down to hospital, went in and told the Sister and the receptionist that I would like to see somebody from the Diabetic Clinic and she read the letter then she told me that I could not get an appointment until a fortnight. At this stage I was really very angry and I started shouting at her. As that started a nurse came out from Casualty and she read the letter. As soon as she read the letter she shouted to a nurse to get a wheelchair, she dumped me in the wheelchair and took me straight upstairs to the Diabetic Clinic. So once I got up there they stripped me off right down to my underpants and started testing me. There was 2 doctors and 3 nurses there and after they stripped me and everything they transferred me over to the hospital. Since the nurse read the letter and took me over to the hospital it only took 22 minutes.*

BH: *When you arrived on the ward at the hospital did the doctors tell you what level your blood sugar was at?*

RG: *No they did not. They only told me it was very, very high and a nurse came over with a jug which held 2 gallons of water and she told me that I had to drink as fast as I could.*

BH = Dr Brian Hurwitz; RG = Patient

actions, events and states of affairs – and revealing causal connections in a way which would not be achieved by a mere collection of propositions, a list, or a chronicle of events – what would otherwise be, in the words of Elbert Hubbard, just one damn thing after another.

The second feature of narrative is *meaningfulness*. Through emplotment, the narrator gives meaningfulness to the raw material by presenting what happened in a way that enables the audience of the narrative to find intelligible the thoughts, feelings, and actions of the protagonists who are part of, or internal to, the content of the narrative, and whose *internal perspectives* are presented in the narrative.[ii] For example, a father might tell the story of Goldilocks and the Three Bears to his young daughter in a way that enables her to grasp the internal perspective of Goldilocks. An audience is able to grasp internal perspectives in this way through empathetically entering into the minds of the protagonists. In this kind of imaginative identification, the audience does not lose sight of its own perspective; rather, the audience so to speak "tries on the other's thoughts for size" – in imagination engaging in a sort of dramatic enactment. For example, the daughter listening to the Goldilocks story might imagine how it would be for her to experience what Goldilocks experienced.[iii]

The third characteristic feature of narrative, in addition to coherence and meaningfulness, is *emotional import*. Emplotment gives emotional import to what happened. To explain this, I need to introduce what has so far been in the background: the narrator's *external perspective*. This perspective is external to the narrative in the sense that, as such, it is not part of the content of the narrative; it is a perspective *on* the actions and events that are narrated.[iv] It follows from this that external and internal perspectives are distinct even when they are the perspectives of one and the same person, as they are in autobiographical narratives. So the external perspective of Winston Churchill, as narrator of *My Life*, is different from the internal perspective of Winston Churchill as protagonist, whilst a young journalist for example, during the Boer War. The process of emplotment undertaken by the narrator, culminating in the act of narration, reveals, from the distance that the narrator's external perspective allows, the narrator's evaluation of, and emotional response to, what happened. This is what I mean by emotional import.

Now let us turn to Robert's story, which I hope the reader has had his or her eye on whilst reading this bit of theory, to see how Robert's emplotment worked on this occasion.

We see coherence. Robert connects events one with the other by revealing causal relations between them: it was having diabetes that caused Robert's water to crystallise; it was being diabetic that caused him to be so weak that he could hardly move.

We see meaningfulness. We find it intelligible that Robert should have gone to the VD clinic (even though, as we now know, he did not have VD); we see, through imaginatively projecting ourselves into his position, just why Robert was so angry with the Sister in the Diabetic Clinic when he was told that he could not have an appointment for a fortnight. His internal perspective and his actions make sense to us, as do the internal perspectives and actions of the other protagonists: for example, we can make sense of the Casualty nurse's actions when she realised how serious Robert's condition was. We may, however, be drawn up short by the doctor who told Robert that he had VD – we can make sense of it (as a misdiagnosis), yet perhaps we cannot help but think "How could he have been so ignorant?" (Empathetic identification might be helped if we remember some of our own stupid mistakes).

And we see emotional import. We grasp Robert's external perspective as narrator (as contrasted to his internal perspective as protagonist). We see that Robert's emotional response to what happened, from the perspective of what he now knows, 30 years after the narrated events, is one of anger and relief: anger in looking back at the misdiagnoses by the two doctors (anger that he did not feel at the time); and relief at having finally found someone who correctly diagnosed his condition. Robert's narration invites his audience also to feel anger and relief at what happened. He is right: we *should* feel these emotional responses, for he really was badly treated (and thus anger is appropriate), although things did come right in the end (and thus relief is appropriate).

Truth in factual narrative

Now I can address the first concern that I raised at the outset. The concern is, roughly, that a factual narrative, such as Robert's autobiographical narrative, is not able realistically to aspire to truth in any robust sense: factual narrative should be assimilated to fictional narrative rather than to discourse about facts. The concern can be put like this: nothing has been said so far to enable us to distinguish, as distinct species of narrative, between, on the one hand, factual and historical narrative, and, on the other hand, fictional narrative. Appeal to structural elements of the narrative – coherence, causal relations, meaningfulness and so on – will not help here, because a narrative just like Robert's could equally well be a work of fiction. So should we just assimilate the two, and accept that factual narratives must float free of the events which they seek to portray and of any possibility of truth, at best achieving some sort of internal coherence and satisfying aesthetic form and genre-type?[v] I think not.

The place to look for the difference is not in the structural dimension, but in the referential dimension. A narrative is fictional not in virtue of its content being false, but in virtue of its being narrated, and read or heard, as part of a practice of a special sort: one which invites the audience to imagine or make believe that what is being narrated actually happened, even when it is known that it did not.[vi] Thus the question of reference and of truth simply does not arise within the "fictive stance": it is just irrelevant.[vii] Fiction, of course, can aspire to be true to life, and to be true in the same way that metaphors are true,[17] and to be much else besides, but none of these aspirations are aspirations to be true *period* – true in the sense in which historical or factual narratives *do* aspire to be true. What sense *is* this exactly? Roughly, in the sense of corresponding to the facts, in the sense that what Robert said will be true just if things were, in fact, as Robert said they were. This might sound trivial, but it is not. It points towards an instance of what philosophers sometimes call the disquotational schema:

> "My doctor told me that I had VD", as uttered by Robert, is true just if Robert's doctor told him that he had VD.

On the left hand side, in quotation marks, we are concerned with language – roughly speaking, with the proposition that is expressed by the quoted words. On the right hand side, not in quotation marks, we are concerned, roughly speaking, with facts – with the way the world has to be for the proposition to be true. So it is a mistake to think of a narrative – which is, after all, a collection of propositions – as *being* a sequence of events; to think of a narrative in this way is in effect to assimilate the left hand side and the right hand side of the schema – to assimilate language and the world. There are, rather, two metaphysically distinct things here, and this is part of what the disquotational schema reveals, trivial as it might initially sound. In this sense, then, the metaphysical notions of reference and truth have application in factual autobiographical narrative, just as they do in, for example, scientific explanation, whereas they have no application in fiction. So, in respect of what I have called their referential dimension, factual narrative and fictional narrative differ.[viii]

Objectivity in factual narrative

Even if the concern about truth (being true *period*) can be dealt with, there remains the concern about objectivity. What can we say here? Let us begin by turning our attention away from the narrator's external perspective, towards the external perspective of the audience, and asking what the audience needs to achieve for there to be a successful narration of a factual narrative – a successful communication.

The audience has a double interpretive task: it needs to interpret the content of the narrative; and it needs to interpret the act of narration itself. I have already considered the first task. In relation to the second task, the audience is interested in the answer to this question: "Why is he relating to me this particular narrative at this particular time, in this particular way?"[ix] Even if the narrative is given in response to a request ("What happened next?"; "Why did your symptoms suggest diabetes to you?"), it is a legitimate question to ask why the narrator is relating this narrative at this time in this way.[x] Relating a narrative is, after all, just a kind of action, done for reasons. Thus, we should as audience seek an explanation of why someone relates a narrative just as we should seek an explanation of other kinds of action.[xi]

In seeking such an explanation, we should look more widely than just to the agent's own reasons for doing (or saying) what he or she did, for we often classify actions and motives, not by reference to the agent's reasons *as such*, but according to our own evaluation. We call an action inconsiderate or heartless or vain without suggesting that the agent was motivated by inconsiderateness or heartlessness or vanity as such. For example, this man has spent the last hour in the gym constantly preening himself in the mirror and checking how he looks as he does his exercises, striving to show off his athletic figure to the best effect: it would be unusual, to say the least, if one of this man's reasons for performing such an action was "doing this would be the vain thing to do", even though it is appropriate to say that his actions were expressive of his vanity.

The same principles apply to explaining an act of narration. Let us assume that someone is relating a narrative with the intention of communicating, in a truthful and sincere manner and without distortion, what happened to him and what he did. For example, I might relate to you a narrative of how I secured some government funding for a research project. I might intend simply to "tell it how it is", but still I might, like the vain man in the gym, unintentionally reveal my vanity: my action – my act of narration – is expressive of reasons that can be appropriately classified as boastful and vain, even though it was no part of my intention to boast in telling you about what happened.

What we have here is a *divergence in evaluation and emotional response* between the narrator's and the audience's external perspectives. I evaluate my securing of government funding as a palpable success, so pride on my part, and admiration on yours, are the appropriate emotional responses. You, on the other hand, see my achievement in a less flattering light, evaluating my act of narration as one expressive of boastful vanity.

So an audience is not bound to accept the narrator's evaluation and emotional responses to the narrative, expressed in his or her external perspective. Indeed, a moment's reflection on the phenomenology of narrative discourse reveals how little we do this: the audience's external evaluation of what happened often diverges from the narrator's evaluation. We are always free to come to a different evaluation of the narrated events, and we often take advantage of this freedom.

There is a further complication – one that is very important. You cannot assume that you yourselves, the audience, are free of bias – perhaps it is your perspective that is distorting and not the narrator's. Thus, your own way of seeing things has also to be taken into account in the interpretive process. For example, you the audience might unknowingly be influenced in your interpretation of my story about getting government funding by your somewhat repressed envy of my success compared with your own efforts. So it is not as though, to quote a remark of Nietzsche's, "reality stood unveiled before you only, and you yourselves were perhaps the best part of it" (*The Gay Science*, Book Two, s. 57).

In the clinical setting too there can be convergence and divergence in evaluation and emotional response. In Robert's story, the narrator's (Robert's) and the audience's external perspectives converge: Robert evaluates what happened as deserving of anger and relief, and we share that evaluation. Whereas if the story were told (by someone else) as a light comedy, the narrator's and the audience's perspectives would diverge. (Perhaps the story could be told as a *bleak* comedy, in the Mike Leigh manner, so that our perspectives converge: there can be a kind of genuine and appropriate humour in human suffering).

Of course we often find divergence of perspective in psychotherapy and psychoanalysis. I would like to take an example from a 2003 article by Vieda Skultans entitled "From damaged nerves to masked depression: inevitability and hope in Latvian psychiatric narratives".[24] In this article Skultans explores the effects of changing social and economic conditions on Latvian thinking about illness and distress. Her research included psychotherapeutic-ethnographic interviews of some 35 patients in a polyclinic in northeast Vidzeme. Skultans says this about these patients: "Of the thirty-five patients who consulted me two-thirds began their narrative by complaining that they could not put themselves in order or that they seemed to have lost control of their lives." One of these patients was Ingrida:

Ingrida is twenty-nine years old, married, and with a nine year old daughter. She feels she is lucky to have a husband who does not drink, a job she likes as a shop assistant, a self-contained two roomed flat and enough money to get by. She knows her circumstances are better than those of her neighbours. And yet, although she evaluates her life as one that should bring about satisfaction and happiness she finds that she cannot contain her anger and exude the calmness that she would like. *When pressed to give an illustration of her failure to live up to cultural ideals she describes coming home from work at eleven at night after a fifteen hour shift and losing her temper because the dishes have been left unwashed and the flat is in a mess. The interesting point relates to the fact that Ingrida blames herself and not her long working hours for her anger. Indeed, she pointed out that she did not have to walk home but that her husband collected her in the family car* (pp 2423–4).

I would like to focus especially on the part that I have italicised. Here we are told that Ingrida related a mini-narrative to Skultans to illustrate what she took to be her failure to live up to her cultural ideals of self-control. In the mini-narrative, Ingrida loses her temper. It is clear from what Skultans tells us that she, Skultans, understands and empathises with Ingrida's internal perspective in the narrative, and specifically with Ingrida's ostensible reasons for losing her temper: the unwashed dishes, the messy flat. But there is divergence in external perspective. Skultans tells us that Ingrida's evaluation of what happened, from her external perspective as narrator, is that she was blameworthy for failing to control her temper. Skultans' evaluation, from her external perspective as audience, diverges from Ingrida's, in that she thinks it is the social and economic conditions, and specifically the horrendous working hours, where the real fault lies.

Here, then, we have a very nice example of the double interpretive task in action, so to speak. Skultans understands the content of Ingrida's mini-narrative, accepting her account of "the facts" (that Ingrida came home from work, that she then lost her temper because of the unwashed dishes and the messy flat). And Skultans also understands Ingrida's external perspective (Skultans understands that Ingrida blames herself for losing her temper). But Skultans also has her own external perspective on what happened, which diverges from that of Ingrida (Ingrida blames herself, whereas Skultans feels that Ingrida is not to blame).

This kind of divergence between clinician's and patient's external perspective on the patient's autobiographical narrative is, as I said, common in psychotherapy and psychoanalysis. And it is common, we can now see, not because there is disagreement about "the facts" – about the truth of the content of the narrative. Rather, the disagreement, or divergence as I call it, arises because the patient and the clinician have divergent evaluations of, and emotional responses to, what is narrated. In a patient's autobiographical memory, as related in an autobiographical narrative, backward-looking emotions of self-assessment, such as feelings of self-blame, shame, guilt, and disgust at oneself or at what one did, can so often be inappropriate, and it is, in part, the clinician's task to help the patient to see that her emotional responses to the past, as revealed in her external perspective, are other than they should be.[xii]

So, finally, I think the right thing to say about objectivity in narrative discourse is something like this. Being objective in narrative discourse (as narrator or as audience) is not a matter of being dispassionate, of being free of all emotion, for narrative discourse is concerned with human values and emotions, and such discourse should not aspire to be dispassionate, like scientific discourse. Rather, being objective in narrative discourse is a matter of having an appropriate external perspective – of having an appropriate evaluation of, and emotional response to, what happened. To echo the words of Aristotle in his *Nicomachean Ethics*,[26] it is a matter of having the right emotions "at the right times, towards the right people, and in the right way".

Acknowledgement

I am very grateful to Vieda Skultans for helpful suggestions and for letting me have access to her unpublished material.

Endnotes

i   I have drawn on a number of sources here, although the overall account is my own: see Ricoeur,[2] Carroll,[3] Velleman,[4] and Goldie.[5,6,7] As my focus in this chapter will mainly be on narrative dialogue, issues that arise in narrative theory concerning the differences in perspective between narrator, implied author, and actual author, and between implied audience and actual audience, will be peripheral; see Booth[8] and the collection of papers in Iseminger.[9] Throughout, where I talk of narrator and audience, I mean actual narrator and actual audience.

ii To be precise, a protagonist is the *central* person in a narrative; I will use the term, harmlessly I hope, to refer to any person in the narrative, whether central or not.

iii For discussion of this way of making sense of others, see Collingwood,[10] Gordon,[11] Williams,[12] Moran,[13] Velleman,[4] and Goldie.[14]

iv For a detailed discussion of the idea of perspective or point of view in literature, see Bal[15] and Genette.[16]

v   For expressions of this sort of view, see, for example, White[17,18] and Fish.[19]

vi A story's being false is neither necessary nor sufficient for its being fictional. Cf Lamarque and Olsen[20] (p 31).

vii Cf Lamarque and Olsen[20] (p 77), Currie[21] (p 30), and Walton[22] (pp 70–3).

viii Sometimes in discussions of narrative-based medicine, I hear the suggestion that an illness *is* a narrative. This surely is absurd: there can be such a thing as a narrative *of* an illness, but to say that an illness *is* a narrative is to run together what is represented with the representation.

ix I presume here that the audience realises that the narrator's intention is to relate a *factual* narrative, and not to relate a fictional narrative as part of a fiction-telling practice.

x This question has a grip on all kinds of communicative act – not just on an act of narration. However, I hope to show that the difficulties in understanding acts of narration demand special attention.

xi As Paul Grice says, about all kinds of communicative act, we should "see talking as a special case or variety of purposive, indeed rational, behaviour"[23] (p 153).

xii I discuss narrative and memory in Goldie.[25]

References

1 Greenhalgh T, Hurwitz B. Why study narrative? In: Greenhalgh T, Hurwitz B, eds. *Narrative-based medicine: dialogue and discourse in clinical practice*. London: BMJ Books, 1998.

2 Ricoeur P. *Time and Narrative*, vol 1 (trans K McLaughlin, D Pellauer). Chicago: University of Chicago Press, 1984.

3 Carroll N. On the narrative connection. In: van Peer W, Chatman S, eds. *New Perspectives on Narrative*. Albany: SUNY Press, 2000. Reprinted in Carroll N. *Beyond Aesthetics*. Cambridge: Cambridge University Press, 2001, pp 118–33.

4 Velleman D. Narrative explanation (unpublished); www-personal.umich.edu/~velleman/Work/Narrative.pdf

5 Goldie P. Narrative and perspective: values and appropriate emotions. In: Hatzimoysis A, ed. *Philosophy and the Emotions*. Royal Institute of Philosophy Supplements Series. Cambridge: Cambridge University Press, 2003, pp 201–20.

6 Goldie P. Emotion, reason and virtue. In: Cruse P, Evans D, eds. *Emotion, Evolution and Rationality*. Oxford: Oxford University Press, 2004, pp 249–67.

7 Goldie P. Narrative, emotion and perspective. In: Kieran M, Lopes D, eds. *Imagination and the Arts*. London: Routledge, 2003, pp 54–68.

8 Booth W. *The Rhetoric of Fiction*. Chicago: Chicago University Press, 1961.

9 Iseminger G, ed. *Intention and Interpretation*. Philadelphia: Temple University Press, 1992.

10 Collingwood R. *The Idea of History*. Oxford: Oxford University Press, 1946.

11 Gordon, R. Simulation without introspection or inference from me to you. In: Davies M and Stone T, eds. *Mental Simulation: Evaluations and Applications*. Oxford: Blackwell, 1995, pp 53–67.

12 Williams B. *Truth and Truthfulness: An Essay in Genealogy*. Princeton, NJ: Princeton University Press, 2002, ch 10.

13 Moran R. The expression of feeling in imagination. *Philosophical Rev* 1994;**103**: 75–106.

14 Goldie, P. Emotion, personality, and simulation. In: Goldie P, ed. *Understand Emotions*. Aldershot: Ashgate, 2002, pp 97–109.

15 Bal M. *Narratology: Introduction to the Theory of Narrative*, 2nd edn. Toronto: University of Toronto Press, 1997.

16 Genette G. *Narrative Discourse* (trans J Lewin). Ithaca, NY: Cornell University Press, 1980.

17 White H. *Tropics of Discourse: Essays in Cultural Criticism*. Baltimore, MD: Johns Hopkins University Press, 1978.

18 White H. *The Content of Form*. Baltimore, MD: Johns Hopkins University Press, 1987.

19 Fish S. How to Do Things with Austin and Searle. In: Fish S. *Is There a Text in This Class? The Authority of Interpretive Communities*. Cambridge, MA: Harvard University Press, 1980.

20 Lamarque P, Olsen S. *Truth, Fiction, and Literature*. Oxford: Clarendon Press, 1994.

21 Currie G. *The Nature of Fiction*. Cambridge: Cambridge University Press, 1990.

22 Walton K. *Mimesis as Make-Believe: On the Foundation of the Representational Arts*. Cambridge, MA: Harvard University Press, 1990.

23 Grice HP. Logic and Conversation. In: Cole P, Morgan JL, eds. *Syntax and Semantics*, vol 3. New York: Academic Press, 1975, pp 41–58. Reprinted in Martinich AP, ed. *The Philosophy of Language*, 2nd edn. New York: Oxford University Press, 1990, pp 149–60.
24 Skultans V. From damaged nerves to masked depression: inevitability and hope in Latvian psychiatric narratives. *Soc Sci Med* 2003;**56**:2421–31.
25 Goldie P. One's remembered past: narrative thinking, emotion, and the external perspective. *Philosophical Papers* 2003;**32**:301–19.
26 Aristotle. *Nicomachean Ethics* (trans T Irwin). Indianapolis: Hackett, 1985, 1106b20.

10: The voice of experience and the voice of the expert – can they speak to each other?

YIANNIS GABRIEL

The facts:

- A nightmare – a computer defies K's instructions and keeps reverting to an old-fashioned snooker game, from which K cannot escape.
- A routine visit to the doctor turns into something more serious. An urgent referral to the hospital, a batch of tests, an anxious wait. Testicular cancer?
- A chance meeting with an old school flame at an airport lobby. Instant revival of relationship. A wedding. A pregnancy.

Three sequences of events involving different persons, or perhaps the same person, simultaneously or in succession. Notice immediately the temptation to discover some meaning in these facts, a purpose, a point. This may be accomplished by seeking additional facts (Who are the protagonists? In what sequence did the events take place? What was the diagnosis?), by looking at the meaning of the events to the protagonists (Why was the computer nightmare upsetting? Was the pregnancy wanted?), and by identifying some key emotions that were experienced by them. It is through the juxtaposition and sequencing of facts, their "engagement" with each other and with the intentions and experiences of their characters, that meaning begins to emerge. For instance, on the day after the nightmare, K went for his routine check-up. Or alternatively – the day after the welcome news of pregnancy, he was diagnosed as having testicular cancer. Facts, even seemingly trivial ones, invite being placed in a story, through the magic of the plot.

Notice too, another temptation – the temptation to silence. Why bother about a case of testicular cancer, a nightmare, or a pregnancy? Why indeed care about them, in the light of personal and world events that cry out for meaning and explanation? Of course, if the protagonists in the above incidents happen to be oneself, or one's spouse, one's son or daughter, one's close friend or acquaintance, then the search for meaning may be burning. But if the subject is one of the anonymous thousands who are diagnosed with testicular cancer, rediscover romance or get pregnant, then the search for meaning may all but vanish. The very requirement that meaning should reside in the facts disappears. They become mere statistics, data, information.

Facts rarely speak for themselves – and never in isolation. Narratives and stories enable us to make sense of them, to identify their significance, and even, when they are painful or unpleasant, to come to terms with them and live with them. This is why many narratives revolve around human misfortune, notably accidents, illness, injustice and loss. As sense-making devices, narratives and stories do not merely help us infuse events with meaning, but also enable us to mould them to our own needs and desires, to comment on them and to contest them. As such, they help us process our experiences, communicate them to others and re-arrange them within larger narratives of identity and selfhood. This chapter reviews how narratives and stories enable individuals and groups to discover their voice, articulate their experiences and even shape their self-identities. I will argue that stories and narratives are shaped within fragile social encounters, in which storytellers and audiences are bound by a psychological contract which regulates legitimate and non-legitimate forms of representation or "regimes of truth". These psychological contracts accord considerable authority to the person who speaks from personal experience, who has witnessed events with their own eyes, an authority that can sometimes be abused, but an authority which stands in direct opposition to the authority of the expert, founded on generalisable and impersonal expertise. The juxtaposition between the voice of first-hand, personal experience and the voice of scientific expertise is played out in many fields, including medicine, law, history, therapy, education; I conclude with some thoughts regarding the possibility of these two voices coming together in a dialogue.

I have deliberately set out to temper some of the current enthusiasm regarding narratives and stories displayed by scholars, researchers, practitioners (medical, management, professional), and others. In the first place, narratives, and particularly stories, are relatively special events, capable of great sense-making feats, but also easily drowned in the din of information, lists, numbers, opinions, rationalisations, and theories that saturate many organisational spaces; or they may remain still-born in environments dominated by relentless preoccupations with efficiency, rationality, and action. In short, stories require time, patience, and trust, qualities that are not in great supply in today's organisations, medical and otherwise. Furthermore, while stories can be vehicles of contestation, opposition, and self-empowerment, they can also act as vehicles of oppression, self-delusion, and dissimulation. Nor do stories, as is sometimes argued, obliterate or deny the existence of facts but allow facts to be re-interpreted and embellished – this makes stories particularly dangerous devices in the hands of image-makers, hoaxers, and spin doctors.

In all of these ways, I would like to reclaim some usefulness for the concept of "ideology", a concept that some authors may have prematurely buried, following the collapse of the Soviet Union and subsequent decline of Marxist scholarship. While I do not claim that ideology is an automatic set of false ideas which is determined by an immovable material base, ideologies, whether political, religious or medical, systematically conceal some of the assumptions which they carry. This applies equally to the ideology of science, which privileges the voice of the expert, and the ideology of personal experience, which seeks to defend and bolster the authority of the person who has lived through certain events at first hand.

Narratives, stories, and experience

Narratives are particular types of text involving temporal *chains* of inter-related events or actions, undertaken by characters. They are not mere snapshot photographic images, but require *sequencing*, something noted by most systematic commentators.[1–10] Stories, for their part, are narratives with *plots*, which "knit events together", allowing us to understand the deeper significance of an event in the light of others.[4,7]

If plot (involving characters, sequencing, action, predicaments etc.) is a crucial feature of stories, a second key feature of many stories is their claim to represent reality (see Goldie, Ch 9). Stories, in other words, purport to relate to facts that happened, but also to discover in these facts a plot or a meaning, by claiming that facts do not "just happen" but that they happen in accordance with the requirements of a plot. Such stories are not "just fictions", nor are they mere chronologies or reports of events as they happened. Instead, they represent poetic elaborations of narrative raw material, aiming to articulate and communicate *facts as experience*, not facts as information.[11] The link between stories and experience is of the greatest significance, since different people may experience the same events in very different ways, or, alternatively, they may experience very different events in the same ways. Experience is shaped by emotions, desire, perception, and interest, all of which have a direct bearing on the stories we tell and our responses to the stories we hear (or refuse to hear).

When a teacher recounts an incident involving a threatening pupil, when a patient recounts the onset of the first symptoms of his illness, when a physician recounts the success or failure of a particular treatment to her peers, some of the requirements for precision are relaxed and the requirements of meaning, sense-making, and communication take precedence. In this sense, such stories are different from the reports that one may give a police investigator or a commission of inquiry, where accuracy of information is of paramount consideration. The same applies to many of the stories that patients tell their doctors, as Kleinman[12] has described it:

> The illness narrative is a story the patient tells, and significant others retell, to give coherence to the distinctive events and long-term course of suffering. The plot lines, core metaphors, and rhetorical devices that structure the illness narrative are drawn from cultural and personal models for arranging experiences in meaningful ways and for effectively communicating those meanings. (p 49)

Thus, storytellers enjoy a unique narrative privilege, *poetic licence*, that enables them to maintain an allegiance to the effectiveness of the story, even as they claim to be representing the truth.

Poetic licence enables the storyteller to buy the audience's suspension of disbelief in exchange for pulling off a story that is communicating something authentic and meaningful. The story is a poetic elaboration on events, one that accords with the needs of the teller and the audience, and one that requires considerable ingenuity on the part of the narrator. Drawing connections, highlighting what is important and unimportant, expressing emotion, commenting on what is bad and what is good, what is accidental and what is typical, attributing motives and emotions, these are all elements of *story work* (or poetic labour), the work that goes into generating a story that both carries meaning and claims to represent reality. This is no easy task. Many events defy containment within narratives, leaving us in a state of confusion – a lack of the resources necessary for making sense of them. This is especially the case with events that leave us in a state of shock, when we may need the help of someone else (a counsellor, a confidante, a friend) in order to construct a convincing and plausible story, or indeed we may "buy" someone else's story as our own story. Think of the meaning vacuum (in much of the UK and the USA, though not in certain other countries) following the events of 11 September 2001, and the importance of those first utterances of world leaders which constructed those events through the use of words like "war", "crusade", and so forth.

There are events that require an enormous amount of story work before they can be accommodated within a meaningful scheme, others that readily fall within a well-established and easily recognisable plot. Yet, stories are quite fragile entities which can be called into question and even destroyed by two deadly questions. The first one is the "So what?" question, the abyss that faces every storyteller[5] (p 360), when the story fails to carry meaning. A story can carry meaning, yet may fail the second test, the test of verisimilitude. In addition to the "So what?" question, which all narrators must face, storytellers must also face the "Did it really?" question, which questions whether the story accurately represents reality. The "So what?" question indicates that the plot is failing to carry meaning, while the "Did it really?" indicates that the plot fails to carry verisimilitude. Between these two questions, storytellers must walk on a tricky tightrope, since meaning may be created at the expense of verisimilitude and vice versa.

Poetic licence is part of a *psychological contract* between the storyteller and his/her audience, that allows the storyteller to twist the material for effect, to exaggerate, to omit, to draw connections where none is apparent, to silence events that interfere with the storyline, to embellish, to elaborate, to display emotion, to comment, to interpret, even as she or he claims to be representing reality. All of these poetic interventions are justified in the name of experience – they are the storyteller's attempt to make sense of events that could otherwise be entirely puzzling, arbitrary, and incoherent. I shall refer to this psychological contract as a *narrative contract*. This is a contract that regulates the terms of a narrative or a story, the acceptable deviations from documentable reality, the drawing of inferences and making of connections, the legitimate exaggerations and omissions. Different types of narrative, such as historical accounts, chronicles, fairy tales, jokes, myths, film, novel, and opera, involve different types of narrative contracts between authors and their audiences or readers. The stories we hear in pubs, hospitals, consultation rooms, schools, business organisations, and other places are governed by their own narrative contracts, establishing their own permissible modes of representation, their own regimes of truth.

Narrative contracts – a small digression to the genre memoir

Small print is a feature of the narrative contract, as it is of all contracts. Its significance becomes clear when the narrative contract is tested, violated or broken. Consider, for example, a recent imbroglio involving a literary memoir, par excellence the literary genre that voices experience. *Fragments: Memories of a wartime childhood* written by Binjamin Wilkomirski,[13] described through the eyes of a child the experience of surviving the horrors of the Holocaust. The book appeared to give voice to the silent sufferings that had scarred the protagonist's entire life. On publication, it was widely acclaimed and showered with awards, in spite of reservations expressed by distinguished scholars like Raoul Hilberg and Yehuda Bauer.

Numerous factual errors in the book were dismissed as insignificant, trivial distortions affecting an adult's recollections of childhood experiences, when compared to the book's moral force. The book presents unspeakable suffering told by a person who was at once a victim, an eye-witness and a survivor, and generates powerful emotions in the reader – compassion for the victims as well as admiration for their courage, outrage against the oppressor, awe at what people are capable of doing to each other.

Gradually, however, and largely through the efforts of Swiss journalist Daniel Ganzfried and historian Stefan Maechler,[14] it became clear that the book was a fake. Wilkomirski (real name Bruno Doesseker, born Grosjean) was neither a Holocaust survivor nor even a Jew and his narrative had been entirely the work of fantasy. "I was there, not you", exclaimed Wilkomirski to his detractors, implying that no historical research, could deny his experience which was authentic through and through. Yet, the damage to the narrative contract between author and audience was already done. The author was seen as someone who abused trust and violated the limits of poetic licence to present fictions as facts. His book was discredited even as a literary document and withdrawn, as were many of the awards that had been given to its author. Some have defended Wilkomirski. Israel Gutman, for example, the director of the revered Yad Vashem and a Holocaust survivor, said that "Wilkomirski has written a story which he has experienced deeply; that's for sure ... He is not a fake. He is someone who lives this story very deeply in his soul. The pain is authentic"[15] (p 61). Others have argued that Wilkomirski spoke not just for himself but with a collective voice, on behalf of a whole class of disempowered and silenced victims. Some indeed have seen this as a perfectly legitimate defence, refusing to acknowledge any difference between factual truth and a presumed symbolic truth.[16,17] The mere contestation of testimonies like Wilkomirski's, according to such defendants, amounts to a denial of every survivor's experience, a virtual blasphemy.

Extreme though the case Wilkomirski may be, it is by no means unique (see Finkelstein[15] for numerous similar ones). What it suggests is in the first place the possibility of grave breaches of the narrative contract, whereby the narrator exceeds the prerogatives of poetic licence and ventures into the field of misrepresentation. Verisimilitude gives way to dissimulation. The narrator is no longer a creditable one and having proven untrustworthy once, he or she remains so for ever – his/her narrative damaged beyond repair. If we hesitate to refer to Wilkomirski as a hoaxer, it is because his deception is, by all accounts, a self-deception as much as a deception of others. (This in itself generates a new type of literary narrative, the literary exposé, which has emerged as the antithesis of the memoir, establishing its own psychological contracts between authors and their audiences. Others may take a less extreme view – they may, for instance, seek to understand why a very strong identification with the experience of someone else may come to be felt as a self-experience).

What makes such breaches of the narrative contract possible? I would contend that the main factor here is the ability of certain narratives to inoculate themselves against criticism, precisely by emerging as the voice of authentic experience, an experience that cannot be denied, without violating the integrity of the narrator. This is especially true when the experience is one of suffering and victimisation, in which case questioning the narrative amounts to compounding the injury through its denial. Wilkomirski's "I was there, not you" rings with an authority that is very hard to contest. This "inoculation" of a claim from legitimate criticism, its elevation to incontestable truth, is not far from what can be labelled ideological, an ideology of unquestioned respect for the personal experience of the victim, whose articulation of this experience enables them to "discover a voice"; it is in this way that the victim ceases to be a victim and becomes a "survivor", the two being very distinct characters in most story plots.

But what if the experience of trauma and injury, as in the case Wilkomirski, is based on events that did not take place or at least did not directly affect the victim? We can no longer believe that the "truth of stories lies in their meaning, not in their accuracy",[18] since the meaning of stories is radically different, depending on whether the facts reported were experienced at first hand or not. The trauma experienced by individuals like Wilkomirski may be real, but the meaning of the trauma is different, depending on whether they actually experienced the brutality at first hand or whether they imagined they experienced it. The argument here is identical to the issue that has long made psychoanalysis a target for criticism, namely that what matters is the experience of trauma, not whether the events causing the trauma actually happened or not.[19,20,21] While the experience of trauma may conceivably be very similar in the cases of individuals who were brutalised by their parents and those who imagined themselves brutalised by their parents, I would contend that the meaning of the trauma is very different. What I am arguing here is that the listener may legitimately then read the meaning of the story very differently from the teller.

What we learn from the Wilkomirski affair is that once the credibility of the storyteller has been corrupted the narrative contract lies in tatters. The storyteller then becomes a story, a story of abuse of trust, of pathological lying or of something else. To the two questions feared by every storyteller, "So what?" and "Did it really?", we must now add a third; one that is never as direct as the other two, yet one that is looming in the background: "Who are you to speak with authority?" Once the authority of personal eye-witness experience has been supplanted, the story becomes absorbed in a new narrative, a narrative of deceit, delusion or manipulation. Poetic licence then must be seen as part of a very complex contract between storyteller and audience which entails the granting by the audience of attention, a temporary suspension of disbelief, a temporary curbing of criticism and enquiry, in exchange for delivering a narrative which makes sense, is plausible, yields pleasure or consolation (entertainment or catharsis), but sustains numerous hidden assumptions about legitimate and non-legitimate forms of representation.

Distortion then can be equally legitimate poetic licence within a narrative contract or a violation of the contract. But distortion is unavoidable within any story, and this includes stories told by patients to their physicians.

Retrospective narratization can readily be shown to distort the actual happenings (the history) of the illness experience, since its *raison d'être* is not fidelity to historical circumstances but rather significance and validity in the creation of a life story.[12] (p 51)

This, of course, does not imply that all or most of what a storyteller says is distorted or inaccurate. Experience is constantly processed, interpreted, and re-interpreted in the light of subsequent events, its meanings re-considered and re-assessed within changing stories and narratives. Truths (literal and symbolic), half-truths and fantasies all have a part in our evolving narrative constructions of experience. Even the foundation of all claims to experience, the claim to have lived through an event at first hand, must be seen in this way. When a storyteller says "I witnessed it with my own eyes" this may be literally accurate and yield strength and authenticity to his/her story; alternatively, it may be legitimate distortion for effect, or, in some instances, entirely fraudulent, relying on sequestered authority. Poetic truth, therefore, becomes a product of this narrative contract, which continuously defines legitimate and non-legitimate deviations from the facts, legitimate and non-legitimate forms of representation.

Who speaks with authority? The voice of the expert and the voice of experience

Over the centuries, various voices have rung with authority. The voice of the prophet with his or her personal line to the divine, the voice of tradition which Burke[22] sought to reclaim, the voices of the artist, the intellectual or the outsider who dare speak their minds with what the Greeks called *parrhesia* (the courage of one's opinion, uninhibited by fear, expediency or tactfulness). Modernity undoubtedly elevated one type of authority, the authority of the expert, the specialist, the scientist above all others. Scientific knowledge seemed to melt other sources of authority away as mere superstition, hearsay, and opinion. Nowhere is the authority of the expert more clear than in the field of medicine, where the scientific treatment of disease was seen as driving away traditional, non-scientific "medicines". It is certainly not accidental that Plato, one of the greatest philosophical apologists of the expert, continuously invoked the metaphor of the physician in his political discourse. If we obey the doctor because we respect the authority of his/her expertise, does it not follow that we would obey our leaders if they could claim a similar indisputable expertise? And if the healthy soul is one in which the different parts are functioning in harmony, does it not follow that a healthy state is one in which the different parts are doing the same?

One of the main casualties of the expert's unassailable authority was "everyday experience". Where the voice of experience was not entirely silenced, it was relegated to the standing of "mere opinion" (Plato called it *doxa*), used in a condescending way by the expert as the raw material upon which to base diagnoses, generalisations, and theories. In medicine the term "anecdotal" was used to this end. Consider for example, the court case, one of the foundations of modernity's claim to rationality which elevates the "expert witness" above the mere "witness" or the "anecdotal evidence". Expert witnesses not only speak with much greater authority, but are entitled to express opinions that are treated as authoritative evidence and accepted with a degree of deference that is withheld from testimony based on mere experience. Within a rational courtroom, submitted to merciless cross-examination, experience is regularly shown to be biased, inaccurate, or even entirely fictitious.

Within modernist medical discourses, experience was further devalued. Who needed to listen to the voice of the pregnant woman or even the midwife's tales of difficult deliveries when the obstetrician knew best how to deliver babies according to the latest medical theories? Who needed to concern themselves with folk medicines, faith healing, and magic cures, given our understanding of placebo effects? It is not surprising that even such an astute commentator of modernity as Benjamin[11] could sixty or seventy years ago seriously believe that storytelling, the voice of "facts as experience", was doomed to permanent silence. The future seemed to belong to information, scientific knowledge and theories. In this sense, we can regard the high noon of modernity as a moment when the ideology of science (that is, its elevation above criticism from alternative ideologies) appeared to eclipse the ideology of personal experience, along with many others.

It is curious then that late modernity has not merely rediscovered an appetite for stories, but has rediscovered authority in personal experience. Where modernity craved for the certainty of theories, late modernity would seem to thirst for the ambiguities of stories. The mass media, far from reporting facts, have turned largely into story-manufacturing factories, equipped with spin doctors and pundits who can directly affect and entertain the public. More specifically, we can argue that, in late modernity, the authority of specialist expertise, the core feature of Plato's political philosophy, is certainly facing a determined challenge from the authority of experience, the authority of the person who lived and witnessed events at first hand. Whether it is as oral history, as medical narrative, as story of self-discovery and growth, personal stories again matter, even to the point of challenging the expert. Numerous documents capture this change of balance – in the field of medicine, it is instructive that the patient can now be referred to as an expert in his/her condition in official Government reports.[23] Thus, late modernity has sought to re-assert the *primacy of experience* over other ways of establishing truth. As Eagleton[24] has argued, "one of the commonest forms of postmodernist dogma, ... the intuitive appeal to 'experience' is absolute because it cannot be gainsaid" (p 67). A result of this has been an argument, implicit or explicit, that *only* he or she who has lived through a certain experience can speak authoritatively about it – thus, only black people can speak authoritatively about race, only gay people about sexual marginalisation, and, more contentiously, only people suffering from cancer about cancer. In this way, the telling of the story becomes a process of discovering a *voice*, through which individuals and groups can build truth on their experience, communicate it, debate it, and share it with other people – in short, build identities.

The experts, for their part, have started to listen to such stories, as contributions to this book testify. And rightly so. Psychoanalysis must be credited with being one of the first disciplines to take a deep interest in the stories of its patients. Yet, its approach to these patient stories was essentially symptomatic – the story was approached as evidence to be interpreted. In so doing, psychoanalysis, since Freud, had laid itself open to three charges: first, that it fails to honour the experiences of its patients, always suspecting ulterior motives and hidden agendas; second, that it is indifferent to the material basis of experiences, notably whether traumas are caused by actual events or are imagined (à la Wilkomirski); and third, that in both of the above, psychoanalysis aligns itself with the discourses of the expert to deprive the non-expert of authority, even as the former listens attentively to the latter. We owe to Foucault the assertive linkage of knowledge and power, knowledge not merely being a tool or an instrument of power but being enmeshed with it. What is defined as knowledge is inextricably linked to the operation of power relations in both an oppressive and an empowering fashion. Foucault[25] also alerted us to a type of discourse, the confessional discourse, whose power agenda is not merely the humiliation or purification of the subject, but the definition of a domain of experience as a domain of surveillance and control:

> The confessional is a ritual of discourse in which the speaking subject is also the subject of the statement; it is also a ritual which unfolds within a power relationship, for one does not confess without the presence (or virtual presence) of a partner who is not simply the interlocutor but the authority who requires the confession, prescribes and appreciates it, and intervenes in order to judge, punish, forgive, console and reconcile .... A ritual which exonerates, redeems and purifies him. (p 61)

I argue in relation to the Wilkomirski case that the confessional discourse in late modernity has assumed a different power/knowledge configuration. As part of the ideology of personal experience, it proclaims aggressively: "Thou shalt not deny my experience; thou shalt not silence my voice!", thus challenging the ideology of scientific expertise.

Where does this ideology of personal experience draw its renewed claim to being authoritative knowledge? It would seem that, in late modernity, science is undergoing a decline in authority not unlike that experienced by religion and tradition as sources of knowledge in earlier times. As we saw, science has undoubtedly been guilty of long disregarding the voice of personal experience. In fields as diverse as medicine, architecture, history, engineering, to say nothing of the social and psychological sciences, the voice of experience was long lost in the midst of the authoritative proclamations of the experts. Now this may be changing.

Even in medicine, a field where the scientist's expertise still earns him/her enormous authority, it is now commonplace to encounter instances when medical science is questioned, challenged and discredited, at times by voices drawn from experience. Instances where physicians err assume wide publicity, seen increasingly as typical of scientific hubris. Consider, for instance, current publicity surrounding medical diagnoses of child abuse or infant death. The case of Sally Clark, a solicitor (and interestingly, a member of the expert classes) is instructive. She was convicted for the murder of her two children, mostly on the grounds of expert medical testimony by an eminent consultant paediatrician who rated the odds of the two children dying from natural causes as "one in 73 million". There was no direct or circumstantial evidence to suggest that the children (aged 8 and 11 weeks at the time of their death) had been "smothered" by their mother – the jury's judgment was largely the result of placing their trust on medical authority rather than on personal experience (which may have supported the view that "normal" mothers do not ordinarily kill their children). Subsequent evidence, however, led to the acquittal of Ms Clark and the discrediting of the medical testimony during her trial – the evidence in this case was also "expert evidence", yet, it underlines the point that the authority expertise (just like the authority of experience) must be seen as provisional. What was "hard science" ten years ago often emerges as mere belief, attitude, and opinion. This is but one of the numerous instances where the authority of the expert comes up against the authority of personal experience and is found to be flawed.

It would be entirely premature to consign the authority of the expert to the obsolete landscapes of modernity. Yet, it seems to me that on numerous battlefields, it is being challenged by the authority of personal experience. Parents challenge social workers and teachers, patients challenge clinicians, students challenge lecturers, sometimes in courts of law. This may be more broadly connected with what has been described as a therapeutic culture, or even the "Oprah-isation" of culture, that is, the increasing hegemony of an incontestable confessional discourse which enables the victim to become a survivor through the magic of finding a voice and having their voice heard. When the knowledge of experts is routinely devalued (and often for excellent reasons), knowledge from introspection, divination or faith is virtually dismissed, and facts become infinitely accommodating of diverse interpretations and spin. We are left with knowledge and truth from authentic personal experience and the different voices that it takes (art, story, memoir, reminiscence), which assumes pride of place.

Suffering narratives

It will not have escaped the reader's attention that the kind of experience ideally suited to the confessional discourse is not that of heroic quest, ironic self-disparagement or romantic affection, but rather that of suffering and oppression; articulating such an experience can help the subject turn shame and rage into defiance and pride – the acknowledgement of victimhood becomes a celebration of survival. Few human experiences call for narrative with the same urgency as suffering. And suffering poses some unique challenges to narrative, unlike many other human experiences. Triumphs, coincidences, conflicts, reversals, revelations, and come-uppances all spawn narratives, but they do not match loss, tragedy, and suffering in narrative urgency – suffering stretches human sense-making capacities beyond most other experiences. Triumphs can be attributed to personal efforts, qualities of character or good fortune; coincidences, reversals, revelations, and come-uppances can be seen as the products of an engineering providence that ensures fairness and justice. Suffering, on the other hand, cannot be accommodated into some sense-making schema quite so easily. And, among different types of suffering, our culture seems most ill-equipped to deal with narratives of illness and pain. Indeed, some extreme forms of pain completely paralyse the human ability to speak, let alone to narrate.[26] And when pain does not paralyse speech, it raises an endless series of questions that are as pressing as they are hard to answer. Why should my child be born with a disability? Why should I be the one who suffers a stroke? Why have I lost my hearing/looks/partner? Can anything be done about my condition? Will I be able to bear it? What is the point of all this?

In a pioneering work, Kleinman[12] explored the different meanings of illness and some of the narratives through which such meanings come to the surface. What was original in that work (and sets it apart from earlier attempts by poets, novelists, and social commentators to identify the meanings of illness (see Sontag[27]), was the exploration of the meanings that illness has for the person who suffers, his/her family, and their wider cultural milieu. As patients seek the deeper significance of their suffering, the illness and its symptoms become embedded in life stories, which Kleinman claimed can tell us a great deal about the nature of the disorder and potential treatments. In many illness narratives, the "pain" emerges as a character in the plot; sometimes it behaves in a consistent way, at others in an unpredictable erratic manner. In some narratives, pain is a fierce enemy which must be fought, in others, more like an unpredictable child one must learn to live with. Of course, people speak about their pain not only to their physicians, but also to their friends, their relatives, and to complementary or alternative therapists. In my own experience as a Greek who has lived most of his life in Great Britain, few issues divide cultures more sharply than the social acceptability of discussing pain and illness. In some countries, including Greece, one finds numerous people who are narrative virtuosos in discussing theirs and others' ailments, always sure to find appreciative audiences. In other cultures, the very mention of a source of pain is virtual taboo. "How is your knee?" my British mother-in-law was asked after returning home following a replacement operation (she had insisted that no one visited her in hospital). "What knee?" was her telling answer. Denying an audience to someone who wishes to narrate their pain is as much a violation as forcing a pain discourse on someone intent on silencing it.

Why do people seek to narrate their pain? Clearly eliciting sympathy is one reason; offering a warning is another. Yet, for the purposes of this discussion, the two functions I want to underline are what I would call the epistemological and the sense-making functions. The former places the pain in a forum where information is sought and given about different treatments, their effectiveness and limitations. In such forums (which resemble what in the case of professionals are known as "communities of practice"[28,29,30] and to which we could refer as "communities fo coping"), people may seek and offer tips, in what exactly amounts to an exchange of "narrative knowledge",[4,31] in quasi-gift transactions. Thus, people suffering from asthma, tinnitus or a whole range of disorders may seek recourse to support groups of fellow sufferers or "alternative medicines" instead of or in addition to the authority of the medical expert.

The epistemological dimension of such stories is not the same as the sense-making aspect. One can very well discuss different ways of dealing with asthma or sinusitis (through scientific or narrative knowledge) without exhausting their sense-making needs, that is, without the sufferers reaching a satisfactory understanding of the ultimate meaning or significance of their condition. In telling a story of their illness, people, beyond seeking sympathy or information, and beyond offering warnings and tips, may struggle to come to terms with a deeper significance. This is perhaps the hardest challenge facing the suffering narrator. There is an arbitrariness in the unequal distribution of suffering, which is far harder to bear than the unequal distribution of money or power. This is why such narratives, that is, those that aim at coming to terms with arbitrariness, are both very pressing and especially difficult. The result is that many narratives of illness are at the same time quests for narrative, in the exact sense described by the much abused term "reflexive". The plot of the story becomes the search for a plot. Thus, for instance, the "quest" narratives[32,33,34] become narratives questing the often evasive meaning of illness ("There must be some meaning to my illness"); the "chaos" narratives are narratives struggling with the chaotic consequences of illness ("My illness does not make sense"). Illness is, after all, an instance where disorder, even chaos, prevails over order. Of course, some narratives undoubtedly and unambiguously discover an underlying plot to illness or to suffering. As Greenhalgh has pointed out, tragic narratives may cast the illness as an evil adversary who is eventually going to be victorious, comic narratives may look at the funny implications of illness while restitution narratives generally look at illness as a test of character, as something that is successfully overcome through courage, fortitude, and medical know-how.[34] Yet, there is something of a chaos narrative in all illness[33]; even where a meaning has been arrived at, it requires a great deal of *story work* to reach it. This undoubtedly makes grave demands on the listener – time, patience, empathy. The story must be drawn out of the suffering person through empathetic listening, supportive interventions, and co-narrating, always building a sense of trust. The listener is suffering with the narrator and part of this suffering lies in the fact that it is not clear whether the narrative will reach the safe harbour of a meaning. The "So what?" question cannot be put safely aside until the end of a narrative that may prove to be interminable.

What happens when the listener is not a fellow-sufferer, a relative or a friend but a figure of authority, a physician? Since the work of Kleinman, much greater recognition is given to patients' stories in their own right rather than as vehicles to diagnosis. Frank[32,33] advocates the role of a physician who maintains a "critical distance" from the narrator, but who listens carefully to the latter's utterances as he/she tries to develop a narrative. Listening is not a task, but part of a gift relationship; instead of listening symptomatically, continuously on the look-out in the narrative for hints as to the "true nature of the illness", (an approach Frank associates with Kleinman[12]), the listener gives unconditional attention to the narrator as part of a gift relationship. Both parties are enhanced by such an experience, as they make their needs known to the other party and see these needs "honoured".

> One listens to ill people's stories not in order to fix them by doing something "therapeutic", but rather to honor them. Again, people tell the stories they need to tell in order to work through the situation they are in.[33] (p 207)

The idea of "honouring" a person by respecting their narrative suggests that the physicians (or researchers) give up any presumption of understanding patients (or storytellers) better than these latter understand themselves and give up any right to "use" the narrative to control the patients or their condition. It also surrenders the premise that the expert's time is more valuable than the patient's, a premise of which all patients are routinely reminded as they wait in long queues before their consultations. It is by surrendering some of the expert authority, that empathetic, non-symptomatic, non-motivated listening enables both physician and patient to escape their respective "iron cages" created by the power/knowledge nexus in which they find themselves.

The narrative contract delineated by this approach is one in which story is itself a gift; it is a gift offered by the teller (it remains his or her story) but one that could not have been produced without the participation of the listener, who offers his/her own gift of time, empathy, and attention. Experience is honoured, emotions are honoured.[35] However, the unqualified honouring of that which is presented as experience, as our digression into the case Wilkomirski suggests, can lead to grave violations of the narrative contract. It seems to me that if science can no longer be trusted to speak on behalf of people and groups to whose voices it is deaf, neither can the voice of experience be elevated to unquestioned and unquestionable authority.

The voice of experience and the voice of the expert – can there be dialogue between them?

It is true that humans suffer. But a mouse too can suffer, not least as the subject of experiments aimed at reducing the suffering of humans. What makes human suffering different is the irresistible search for meaning, which, in all its undoubted grandeur, may bring grace or may lead us to delusion. It is the combination of suffering and delusion that lies at the heart of humanity's uniquely tragic condition. Honouring the suffering, honouring the narrative, and honouring the storyteller, does not mean accepting unconditionally the truth of the story.

Where does this leave us? Undoubtedly, experience as a source of authoritative knowledge is here to stay. There is much to learn from direct experience and science can no longer disregard it or take automatic precedence over it. We are now aware that much of the knowledge on which we rely for our daily activities is narrative knowledge, that is, knowledge deriving from ours and other people's experience and disseminated through stories. Equally, however, knowledge from experience cannot be accepted without interrogation, verification, and criticism. While Descartes' rationalism has lost much of its appeal in our time, we would do well to remember his warning about the "deceiver, supremely powerful, supremely intelligent who purposely always deceives me" (Meditation 2) and approach experience with a healthy dose of scepticism. Our own experience, no less than that of others, can deceive us, and, in our self-deception, we may deploy it to deceive others. The very narratives that help us make sense of our suffering and live with it can be deceiving us.

Instead of accepting all voices of experience as equally valid and equally worthy of attention, I would argue that it is the job of researchers to interrogate experiences, seeking to examine not only their origins, but also those blind spots, illusions, and self-deceptions that crucially and legitimately make them up. Far from being an unqualified source of knowledge, experience must be treated with the same scepticism and suspicion with which we approach all other sources of authoritative knowledge. Joining the postmodern choirs of ever smaller voices does little credit to academic research. Disentangling these voices, understanding them, comparing them, privileging those which deserve to be privileged and silencing those that deserve to be silenced, questioning them, testing them, and qualifying them – these seem to me to be essential judging qualities that mark research into storytelling and narratives as something different from the acts of storytelling and narration themselves. Deception, blind spots, wishful thinking, the desire to please or to manipulate an audience, lapses of memory, confusion, and other factors may help mould a story or a narrative. It is the researcher's task not merely to celebrate the story or the narrative but to seek to use it as a vehicle for accessing deeper truths than the truths, half-truths, and fictions of undigested personal experience.

Acknowledgement

Many thanks to Trisha Greenhalgh, whose extraordinary enthusiasm for medical narratives was a great source of inspiration for me in looking at stories and storytelling from an angle that I had not considered earlier. All three editors of this book have been extremely helpful with suggestions and comments on earlier drafts of this chapter. My thanks to them all.

References

1 Bruner J. *Acts of meaning.* Cambridge, MA: Harvard University Press, 1990.
2 Culler J. *The pursuit of signs: semiotics, literature, deconstruction* (Routledge Classics edn). London: Routledge, 1981/2001.
3 Czarniawska B. *Narrating the organization: dramas of institutional identity.* Chicago: University of Chicago Press, 1997.
4 Czarniawska B. *Writing management: organization theory as a literary genre.* Oxford: Oxford University Press, 1999, p: 64f.
5 Labov W. *Language in the inner city.* Philadelphia: University of Pennsylvania Press, 1972.
6 MacIntyre A. *After virtue.* London: Duckworth, 1981.
7 Polkinghorne DE. *Narrative knowing and the human sciences.* Albany, NY: State University of New York Press, 1988, pp 18–19.
8 Ricoeur P. *Time and narrative,* vol 1. Chicago: University of Chicago Press, 1984.
9 Van Dijk TA. Action, action description, and narrative. *New Literary History* 1975;6:275–94.
10 Weick KE. *Sensemaking in organizations.* London: Sage, 1995.
11 Benjamin W. The storyteller: Reflections on the works of Nikolai Leskov. In: Arendt H, ed. *Walter Benjamin: Illuminations.* London: Jonathan Cape, 1968.
12 Kleinman A. *The illness narratives: suffering, healing, and the human condition.* New York: Basic Books, 1998.
13 Wilkomirski B. *Fragments: memories of a wartime childhood.* New York: Random House, 1996.
14 Maechler S. *The Wilkomirski Affair.* Basingstoke: Picador, 2001.
15 Finkelstein NG. *The Holocaust industry: reflections on the exploitation of Jewish suffering.* London: Verso, 2000, p 61.
16 Binford L. Empowered speech: social fields, testimonio, and the Stoll–Menchu debate. *Identities – Global Studies in Culture and Power* 2001;8(1):105–33.
17 Gledhill J. Deromanticizing subalterns or recolonializing anthropology? Denial of indigenous agency and reproduction of northern hegemony in the work of David Stoll. *Identities – Global Studies in Culture and Power* 2001;8(1):135–61.
18 Reason P, Hawkins P. Storytelling as inquiry. In: Reason P, ed. *Human Inquiry in Action: Developments in New Paradigm Research.* London: Sage, 1988, pp 71–101.
19 Crews F. *The memory wars: Freud's legacy in dispute.* New York: New York Review of Books, 1995.
20 Forrester J. *Dispatches from the Freud Wars.* Cambridge, MA: Harvard University Press, 1997.
21 Gabriel Y. *Organizations in depth. The psychoanalysis of organizations.* London: Sage, 1999.
22 Burke E. *Reflections on the Revolution in France.* Harmondsworth: Penguin Books, 1790/1998.
23 DoH. *The Expert Patient: A New Approach to Chronic Disease Management for the 21st Century.* London: Department of Health, 2001.
24 Eagleton T. *The illusions of postmodernism.* Oxford: Blackwell, 1996.
25 Foucault M. *The history of sexuality: an introduction,* vol 1. Harmondsworth: Penguin, 1978.

26 Scarry E. *The body in pain*. Oxford: Oxford University Press, 1987.
27 Sontag S. *Illness as Metaphor/AIDS and Its Metaphors*. Harmondsworth: Penguin, 1991.
28 Brown JS, Duguid P. Organizational learning and communities of practice: toward a unified view of working, learning and innovation. *Organization Science* 1991;2(1):40–57.
29 Wenger E. *Communities of practice: learning, meaning and identity*. Cambridge: Cambridge University Press, 1998.
30 Wenger E. Communities of practice and social learning systems. *Organization* 2000;7(2):225–46.
31 Tsoukas H. Forms of knowledge and forms of life in organized contexts. In: Chia RCH, ed. *In the Realm of Organization: Essays for Robert Cooper*. London: Routledge, 1998.
32 Frank AW. *The wounded storyteller: body, illness, and ethics*. Chicago, Il: University of Chicago Press, 1995.
33 Frank AW. Just listening: Narrative and deep illness. *Families, Systems and Health* 1998;16:197–216.
34 Greenhalgh T. *Narrative and the primary care consultation*. London: University College, 2002.
35 Meyerson DE. If emotions were honoured: A cultural analysis. In: Fineman S, ed. *Emotion in Organizations*, 2nd edn. London: Sage, 2000, pp 167–83.

Section 2:
Counter-narratives

11: Wounded or warrior? Stories of being or becoming deaf

LESLEY JONES, ROBIN BUNTON

Different stories are told about the experience of being deaf. For some people, becoming deaf is an interruption of their story, for others being deaf becomes the point of the story itself. This chapter explores some of the ways in which people describe being or becoming deaf and how their stories relate to medicine. Medicine can be an integral part of the story, or simply a sub-plot. Knowing the various ways that deaf people see their deafness, will help provide better understanding of the impact of clinical practice on deaf people.

Although the consequences and meaning of being deaf vary, research shows how closely deafness and personal identity can be linked. Some people describe themselves as Deaf with a capital D, denoting membership of the "Deafhood" community and culture, and conceive of themselves as a linguistic minority which uses a national sign language. These people generally claim citizenship of the "Deaf Nation" as almost an ethnicity. But for others, deafness is not a defining feature of their self identity; these people never use the word "deaf", or may, in effect, say: "I don't hear so well on that side" or "I miss things when people mumble". For these people, their sense of identity is more akin to that of hearing people.

Two salient narratives can be identified in relation to being and becoming deaf: one that can be termed "wounded", and another we have called the "warrior" narrative. The wounded narrative corresponds to Arthur Frank's account of "illness narrative".[1] Our research suggests the existence of another related narrative, that of warrior. Like illness narratives, these narratives may be taken up and used in various ways throughout people's lives. Illness narratives can help to order experience over time as illness-related events unfold. They give expression to changes in one's body and relationships with others.[2]

Several narrative "genres" can be discerned including the epic or heroic, the tragic, the comic or ironic, disembodied or romantic, and the didactic[3] framed in relation to medical diagnosis and intervention. Deaf people endeavour to shape their accounts in response to contact with others, including the medical profession. Medicine has its own discourses about deafness, and its own "remedies", such as cochlear implants and emerging genetic technologies. The authors are both

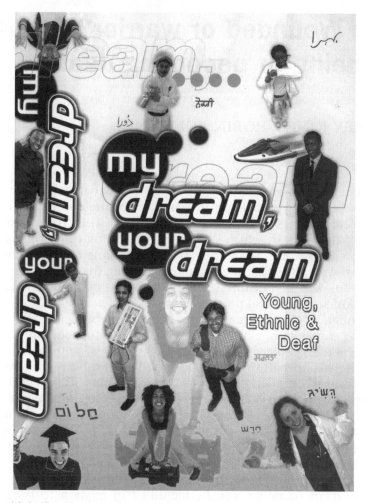

Figure 11.1 Positive identities

hearing and base this chapter on their research and practice. It attempts to bring together research interests on the experience of deafness and medicine by Lesley Jones,[i] with work on the social aspects of health and the body by Robin Bunton.

We begin this study by contrasting two views of the experience of deafness taken from two videos made by young people in the UK, both of which are designed to share the experience of being deaf with other deaf young people. The first image comes from a video titled "My Dream, Your Dream: Young, Ethnic and Deaf" made by a group of young deaf people from minority ethnic communities in Britain.[4] The young people who made this video were largely users of British Sign Language and identified with the Deaf community. Figure 11.1, showing the flyer for this "warrior" video, contains positive images of achievement and hopes for the future, reinforced by the video itself which gives young deaf people the message that "you can do anything you want to". This is typified by a young deaf Karate champion, who says: "I wanted to show hearing people, I was better than them."

This contrasts with another video made by young people who became deaf in their teens, and was designed to be helpful to those in the same situation.[5] Despite its positive title, "It's Not the End of the World", this video presents a series of "talking head" shots of young people, and images of broken lives and damaged futures. One young woman said:

My life had changed completely. I live with my Mum and it was very hard for her. She just couldn't accept that she'd got a deaf daughter instead of a hearing one. ... She couldn't accept that I couldn't use the phone and couldn't bear to use the phone for me. It was like (she thought) "Oh God, she really is deaf and if I do that for her, she is going to be even deafer."

Another young woman who appears in the video repeatedly talked about the desire to return to the status quo after her "drastic reduction in hearing".

I thought I would go into hospital and I would be normal again.

She spoke of her suicidal depression after a failed operation and the realisation that she could "never be normal again".

Both videos were made by young people for others in the same or similar situation and are intended to empower and encourage by "letting people tell their own stories". The videos are in different languages. The warrior video was made in the visual language of British Sign Language (BSL), a language with no accepted written form. The "wounded" video is in spoken English, with subtitles. Differences in languages reflect differences in the narrative.

The two narrative structures are illustrated in Figure 11.2.

Warrior narratives tend to be used by those born deaf or who became deaf in early childhood and identify with British Sign Language and the Deaf community. We have added the term Born (Again) Deaf for those people who decide to move from an earlier identification with the hearing world and the spoken language (perhaps because of an oral education or upbringing) to that of the Deaf world.[6] Often this may involve a switching of narrative. This model speaks of citizenship, nationhood, and human rights, and of being part of a linguistic minority. It is opposed to a "deficit model" of deafness as impairment, which is a feature of the wounded narrative. This wounded narrative constructs a picture of identities experiencing "loss" or "damage" by the onset of deafness. The wounded and the warrior accounts in some ways resemble elements of comic/ironic and epic/heroic narratives identified by Kelly and Dickenson in discussing

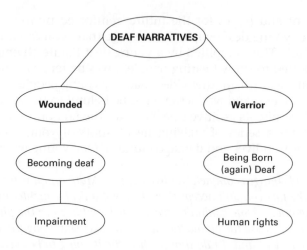

Figure 11.2   Wounded and warrior meanings

ulcerative colitis.[7] Pain and discomfort are dealt with from a humorous and positive viewpoint. The warrior narrative also contains strong images of war and fighting against oppression.[8,9]

These two narratives by no means exhaust the wide range of deaf people's experience. They are presented here only as two particularly interesting and widely available narratives offering accounts of some of the variety of responses to being deaf. Deaf people are too often lumped together by health professionals such that hard of hearing people (who may use amplification) are placed alongside those who do not use speech at all, and together with those with a dual sensory impairment, such as deaf–blind people. Across these distinctions is the usual diversity of human beings who differ by gender, race, religion, age, sexuality, class, income, and education. Such contextual, cultural, and language diversity influences how deaf people's body and identity narratives unfold, as they do for the hearing. Though the language used for these narratives varies (BSL for the warriors and speech for the wounded), as do the heroes and villains of these narratives, a positive interpretation of events is a continued theme throughout.

The wounded narrative

In his book *The Wounded Storyteller*,[1] Arthur Frank takes up Kleinman's statement that cultures "unfold" into bodies. By this expression the authors refer to the processes of bodily understanding and body maintenance. During illness people face difficulties maintaining previous understandings of their bodies and themselves because of the physical changes they are experiencing. They develop, Frank tells us, difficulties in continuing to be the body they have been used to being, and must come up with new strategies for maintaining their relationship to, and control of, their bodies. Humans face not dissimilar problems at times of physical transition – adolescence, pregnancy, and ageing for example. During such times of change people are likely to become more reflexive about their bodies, and may often re-work their relationships to their own bodies. Illness narratives are also narratives about bodies. They are a resource to help account for physical changes.

Illness narratives often appear as stories of the "wounded" and have much in common with other experiences of loss and damage to the body. Loss of a limb or a sense, for example, requires more than physiological adaptation, it requires a new body narrative and adaptation to a different social status. The wounded deaf narrative illustrates some features of the stories which Frank refers to. The wounded narratives focus on:

- **Damage** – loss and limitation
- **Exclusion** – from Deaf and hearing worlds
- **Integration** – re-assimilation or "passing"[1]

Stories told using the idea of impairment and loss describe becoming deaf as a threat to competency and, in the words of a young British woman in her early thirties:

I could have quite happily strung myself up when I first went deaf. If I'd had any sort of courage I would have. I couldn't see that I was going to be any sort of mother to them, I couldn't understand them. Something that really brought it home to me happened – I was sitting here, we'd had breakfast … [one child had fallen down the stairs and came in crying with his nose bleeding] I'd not heard and he'd had to pick himself up to come and tell me.

Interestingly, when visited a year later this woman's views had shifted slightly. She spoke of hearing people's lack of effort in communication and she seemed more assertive about her own predicament:

Don't let the sods [uncommunicative hearing people] get you down!

The despair and shame she had felt at her deafness had turned to anger and resistance about the behaviour of others towards her

Wounded narratives frequently focus on damage, the fragility of the body, and exclusion from other communities of bodies. Integration into non-stigmatised interaction is valued and such accounts often mention the desire to belong and to "pass" as hearing. We might recognise a classic tactic of the stigmatised.[10] There is a desire to return to a previous embodied state: to be "the same as I was before I became deaf", which Arthur Frank refers to as a "restitution narrative". The pattern is, yesterday I was well, today I am ill, tomorrow I will be well.

The following quote illustrates one woman's concern with these matters:

I used to feel I was deformed. It's a deformity, something to be ashamed of. Now I class it as the same as wearing spectacles. What's the difference between having bad eyes and bad ears? (British woman in her thirties)

This account suggests a transition, though it still uses imagery of a damaged body; over time this woman adopts a more pragmatic view, playing down the damaging significance of being deaf. Such reasoning is often aligned with descriptions of the body's "wearing out" and growing older, rather like "wear and tear" analogies commonly used by both patients and professionals about arthritis.

The image in Figure 11.3 of the old man in Sutcliffe's photograph suggests that it may be all right to be deaf, if you are old. You may be surrounded by attentive hearing people who engage in the joint enterprise of communication with you. The posed scene of Victorian Whitby presents an image of respect for older people and for cross-generational attempts to understand one another. As one respondent of a study of people who became deaf said, "It is OK to be deaf if you are old. I would wear my hearing aid if I was old." This stereotype is at odds with angry demonstrators for the acceptance of British Sign Language as an official language, the subject of three national demonstrations outside the House of Commons.

As a part of the ageing process, hearing loss may be seen as acceptable. By contrast, another woman, deafened in her teens, writes of her experience:

We want the hearing person I once was back again because she had control of her life. We think that this is all happening because of some tiny fault in our ears. But we aren't faulty people, if we could get our hearing back all the problems would go away. So we shop around for cures for a bit until finally giving up except to monitor cochlear implant experiments.[11]

She goes on to comment on what medicine offers:

We are stuck with pathological models and medical definitions of who we are when in reality we are not sick or ill people.

Social models of disability are no better than medicine at offering a positive view. The wounded stories emphasise isolation and loss and the different experience of those who become deaf rather than grow up deaf. This initial reaction (as we have seen above) can change when a reinterpretation of the situation usually takes place. At other times the narrative becomes fixed and the main theme of the story, and the sense that is made of their lives, centre on features of loss, isolation, damage. This view, of course, is reinforced by much of psychological/psychiatric literature on the effects of deafness, which

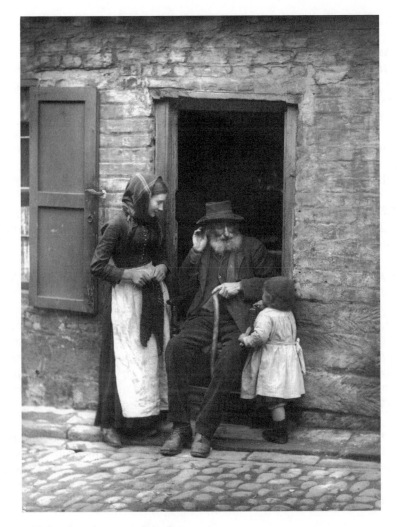

Figure 11.3 Past images of deafness

focuses on psychiatric morbidity and deafness. The wounded stories, then, focus on overcoming damage, humiliation, and the desire for integration and contrast with the warrior stories.

Warrior narratives

The warrior narratives we identified focus on the following features:

- **Fight** – for human rights and citizenship
- **Belonging** – to a nation, a culture, a community
- **Separatism** – segregation, being a part of a linguistic minority

This 40-year-old Portuguese man illustrates well the fight analogy:

Deaf people should get together and tell governments about their situation ... I would like the government to treat Deaf people the same as hearing people. I don't like to see them thinking that to be deaf is also to be unintelligent – inside we are all equal.

He also emphasises the need to belong, to get together to be stronger in order to withstand the way in which people unable to hear are treated by society. This reinforces a sense of belonging, as shown by the following quotes from respondents in other studies:

I'd like to have a Deaf town, a Deaf community. I want to be involved in a deaf community. I'd like to feel welcomed and part of a deaf community. I don't want to be on my own. (26-year-old British-Indian man)

It feels like home – It's a Deaf community it's the Deaf world. I felt this was great. (20-year-old British-Pakistani woman)

The cohesion sometimes comes from a response to outside forces:

The teachers at my school did not like sign language. They used to tie my hands behind my back and hit my hands if I signed but I didn't care – my father was deaf like me and we used sign language at home. (49-year-old Spanish woman; quoted in Jones and Pullen[12])

Some hearing people are very cruel and they say oh you're crap, and you're no good and you don't know anything, that's why hearing people are cruel. I tell them, Oh shut up, stop being stupid you don't know anything about deaf people, you are not learning about deaf people. (11-year-old Pakistani-British schoolgirl describing bullying[13])

Being drawn together in reaction to discrimination and disadvantage leads to community solidarity, though not always a political one. The political element is one, however, which shapes many of the warrior stories. Up until the end of the 1990s, Deaf people in the UK kept themselves apart from the Political Disability Movement, and saw themselves as a linguistic minority not as disabled. This has changed through the lobbying for the Disability Discrimination Act and the mixed benefits of recognition in the benefit system – for communication support for example. It has also changed because of the political Disability Movement's backing of the fight for the recognition of British Sign Language. There is still an uneasy alliance between the disparate groups. The social model of disability stresses the barriers to access, as opposed to the "medical deficit" model which focuses on the person with the impairment. The social model fits in well with the lack of access experienced by Deaf people in everyday life, for example, a sign language interpreter is there for the benefit of both the deaf person who uses sign language and the hearing person who does not.

There is an emphasis on separatism in order to build strength to fight in this warrior rhetoric. Attitudes to integrated schooling illustrate this process. Integration is seen as undermining BSL, and the Deaf community. Community closeness is valued as it was in the past, with deaf children being educated together in residential schools but usually born to hearing families. This meant that they lived together learning BSL from one another, and usually marrying other deaf people. Giving birth to a deaf child is often seen as desirable, "as it is so much easier" for deaf parents. Integration and medical attempts to cure deafness are seen as a threat.

Differences in the two accounts of being deaf are highlighted in the ways in which they relate to the following elements of their lives: integrated education, medicine, British Sign Language, Deaf culture and the Political Disability Movement. In each case opposite view points are expressed. We previously mentioned differences in attitudes towards medicine and towards integrated education. The same differences are apparent in relation to the use of BSL or speech. BSL is supported in warrior narratives and is a crucial part of identity and struggle, but it is viewed with suspicion in the wounded narratives, where speech is essential to membership of the hearing world. The same oppositions are there in relation to Deaf Culture, which is seen as integral to warrior narratives though often irrelevant to wounded accounts. Only in attitudes towards the Political Disability Movement do both groups share a common attitude: that of ambivalence. Neither group feels at ease about identifying unconditionally with these aspirations. Warriors because they do not see themselves as disabled, but rather as a linguistic minority: the wounded because they wish to identify with the non-disabled community.

Once again oppositions are very clear in the way in which the storytellers relate to important elements of their lives. The relationship between deaf stories and medicine will be the focus of the next section.

Medicine

Medicine is one of the main providers of narratives about deafness, but it is not the only one. As we shall see, when people experience being or becoming deaf they can draw upon many different narratives to make sense of their place in the world, and their physiological predicament. Deaf people make sense of their world and themselves by drawing on a range of narratives, some medical, some religious, some of a non-systematic nature. Sometimes these narratives are limiting and negative: other times they are not. Nora Groce's study of hereditary deafness in Martha's Vineyard, observed that deaf people in these communities experienced little or no stigma or marginalisation because of the large numbers of deaf people in that community.[14] The relative isolation of that population and the presence of hereditary deafness resulted in the community adapting positively to the presence of deafness. For 200 years or so, everyone in this community could use sign language. Being deaf carried little or no social disadvantage. In Martha's Vineyard at this time, deaf people's understanding of their bodies and themselves was little different to hearing people's. Numerous examples such as these illustrate the ways in which body narratives develop and change with social and cultural developments. The example of the two deaf women in the United States who chose to have a deaf child using the donated sperm of someone with a history of genetic deafness in the family[15] was described in the *BMJ* as "designer disability" and shows the difference in interpretation of deafness amongst different groups of people. Not only does medicine make distinctions between views of technology and deafness, there are also distinctions made between different groups of deaf people. Part of the warrior narrative is the history of struggle against "oppression". Blume highlights this struggle in his examination of one technology.

Deaf people have located cochlear implants within a history of their own oppression, rather than in a history of their own progress. Each historical rendering is used to try to influence policy. The contest, however, is an unequal one.[16]

The two narratives we are describing have very different relationships to medicine. The warrior narrative often rejects medicine completely (and modernism), appearing, in the past, almost pre-modern. Commentators have argued that we have never been totally modern and that throughout the modern period in the West non-scientific systems of thought and belief have continued to exist alongside the discourses of modern science.[17]

The wounded storytellers, however, often embrace medicine and technology in varying degrees. This can be seen in their attitudes both to medicine and medical technology, and to that based on talk.

Table 11.1 shows the differences between the two narrative views in relation to medical technologies used with deaf people.

The attitudes towards surgery and technology designed to enhance hearing are interpreted in completely opposite ways. This same pattern is also evident in the views of the clinical interventions based on speech. It would seem to be obvious that speech-based therapy is immediately at odds with users of BSL and other sign languages coming as they do from within an education system which has been based for most of the twentieth century on the acquisition of speech

Table 11.1   The different views of techno medicine

	Wounded	Warrior
Cochlear implants	Cure	Invasion
Surgery	Repair	Eradication
Genetics	Prevention	Genocide
Amplification	Life-line	Interference
Audiology	Support	Surveillance

Table 11.2   Different views of medical practice based on talk

	Wounded	Warrior
Speech and language therapy	Vital	Irrelevant
Hearing therapy	Support	Irrelevant
Counselling	Support	Inaccessible

and the suppression of their language. Table 11.2 shows the views of these therapies.

Techno medicine

Thus there are two very different accounts of cochlear implantation, for example, embedded in two very different histories. One is a tale of medicine's triumph, akin to many other such tales: a tale of courageous pioneers, of the wonders of medical science and technology. The other is a genre that has emerged only in the past two decades and which highlights the subordination of medicine to surveillance, social control, and normalisation. This tale is of one of the oppression of Deaf people and of hearing people's inability to accept deaf people as they are.

Blume[16] writes of this division:

> ... Both [accounts] are mobilised in the attempt to influence the way in which the technology of cochlear implantation is to be used. (p 1265)

As Blume points out, techno medicine offers the hope of a cure and repair and correction for the wounded storyteller, through hearing aids, surgery, and cochlear implants. For the warrior narrator it offers only genocide or humiliation. The sign used by deaf people for cochlear implants in the 1980s was a gun held to the head. It was seen as a threat to the Deaf world "to get rid of the Deaf." This same threat has been perceived in the genetic advances in pre- and neonatal screening. Again the rhetoric of the Political Disability Movement has been employed to highlight the human rights issues about the value of each individual and the folly of controlling populations. The search for the Deaf Gene is described as "the final solution" by leading Deaf academic and activist Paddy Ladd,[8] echoing the language of National Socialism in Germany in the 1930s, which is also found in the wearing of blue ribbons at national and international events as a symbol of solidarity. Blue was used by the Nazis to identify deaf and/or disabled people.

However, technology in these narratives now has a more complex role with improvements in information technology. Technology has provided improved access for deaf people through text communication, video, and the computerisation of knowledge as well as through better environmental aids. The pre-modernism of the past warrior stories has given way to enthusiasm for some aspects of technology which act as agents of equity, particularly amongst young deaf people. The joy of text messaging is a great equaliser for deaf and hearing people. The sharing of subtitled access to popular culture in the form of soap operas and videotapes of Hollywood films can only be breaking down barriers between the deaf and hearing world. The relationship with biotechnology seems much more problematic and complicated now for warriors, not just a straightforward rejection.

Discussion

Our analysis of deaf narratives highlights a number of features of the relationship between deafness, the body, and self identity. People's bodies seem to represent fundamental aspects of their cherished sense of self and when changes occur in their physical bodies then it has implications for their sense of self, their well-being and happiness. Whilst the physiology of deafness has a number of common features, the experience of being and becoming deaf is highly varied and far from predictable. The stories deaf people tell reflect a wide variety of experiences of selfhood, citizenship, social, ethnic, and cultural diversity. For some, deafness can mean marginalisation and exclusion, for others acknowledging one's Deafness is a key issue of belonging and collective action in the battle for linguistic and cultural equality. Whilst medical science may be involved in mediating much of the experience of deaf people, it is only one of many influences over the experience of deafness. It can have much to learn from study of the social understanding of deafness, just as it continues to learn from the related field of the social study of health and illness. It may be that Deaf people "may choose to situate their worldview around cultural and linguistic perspectives, rather than audiological perspectives".[8]

The warrior narrative, which we have presented here, relies upon the use of words like strength, pride, struggle, and fight. This is clearly shown in the text of the "Blue Ribbon" Ceremony, World Congress of the World Federation of the Deaf, Brisbane, July 1999,[8] which declared:

> We are here to bear witness ... to Deaf people from every part of the world, of all ages and all colours, this diversity joined in unity. We celebrate our proud history, our arts and cultures. And we celebrate our survival. Despite adversity and oppression, we are still here and stronger than before.

There are elements of international strength through numbers, an almost tribal pride in belonging to a marginalised group, which characterises the warrior view of being deaf. The emphasis is upon battle, as articulated by Ladd, who defines scientific/medical/education oppression as a feature of "war-time" as opposed to "peace-time" agendas. They are seen as an external threat to deaf people.

The wounded storyteller's narrative progresses from order to chaos and back to order again. For someone who becomes deaf as an adult, having already become accustomed to being a part of the hearing world, this may well be how they see their "hearing loss". It may also describe the experience of someone born into a hearing family where their deafness is seen as a tragedy (encouraged perhaps by the way in which the diagnosis is presented by clinicians). Medicine and science offer the possibility of order through correction. There remains the risk of techno-chaos with the threat of technology's inherent capacity to fight back. Operations may fail, implant or amplification aids may fail to restore hearing to the level anticipated, a cochlear implant may stop working when wet. There is still the fear of medical mistakes and of misfortune – after implantation a child may be neither fully a part of the Deaf world nor of the hearing world. The wounded narrative is, however, still a narrative of progress and ongoing search for something that has been lost, or for enhancement of a perceived inadequacy. The arrival of laser treatment for astigmatism in the High Street suggests that some similar "ear tinkering" may well be seen as desirable or available in the future.

The warrior narrative seems to have no such simple progression from chaos back to order. It promises only struggle compensated for by a sense of belonging, to an increasingly small group. Warriors may have simply learned to live with the changing rules of disorder in a world of uncertainty. Biomedicine seeks to eradicate deafness just at the point where Deaf nationhood seems to have been declared, making it all the more necessary for the full variety of deaf narratives to be understood.

Endnote

i   The research was undertaken with deaf and hearing researchers over a period of 20 years: Waqar Ahmed, Aliya Darr, Raymond Hetu, Michael Hirst, Louise Getty, Jim Kyle, Ghazalla Mir, Karl Atkin, Sally Baldwin, Rampaul Chamba, Gohar Nisar, Gloria Pullen, Tasnim Sharif, Ranjit Singh, and Peter Wood. The research was funded by the DoH, ESRC, JRF, European Union, and the Leverhulme Trust. The practice is in the collaboration and friendship of working with deaf researchers and teaching in Deaf Studies, and growing up in a hard of hearing family. The theory comes from reading and thinking about concepts of storytelling in health and medicine. We acknowledge with gratitude the work of our co-researchers and all those involved as participants, to whom we are indebted.

References

1   Frank A. *The Wounded Storyteller: Body, Illness and Ethics.* Chicago: Chicago University Press, 1995.
2   Bury M. Illness narratives: fact or fiction? *Sociol Health Illness* 2001;**23**(3):263–85.
3   Gergen KJ, Gergen MM. Narrative form and the construction of psychological science. In: Sarbin RT, ed. *Narrative psychology: the storied nature of human conduct.* New York: Praeger, 1986.
4   Joseph Rowntree Foundation. *My Dream, Your dream: Young, Ethnic and Deaf.* Video made by a group of young Deaf people from minority ethnic communities in Britain. York: Joseph Rowntree Foundation, 2000.
5   Department of Health. *It's Not the End of the World.* London: Visual Motions for the Department of Health, 1989.
6   Lane H, Hoffmeinster R, Bahan B. *A Journey in the Deaf-World.* San Diego: Dawn-Sign Press, 1996.
7   Kelly M, Dickenson H. The narrative self in autobiographical accounts of illness. *Sociol Rev* 1997;**45**(2):254–78.
8   Ladd P. *Understanding Deaf Culture: in search of deafhood.* Clevedon, UK: Multilingual Matters, 2003.
9   Blume S. Land of Hope and Glory: exploring cochlear implantation in the Netherlands. *Sci Technol Human Values* 2000;**25**(2):139–66
10 Goffman E. *Stigma.* London: Penguin, 1967.
11 Woolley M. Acquired hearing loss, acquired oppression. In: Swain J, Finkelstein V, French S, Oliver M, eds. *Disabling Barriers, Enabling Environments.* London: Sage, 1994.
12 Jones L, Pullen G. *"Inside We are All Equal": deaf people in Europe.* Brussels: ECRS, 1990.
13 Ahmed WIU, Atkin K, Jones L. Being deaf and other things: young Asian people negotiating identities. *Soc Sci Med* 2002;**55**:1757–69.
14 Groce N. *Everyone Here Speaks Sign Language.* Cambridge, MA: Harvard University Press, 1985.
15 Savulescu J. Deaf lesbians, designer disability and the future of medicine. *BMJ* 2002;**324**(7367):771–3.
16 Blume S. Histories of cochlear implantation. *Soc Sci Med* 1999;**49**:1257–68.
17 Latour B. *We Have Never Been Modern.* Hemel Hempstead: Harvester Wheatsheaf, 1993.

Commentary

PHILIP ZAZOVE

Lesley Jones and Robin Bunton do a wonderful job of discussing the response some people get to losing their hearing. They tell two stories related to this – which they call the "wounded" and the "warrior". The tale of the wounded is about a group of deaf people who despair about their disability, feel outcast from society, and wish they could hear. For the most part, the wounded narrative focuses on those who lose their hearing later in their life, that is to say, not those born deaf.

Then the authors talk about the "warriors", people at the opposite extreme. These individuals are proud to be Deaf, and capitalise the D in Deaf to denote this pride as well as their membership in the Deaf community. They resent any implication by medical professionals, however well meaning, to "reduce" their hearing loss. Studies have documented that the Deaf community is a true minority population, the equal of any other, with its own language, culture, and traditions.

Both these stories apply to numerous d/Deaf persons, regardless of where in the world they live. However, the reader should keep a few important points in mind. First, despite popular misconception, most deaf and hard of hearing (D&HH) people with a hearing loss, even those with a profound loss, are deaf, not Deaf. The misconception exists because the latter have done a much better job publicising their values. Second, those who lose their hearing at birth and grow up deaf, are quite different from those who lose their hearing later in life. The former never knew it any other way, and though they likewise may seek technology (for example, cochlear implants) to hear better, they are also more likely to be coping well in a hearing world. Major organisations exist, such as the Alexander Graham Bell Association, which are composed of these individuals. Nevertheless, there are many d/Deaf persons who for whatever reason do not learn to communicate orally; this has nothing to do with their intelligence but rather is an outcome of a complex set of factors. The warrior mentality of the Deaf community provides enormous support for these individuals by giving them a sense of community and self worth that they otherwise wouldn't get.

Third, society treats people with a hearing loss poorly, regardless of its intention. This has been shown again and again. Even people like me (I have a profound, bilateral, sensorineural, congenital loss) who have been as successful as any hearing person, regularly experience this unconscious bias. For example, people often forget to face me even though they know I depend on lip reading to communicate.

Likewise, I've been on the London Underground several times when there have been problems; the situation has always been communicated only by loudspeaker, which I cannot understand.

A few other facts should also be highlighted. It is extremely difficult to define who is deaf and who is hard of hearing. Unlike with visual loss, there are no good criteria to separate the two. Moreover, communication is *the* underlying issue with hearing loss, regardless of the severity. Every deaf–blind person I have talked to (and Helen Keller reportedly concurred) has said that being deaf is worse than being blind because deafness cuts them off from people whereas blindness cuts them off from things. And since 90% of d/Deaf persons are born to hearing parents, who clearly desire their children to communicate orally as much as possible, these parents embrace technology to help ensure this. Thus I can see the Deaf community, despite its obvious strengths, growing smaller as cochlear implants, genetic testing, and other interventions become more widespread. Of interest, many Deaf people are no longer against cochlear implants, so long as the decision for it is made by an informed adult.

Finally, but not least, d/Deaf people comprise only 2–3% at best of all D&HH persons. The hard of hearing are the vast majority. These people actually may suffer the most socially because they too have significant communication difficulties, the extent of which is not appreciated by most hearing persons. They are truly a silent majority.

So D&HH persons comprise a complex and diverse group of individuals. Nevertheless, despite focusing on the two extremes of deafness, this chapter is well worth the read. It provides a glimpse into the spectrum of individuals with this disability. Hopefully, the reader will then be more attuned to potential issues the next time they see a deaf patient.

12: Narrative analysis and contested allegations of Munchausen syndrome by proxy

CLIVE BALDWIN

Munchausen syndrome by proxy (MSbP) is said to be a form of abuse in which a carer (usually a mother) feigns, fabricates or induces illness in another (usually a child) in order to seek medical attention. It is a controversial diagnosis that evokes strong reactions. Its proponents hold that it has a respectable history and has saved many children from significant harm, if not death.[1] Its critics point to its internal incoherence and lack of scientific basis and an increasing number of cases of false allegations of abuse.[2,3,4] Given that there can be fundamental disagreement over such apparently simple things as who won a horse race,[5] it is not surprising that incommensurable narratives arise when the stakes are the safety of a child or the protection of family life.

This paper is about just that incommensurability. The research on which it is based was funded by the Economic and Social Research Council (ESRC) and included in-depth interviews with eight mothers who contested the accusations of MSbP and examination of extensive case documentation. These were supplemented by research notes and case documents from four further families and a number of publicly available stories were drawn upon to illustrate points arising from the analysis. Here I will outline how each side in the debate deploys a range of narrative tactics in order to silence, negate or manage the challenge thrown up by the opposing narrative. The range of tactics available to each side and the ability to deploy them are, however, unevenly distributed in favour of those constructing a narrative of abuse.[6] Some of the implications for the conceptualisation and operationalisation of MSbP are then drawn out.

Narrative analysis and the sociology of stories

Narrative analysis

This chapter is based on research that linked two forms of analysis: narrative analysis as outlined by Polkinghorne[7,8] and Barone[9] and Plummer's sociology of stories.[10]

Narrative analysis (as distinct from the analysis of narratives) proceeds from the basis that narratives constitute the social reality of the narrator, life and narrative being inseparable and narrative not only shaping experience but also becoming experience.[11–15] The focus here is the dynamics of narration and the process of production,[16] treating narratives as facts in themselves, rather than for the facts they might contain. By bringing disparate elements together into a coherent story the aim of the analysis is to capture the lived experience of others.[8] Such analysis attempts to provide an internally coherent narrative[5,17] that expresses the narrative truth of lived experience.[15,18] In so doing, because it is the narrative itself that brings facts into being and binds them together in a persuasive whole, competing narratives that express different social realities cannot be evaluated using "simple-minded 'triangulation'... [which] fails to do justice to the embedded, situated nature of accounts".[19]

The sociology of stories

One way of analysing the interaction between competing narratives is Plummer's "sociology of stories",[10] which consists of five elements.

The nature of stories addresses the issue of whether a particular narrative seeks to empower and facilitate or to degrade, control or dominate another. Some stories, such as those found in the reports of experts, tend to pathologise the voices of the mothers. These stories are told both from above and within a world view and investigative framework that advantages their telling and they are thus given priority and more credibility. This in turn helps to marginalise or exclude the mothers' talk from "below".

The making of stories deals with the strategies that are employed in order to tell one's own narrative and to silence others: "Does a coaxer, for example, facilitate stories (enabling new stories to be heard) or entrap stories, into a wider story of his or her own?"[10] In cases of MSbP the mother's story is usually solicited by a variety of professionals, each with their own approach, and is thus subsumed into a wider story of child protection which forms the basis on which the mother's narrative of innocence will be judged.

The consuming of stories involves issues of who has access to particular narratives, whether such stories are widely available or restricted to narrow groups and whether access to stories is extended or curtailed. In this "a significant factor affecting the plausibility of a newly-communicated story is the degree to which it fits a narrative which already exists within this stock of social knowledge".[20] It is difficult, in other words, to gain support for a story that does not relate to an existing stock of stories or, perhaps, that does not have an existing stock of stories to draw upon. For the narrative of abuse the MSbP literature provides a large stock of stories.[21] For the narrative of innocence there are far fewer stories in the literature to draw upon[22] and the development of a stock of such narratives is constrained by the secrecy of the courts that prevents these stories entering the public arena.

The strategies of storytelling examine the ways in which narrators employ certain devices in order to open up their own story and close down the competition. O'Barr[23] has shown that in the courtroom narrative testimony is deemed more persuasive than fragmented testimony, while cross-examination is the opportunity for advocates to fragment the telling of a narrative.[20] In cases of suspected MSbP the mother is subjected to a number of assessments by different professionals (each with their own intent and orders of evidence), which fragment her narrative by setting different agendas and taking the narrative initiative. In contrast there is little opportunity for the mother or her legal team to fragment the narrative of abuse prior to cross-examination in court.

Finally, stories in the wider world: "Some voices – who claim to dominate, who top the hierarchy, who claim the centre, who possess resources – are not only heard much more readily than others, but are also capable of framing the questions, setting the agendas, establishing the rhetorics much more readily than the others".[10] The wider world in which narratives of abuse and innocence are told is one of child protection and criminality. The investigative process is built upon accepted bodies of professional knowledge against which competing narratives are evaluated. The framing of the investigative process, however, is not neutral but provides an advantage to narratives that are familiar, have a common stock of stories to draw upon, are told by approved narrators, and have the wider range of narrative resources.

A note on incommensurability

Where two narratives told about the same event cannot both be believed they can be said to be incommensurable. Incommensurability is accepted in the literature of the sociology and anthropology of medicine (see, for example, Good,[24] Tsouyopoulos,[25] Montgomery Hunter,[26] Veatch[27]). Narratives, by their very nature, call forth the possibility of other, competing narratives. In social work: "Throughout the story there are alternative versions lurking in the background which threaten to disrupt the balance of blame and responsibility. One alternative version lies in the mother's own account of what has happened. For any of the episodes which the social worker reports there is the possibility to construct an alternative mother's version".[28]

Narrative 1

It all started shortly after I made a complaint against the hospital. My daughter had been ill for years but the doctors couldn't find what was causing it. Sometimes she'd be terrible at home but by the time the doctor came out or by the time someone saw her in the hospital she was OK. And each time the tests came back negative. I reckoned she was allergic to all sorts of things and read up about it but they didn't take me seriously. Chloe just got worse and worse and so I made my own arrangements to see a specialist in the hope that she might be able to do something. She was great. She got Chloe tested and it turned out that she was allergic.

And then I thought about all the times I'd been to the other hospital and how they had failed to find out what was wrong. They'd given her all sort of tests and unnecessary drugs that she'd reacted to and basically I thought they'd mismanaged the whole affair so I put in a complaint.

A few weeks later I got a letter from the child protective services saying that they had concerns for my daughter's safety. It appears that on reviewing Chloe's records – records by the way that can't now be found – the doctor at the hospital thinks I was making everything up and thus harming her. Munchausen's by proxy they call it. A bunch of bollocks I call it. I read up on it, as you would, and you wouldn't believe the nonsense – I mean it can hardly be called a reliable diagnosis and that's being generous.

There was a case conference at which a so-called expert I'd never seen and who had never seen Chloe reckoned that there were all the signs of child abuse. Everyone went along with him, even though he was already in trouble because of other cases he's been involved with. You'd think he was God Almighty. Chloe was taken into foster care.

And then things got worse. Everything I did or said was taken as being Munchausen's. I was too cooperative or uncooperative, every mistake I made was taken as being a deliberate lie, they even went into my sex life saying that I had a history of conflict in my relationships. They didn't seem to care that my ex used to beat up on me, as far as they were concerned I was the problem. At the same time they weren't interested in even looking at the fact that the social worker had made up things in her report or that the original allegation came in response to my complaint.

Anyway I started finding things out on the Internet and there's loads of families that have been torn apart by this. I contacted the local press 'cos I was desperate no one was listening. They wanted to run the story but before they could the authorities got a restraining order or an injunction or something that meant they couldn't do it and telling me that if I talked to the press again they'd do me for contempt of court.

And then I was told that talking to the press was further evidence of my "attention-seeking behaviour". You just can't win.

It was really difficult to argue against them because I wasn't allowed to see a lot of the documents – confidentiality they said, protecting their backs I say. In the end my lawyer got them and there were all sorts of things wrong in the medical records and pages missing. Fortunately my lawyer got an expert in allergies to stand up and say that he thought Chloe's care at the first hospital was dodgy and that I wasn't to blame. I think that's what did it but I was so lucky 'cos usually they stick together. Chloe came home after that but I'm dead scared that that expert won't let go, it's happened before, you know, and they come back and try again.

Narrative 2

She was forever taking Chloe to hospital. If it wasn't one thing it was another but mainly because she claimed that Chloe was allergic to anything and everything. Chloe had all sorts of tests but these all came back negative and quite often what the mother said about Chloe didn't really square with what the doctor saw. At first she was very, and I mean very, cooperative with the doctors; they couldn't do anything wrong. But after a while she'd fall out with them and go to a different one. This happened a few times.

Anyway, one of the doctors at the first hospital notified the child protective services because he suspected that this might be a case of Munchausen's syndrome by proxy. There were a number of signs there and we had to investigate just in case. I mean, at this stage, it could have gone either way but as we found out more, it emerged that she must have been doing something to Chloe or at least making things up, there's no other proper explanation for it.

Anyway we started to investigate and it was like pulling teeth. She was so uncooperative and started playing us off against each other. Really manipulative like.

We asked an expert to look at the records, I mean a top notch expert, and he went through them with a fine tooth comb. The bottom line was that there were so many discrepancies in the medical records where she'd told one doctor one thing and another another and these had resulted in Chloe being treated for all sorts of things that she simply didn't have. And the number of presentations! I mean there wasn't a week went by without some attendance at the doctor's.

We had a case conference and it was perfectly clear that Chloe was at risk. Everybody agreed. And so we took her into foster care. The mother went ballistic accusing us of all sorts, of making things up, of lying to her, hiding records, everything under the sun. She made more official complaints than I care to remember but they were all unfounded. She then went to the press and on the Internet. She was just out of control so we had to do something. We tried talking to her but it just went on so eventually we had to get an injunction against her. It also turns out that all this sort of behaviour is suggestive of MSbP anyway.

The case went to court where her legal team first tried to argue that MSbP isn't a recognised diagnosis. It was touch and go but eventually the judge said he'd hear the arguments. The mother and her legal team had done this long statement going through all the medical records pointing out what happened when in mind-boggling detail. Our legal team thought this was a typical ploy trying to confuse the matter and they focused on the pattern. That's what's important in these cases, the pattern. Then the mother produced an expert who said that he reckoned that the first hospital had mismanaged the affair. I don't know where they dug him up from but we were gobsmacked that the judge took him seriously enough to order the return of Chloe. Our expert had said that there's a lot of disbelief that mothers can do these sort of things but I thought that the judge would have been better informed.

Anyway, Chloe went back to her mum but we're keeping an eye on her. The doctors round here know of her now so if anything untoward happens we'll be informed immediately. I guess that's the best we can do.

When narratives are in competition, Plummer[10] identifies three possible responses. First a fundamentalism which adheres to the truth of one story, thus denying the legitimacy of the voice of the other; second, a communitarianism in which differing stories co-exist, without assuming moral superiority, provided they are told within a common framework; and third, a constraint and limiting of differing stories in which it is tacitly agreed not to speak of such things.

In cases of MSbP, the latter two strategies are inadmissible. Social work, especially child protection, is a moral activity[28] and requires an evaluation of the moral superiority of one narrative over another: either the child is at risk (whether or not that risk is manageable) or not. It is simply not possible to allow a narrative of innocence to co-exist on equal terms with a narrative of abuse or to enter into a silent agreement not to speak of such things; a decision has to be made one way or the other. In cases of alleged MSbP, one narrative is of an abusive mother presenting her child for unnecessary medical intervention, the other of a sick child for whose illness the doctors have not been able to find the explanation or a cure (see example narratives). These narratives cannot be reduced one to the other and the question thus becomes how the respective narrators attempt to manage this incommensurability to their own advantage.

Narrative analysis and the sociology of stories provide ways of addressing this problem in that they allow for an examination of how the persuasive power of a particular narrative "does not lie so much in its truth but in an ability to counter the accounts and ploys of the opponent".[29]

Narrative tactics and the pursuit of privilege

How then do the respective narrators attempt to silence, manage or negate the challenge thrown up by the opposing narrative? The first part of this section will examine those tactics, identified in the emerging narratives of abuse, used by professionals in the pursuit of privilege; the second examines those tactics used by mothers attempting to present their narratives of innocence.

Narrative tactics in allegations of MSbP

Within the narratives of abuse a number of tactics can be identified whereby it was attempted to silence, negate and/or manage the mother's rival narrative of innocence. These narrative tactics included silencing and narrative constraint, recuperation, asymmetry, and character work.

Silencing and narrative constraint

The mothers' accounts were silenced in a number of ways, most commonly through injunctions and forced undertakings that prevented them from talking to the media or other people. These injunctions and forced undertakings were based on the professional interpretation of the child's best interests but they silenced the mothers' narratives, thus allowing the professionals' narratives to prevail. Such tactics, Morgan argues, serve the interests of the professionals more than the interests of the child.[30]

This form of silencing has two consequences for the mother's narrative of innocence. First, the audience for the mother's story is limited to those involved in the case and thus development of a publicly accessible stock of stories of innocence and wrongful allegations is effectively prevented. Second, the mother is limited to telling her story within the alien framework set by the child abuse investigation, which also limits what she can say and who listens. As Plummer[10] says: "Telling a story face to face around a log fire is very different from telling a story through a pulp-paperback book, telling a story to a therapy group that engulfs you in its twelve-step programme, or to telling your story in full frontal glare on *Kilroy* or *Oprah.*"

A further form of silencing or hindering the development of a narrative of innocence is to exclude any reference to the alternative narrative. In virtually all the expert reports seen during this research there is little, if any, mention of the controversy and empirical and conceptual problems surrounding the diagnosis of MSbP. The assumption is that the concept is both valid and generally accepted. This frame is very important because by controlling how a narrative can be told it is possible to hinder, fragment or marginalise an alternative narrative,[10] thus making it less persuasive.[23]

Recuperation

Recuperation is the process whereby one narrative interprets aspects of the other narrative as indicative of its own validity, that is, interpreting the person's story as indicative of pathology.[31] For example, a narrative that is not clear and polished might be labelled as evidence of "confusion". Four points of recuperation were identified in the narratives in this study.

First, some of the mothers in the study chose to tell their story to the media because they felt that they were not being listened to by those undertaking the investigation. Such actions were recuperated into the narrative of abuse as further examples of attention-seeking and thus indicative of MSbP.

Second, a number of mothers sought second opinions after what they perceived as the failure of the doctors to accurately diagnose and treat their child's illness. While seeking a second opinion might be viewed as a wise decision,[32] such action on the part of an accused mother might be described as pathology. For example, one mother who sought out different psychological and psychiatric experts was accused of subjecting her son to a variety of differing therapeutic regimes, so creating and maintaining his psychological problems.

Third, while networking and group support can be seen as a normal part of dealing with a personal crisis such behaviour on the part of mothers who have been accused of MSbP has been interpreted as further evidence of pathology[33] and thus recuperated into the professional narrative of abuse.

Fourth, some mothers chose to fight their battle for their children within the court system, a choice that was recuperated into the narrative of abuse. By opposing the medical narrative and seeking legal redress, those accused were described as acting in ways that simply corroborated the allegations. Having been caught and thus no longer able to avail themselves of medical attention, they turn to litigation.[34,35,36] In suing the hospital or the individual doctor, the individual is seeking attention and thus displaying MSbP behaviour.

In some cases even the act of appealing court decisions (usually accepted as a person's legal entitlement) was interpreted as indicative of MSbP abuse. From the mother's point of view, however, the only way to have her children returned and to maintain her integrity (that is, be able to identify with being a good mother) was to clear her name through the proper or available channels.

Finally, even the attempt by mothers to defend themselves against the accusations has been recuperated as indicative of MSbP behaviour. For example, one MSbP expert dismissed the mother's detailed examination of the medical records, which challenged his interpretation, as "typical of an MSbP mother" without dealing with any of the disputed facts or interpretations contained within her defence statement.

Asymmetry

In the cases in this study there was a marked asymmetry between how professionals viewed the narratives of the mothers and the narratives of other professionals. Usually, the mother's narrative was viewed with suspicion and the narratives of other professionals accepted uncritically. For example, in one case, the social worker reported that the mother falsely claimed there had been a house fire (another indicator of MSbP behaviour[33]). Even though the social worker reported this as fourth hand information, without checking the story with the mother, any family member or indeed the relevant fire department, other professionals accepted her report as factual.

On the other hand, when mothers made allegations about professionals (for example, allegations of perjury, abuse of their children while in foster care, and the selective disclosure of documentation) these were either ignored or dismissed without investigation.

Similarly, where there were discrepancies between the mother's account and medical records, or within the medical records, the medical records were accepted as objective fact and mistakes and discrepancies were explained in terms of the mother's deceitfulness rather than arising from contextual features of time and place and how the narrative was solicited and told.[37] Furthermore, the focus on errors and discrepancies in the medical records as evidence of MSbP behaviour ignores the lack of baseline research on the frequency of errors in medical records generally and research that indicates that errors are part and parcel of everyday medical practice.[38,39,40] This unreflexive, asymmetrical approach avoids the difficult questions that can be asked of the narrative of abuse by placing responsibility for errors firmly with the mother.

Asymmetry in evaluating evidence claims disadvantages the mother's narrative by framing the questions that will be asked and of whom. In general terms it is only the mother's narrative that is to be automatically viewed as suspect and it has been shown that in cases of false allegations of sexual abuse this assumption of guilt can result in perpetuating mistakes.[41]

Character work

Character work involves the uncovering of a person's moral essence.[42] While Strong views character work as being rarely used in the cases in his research, it appears as a regular feature of MSbP abuse and, indeed, is written into its very conceptualisation. Schreier and Libow "believe that the mother's relationship with her pediatrician is paramount in the development and continuance of what is a process of mother imposturing ... in which lying is the essential mode of interaction and represents a particular form of 'character perversion' ...".[34] In this view, the mother is highly dangerous because, contrary to her appearance as a loving mother, who cooperates, the "reality" is that she is attempting to deceive the doctors using the child as the means to accomplish this end. All the mothers interviewed could recount stories, found in the case documentation, of how their character was called into question (ranging from their sexual activity to their diet).

A recent case before the European Court of Human Rights (ECtHR) – *P, C & S* v *the United Kingdom* – clearly illustrates the use of character work in an attempt to discredit the parents' narrative. During the hearing the UK Government made various claims about the behaviour of both parents during the original care proceedings. These included, amongst others, a lack of cooperation with the authorities, a complete denial of the concerns of the local authority, restraining orders being issued against the mother and the father impersonating a therapist. The parents' legal team challenged these allegations and neither the Government nor the representative of Rochdale Social Services could provide evidence in support of their claims. In addition, the Government re-iterated claims that the mother had attempted to harm the child, despite the fact that the domestic courts had already ruled "there was nothing to be said against this mother in relation to anything that she had done or in relation to her approach to child care in her interaction through contact with S".[43] These attempts to negate the parents' narrative through character work were rejected by the ECtHR who ruled that the "draconian step of removing S from her mother shortly after birth was not supported by relevant and sufficient reasons and that it cannot be regarded as having been necessary in a democratic society for the purpose of safeguarding S".[44]

The denial of due process

P, C & S v *the United Kingdom* also illustrates how the mother's narrative was hindered by the failure of due process. In this case the mother was forced to act without legal representation throughout the final hearing because Justice Wall refused her request for a short adjournment to seek legal counsel after her original team withdrew without notice. In his judgment Justice Wall provided a lengthy self-justification and attempted to silence the mother from challenging his actions by refusing her leave to appeal. Nevertheless the mother, again without legal representation, applied to the Courts for permission to appeal. This was refused with the Appeal Court Justices, Thorpe and Roch, ruling that Justice Wall "was throughout meticulous in ensuring fairness, and scrupulously careful to consider any points that went to the advantage of the mother".[43] The ECtHR, however, did not agree and ruled that the domestic court had seriously disadvantaged the parents and violated the right to a fair hearing (Article 6 of the Human Rights Act) a violation that might have had an effect on the outcome for the family as a whole.[44]

Countering the narrative of abuse

Narratives of innocence are by their very nature reactive narratives. By the time the mother is confronted with the allegations of abuse, there have usually been numerous meetings and consultations between professionals at which the narrative of abuse has been worked up into a reasonably firm persuasive hypothesis. The mother is thus faced with having to counter both the allegations of abuse and the trajectory already established by that narrative of abuse.[6] In attempting to counter the allegations, mothers in the research deployed tactics of silencing, the redistribution of responsibility, character work and the failure of due process.

Silencing

In the US there have been successful attempts to silence the professional narrative of abuse by arguing that evidence regarding MSbP fails the test for the reliability of evidence – the Daubert analysis (see Box).

Daubert v Merrill Dow Pharmaceuticals Inc., 509 US 579, 597 (1993)

The petitioners alleged that the children's serious birth defects had been caused by the mothers' prenatal ingestion of a prescription drug marketed by Merrill Dow Pharmaceuticals. The District Court found in favour of the respondent based on an expert's affidavit that concluded that a mother's use of the drug had not been shown to be a risk factor for human birth defects. The petitioners' argument was supported by eight other experts, who based their conclusion that the drug can cause birth defects on animal studies,

(Continued)

(Continued)

chemical structure analyses, and the unpublished reanalysis of previously published human statistical studies. The court, however, determined that this evidence did not meet the applicable "general acceptance" standard for the admission of expert testimony. The Court of Appeals upheld the District Court's decision and the Federal Rules of Evidence that provide the standard for admitting expert scientific testimony in a federal trial.

Under these rules the trial judge must make a preliminary assessment of whether the testimony's underlying reasoning or methodology is scientifically valid and can be properly applied to the facts at issue. Many considerations will bear on the inquiry, including whether the theory or technique in question can be (and has been) tested, whether it has been subjected to peer review and publication, its known or potential error rate, and the existence and maintenance of standards controlling its operation, and whether it has attracted widespread acceptance within a relevant scientific community.

Adapted from: Legal Information Institute, http://supct.law.cornell.edu:8080/supct/html/92–102.ZS.html (Accessed 8 July 2003)

It has been successfully argued that evidence regarding MSbP fails the test for the reliability of evidence because:

(a) in view of serious disputes about whether MSbP is even properly categorised as a syndrome[45] and about the supposed characteristics of MSbP,[46] it likely cannot be tested;

(b) rather than establishing the reliability of the diagnosis, publications about the syndrome demonstrate that controversy surrounds the diagnosis and MSbP theory generally and peer review of MSbP theory has found it to be unreliable and problematic;

(c) the potential rate of error in MSbP theory is unknown and that diagnoses of MSbP have led to false accusations;

(d) the current literature on MSbP, for example, Morley[47] and Donald and Jureidini,[46] fails to reveal any standards or controls for diagnosing MSbP, or even for establishing that such a syndrome actually exists;

(e) MSbP is a controversial diagnosis and there is significant debate about whether MSbP is a paediatric or psychiatric diagnosis; thus, it cannot be said to be "generally accepted" within a relevant community.

So serious is this challenge to the admissibility and credibility of MSbP that a number of authors have published advice to prosecution lawyers on how to present MSbP evidence in court and how to respond to the defence case.[33,48]

The redistribution of responsibility

In the narrative of abuse the responsibility for the alleged harm to the child is clearly laid at the mother's door. Successful responses have been to redistribute that responsibility, arguing that children have been iatrogenically harmed and the child's illness was poorly managed by the doctors.

Second, accusations of MSbP do not always focus on individual events but on the pattern of their presentation. One method of countering this argument is to analyse the type of and reason for presentation: in other words to redistribute the responsibility for the presentation and thus counter the alleged pattern. For example, while there may be a pattern of frequent presentation this may be as a result of regular, scheduled appointments, appointments initiated by the doctors, referrals, appointments deemed to be necessary and those deemed to be unnecessary, appointments where the child has been presented by another person in the absence of the mother or appointments made because the mother was over-anxious or uneducated. It must be noted, however, that such an attempt at redistributing responsibility can be recuperated into the narrative of abuse as being "typical of a Munchausen mother".

Sometimes the mother is charged with having an unusual degree of medical knowledge and this is taken as one factor in the profile of the MSbP perpetrator. However, at least one mother in the research had learnt about her child's illness at the prompting of the health professionals rather than it being indicative of anything suspicious (even assuming that a lay person having medical knowledge is something to be suspicious about).

Character work

In response to the attacks on their moral character as presented in the narrative of abuse, a number of mothers have attempted to engage in their own character work. For example, one mother claimed that the expert was not above exploiting his position for pecuniary gain and by fabricating additional dramatic evidence to sustain his diagnosis of the mother was titillating his audiences with an exciting case study.

This course, however, is difficult to pursue due to the established view that professionals are generally seen as beneficent and benign[49] and the official stance is that expert witnesses should be "treated with courtesy and respect by judges" and "cross examination which is hostile, discourteous, or personal is simply not admitted".[50] This is, of course, in direct contrast to how the courts allow the mother to be treated.

The failure of due process

Several of the mothers in the research attempted to cast doubt on the narrative of abuse by arguing that they had been hindered in telling their story through a number of "dirty tricks": the loss of medical records and notes by the professionals involved thus making it impossible to challenge their interpretations and allegations, the alteration of records and documents, the lack of and delays in disclosure and the deliberate withholding of medical reports thus preventing the mother and her legal team from having time to examine them. The implication is that the expert's narrative of abuse would not have withstood due process and it is open to question why such activities should be deemed necessary if the narrative of abuse is thought robust enough to withstand cross-examination in the courts.

Concluding remarks

The application of narrative analysis and the sociology of stories to the study of cases of MSbP raises issues that have not yet been adequately addressed in the literature. In this final section I want to outline the challenges raised by such an analysis.

The first challenge posed by narrative analysis is to the abstractions of both the perpetrator profile and patterning of presentations. The deep contextualisation, fluidity, and ambiguity of narratives, embedded as they are in the flux of everyday life, challenge the neatness of the concept. Proper risk assessment necessarily involves an understanding and evaluation of the situation, including its context, history, and potential future and needs to explore the alternative, non-suspicious, and credible explanations for events and behaviours available in the mother's narrative. In this, narrative analysis can provide an in-depth and engaged understanding and identify the narrative tactics used by each side, pointing to areas in which narrative techniques may have supplanted forensic examination. Such detailed sociological analysis, although time consuming and perhaps unfamiliar may serve to protect both children from abuse and professionals from making diagnostic mistakes.

Secondly, the nature of narratives challenges the approach that privileges one narrative over another from the outset as this is prejudicial to the least powerful narrator. Indeed, it has been agued that the first task when things go wrong is to attempt to see the point of the other's story and to grasp the other's vision; a task that lies more heavily on the professional because of the vulnerability of the other.[51] It is incumbent upon those charged with child protection investigations to ensure that the process of narrative construction and evaluation is as even-handed as possible.

Such an approach challenges the a priori pathologisation of the mother and her narrative and the asymmetry of approach between the professional and lay narrative. It challenges the pathologisation in the sense that the construct of the mother as pathological is an outcome of accepting the professional narrative of MSbP rather than a basis for that narrative (see Latour[52] for this discussion applied to scientific debates) and thus puts the cart before the horse. It challenges the asymmetry of approach because competing narratives can be equally true in Spence's sense[15] – that is, contain both historical and narrative truth.

While this poses a challenge to professional knowledge and practice that is outside the scope of this chapter, a more disinterested examination of the competing narratives may help both professionals and the courts in their evaluation of the case and provide a basis for more confidence in the outcome.

Thirdly, the science of MSbP is called into question. Narrative truth and historical truth interact in complex and dynamic ways. MSbP does not exist outside of the persuasive hypothesis that calls it into existence. Professional narratives are a mixture of history and narrative and if professional narrators of abuse wish to use a claim to objective evidence as a basis for the persuasiveness of their narrative then two things become necessary. First, there is a need to reject the tactics of narrative privilege that cannot be linked directly to substantiating evidence, that is, silencing and narrative constraint, recuperation, asymmetry of evidence, and character work. Neither can they rely on narrative techniques to bolster weaknesses in their forensic analysis. Second, there is a need to provide baseline research which, in their own terms, supports their claims – for example, what is the level of discrepancies in the medical records of the population generally; what is the occurrence of features of the perpetrator profile in the population generally; what is the exact pattern of presentations when different types of presentations are analysed.

Fourthly, there is a need for increased reflexivity. Narratives are both dynamic and interactive. They are constructed in contexts and relationships. They are individually, co- and collectively constructed. As such they can be seen as a dance with one or more partners. In cases of alleged MSbP abuse the stakes are so high that it is incumbent upon the professional narrators of abuse to be reflexive as to their part in creating the situation rather than simply pathologising the mother. While there is some literature on how a lack of reflexivity on the part of medical professionals may contribute to further harm being inflicted upon the child,[53] there is nothing, at present, on how this same lack of reflexivity may contribute to false allegations of MSbP abuse. Such reflexivity would give more credence to the remaining narrative of abuse and credibility and respect to the narrators.

Finally, there needs to be an appreciation of the interaction of the narratives of the medical world and those of the lifeworld. The medical encounter is one of narrative translation[25] and as such is open to mis-hearings and misunderstandings. Patients do not present their symptoms in a clinical manner, present only those symptoms they think important, can respond to the same question differently depending upon their relationship with the questioner and so on. This translation process is fraught with difficulty and can be used, if uncritically accepted as neutral and benign, against the mother in allegations of MSbP. A thorough understanding of narrative allows one to notice that "a powerful clique can grasp the narrative podium and privilege its way of telling the story"[54] and thus take steps to balance the narrative scales.

All of this, I am very aware, makes life more difficult for medical practitioners and other professionals in cases of suspected MSbP abuse. However, the stakes are high and such work can reduce both the chances of "getting it wrong" and the level of ambiguity and uncertainty experienced by professionals in making such a diagnosis.

References

1 Wilson RG. Fabricated or induced illness in children: Munchausen by proxy comes of age. *BMJ* 2001;**323**:296–7.

2 Allison DB, Roberts MS. *Disordered mother or disordered diagnosis?: Munchausen by proxy syndrome.* Hillsdale, NJ: Analytic Press, 1998.

3 Mart EG. *Munchausen's syndrome by proxy reconsidered.* Manchester, NH: Bally Vaughan Publishing, 2002.

4 Earl Howe, House of Lords official report (Hansard) 2003 5 February: col 316. http://www.parliament.the-stationery-office.co.uk/pa/ld199900/ldhansrd (accessed 10 Mar 2003).

5 Riessman CK. *Narrative analysis.* Newbury Park, CA: Sage, 1993.

6 Baldwin C. Munchausen syndrome by proxy: Telling tales of illness. Unpublished PhD thesis, University of Sheffield, 2000.

7 Polkinghorne DE. *Narrative knowing and the human sciences.* Albany, NY: State University of New York, 1988.

8 Polkinghorne DE. Narrative configuration in qualitative analysis. In: Hatch JA, Wisniewski R, eds. *Life history and narrative.* London: The Falmer Press, 1995.

9 Barone T. Persuasive writings, vigilant readings, and reconstructed characters: the paradox of trust in educational storysharing. In: Hatch JA, Wisniewski R, eds. *Life history and narrative.* London: The Falmer Press, 1995.

10 Plummer K. *Telling sexual stories: power, change and social worlds.* London: Routledge, 1995.

11 Bruner J. Life as narrative. *Social Res* 1987;**54**:11–32.

12 Bruner J. *Acts of meaning.* Cambridge, MA: Harvard University Press, 1990.

13 Bruner J. The narrative construction of reality. *Critical Inquiry* 1991;**18**:1–21.

14 Frank AW. *The wounded storyteller. Body, illness and ethics.* Chicago: University of Chicago Press, 1995.

15 Spence DP. *Narrative truth and historical truth: Meaning and interpretation in psychoanalysis.* New York: WW Norton, 1982.

16 Booth T, Booth W. *Parenting under pressure: mothers and fathers with learning difficulties.* Buckingham: Open University Press, 1994.

17 Bennett WL, Feldman MS. *Reconstructing reality in the courtroom.* London: Tavistock Publications, 1981.

18 Blumenfeld-Jones D. Fidelity as a criterion for practicing and evaluating narrative inquiry. In: Hatch JA, Wisniewski R, eds. *Life history and narrative.* London: The Falmer Press, 1995.

19 Silverman, D. *Interpreting qualitative data: methods for analysing talk, text and interaction.* London: Sage, 1993.

20 Jackson BS. *Law, fact and narrative coherence*. Roby: Deborah Charles Publications, 1988.

21 Feldman MD, Brown RM. Munchausen by proxy in an international context. *Child Abuse Negl* 2002;**26**:509–24.

22 Feldman M, Rand D. Misdiagnosis of Munchausen Syndrome by proxy: a literature review and four new cases. *Harv Rev Psychiatry* 1999;**7**:94–101.

23 O'Barr, WM. *Linguistic evidence*. New York: Academic Press, 1982.

24 Good BJ. *Medicine, rationality and experience: an anthropological perspective*. Cambridge: Cambridge University Press, 1994.

25 Tsouyopoulos N. Postmodernist theory and the physician–patient relationship. *Theor Med* 1994;**15**:267–75.

26 Montgomery Hunter KM. *Doctors' stories: the narrative structure of medical knowledge*. Princeton, NJ: Princeton University Press, 1991.

27 Veatch RM, Stempsey WE. Incommensurability: its implications for the patient/physician relationship. *J Med Philos* 1995;**20**:253–69.

28 Hall C, Sarangi S, Slembrouck S. Moral construction in social work discourse. In: Gunnarsson B-L, Linell P, Nordberg B, eds. *The construction of professional discourse*. London: Longman, 1997.

29 Thomas J. Prisoner cases as narratives. In: Papke DR, ed. *Narrative and the legal discourse*. Liverpool: Deborah Charles Publications, 1991.

30 Morgan B. Munchausen syndrome by proxy: A study in secrecy. *Child Exploitation and the Media* 1997;**July**:91–5.

31 Hyden L-C. Illness and narrative. *Sociol Health Illness* 1997;**19**:48–69.

32 Meadow R. What is, and what is not "Munchausen syndrome by proxy"? *Arch Dis Child* 1995;**72**:534–8.

33 Artingstall K. *Practical aspects of Munchausen by proxy and Munchausen syndrome investigation*. Boca Raton, FL: CRC Press, 1998.

34 Schreier HA, Libow JA. *Hurting for love: Munchausen by proxy syndrome*. New York: Guilford Press, 1993.

35 Levin AV, Sheridan MS, eds. *Munchausen syndrome by proxy: issues in diagnosis and treatment*. New York: Lexington Books, 1995.

36 Parnell TF, Day DO, eds. *Munchausen by proxy syndrome: misunderstood child abuse*. Thousand Oaks, CA: Sage, 1997.

37 Morley C. Experts differ over diagnosis criteria for Munchausen syndrome by proxy (Letter). *Br J Hosp Med* 1992;**48**:197.

38 Kaushal R, Bates DW, Landrigan C, McKenna KJ, Clapp MD, Federico F *et al.* Medication errors and adverse drug events in pediatric inpatients. *JAMA* 2001;**285**:2114–120.

39 Kozer E, Scolnik D, Macpherson A, Keays T, Tshi K, Luk T *et al.* Variables associated with medication errors in pediatric emergency medicine. *Pediatrics* 2002;**110**: 737–42.

40 Goldmann D, Kaushal R. Time to tackle the tough issues in patient safety. *Pediatrics* 2002;**110**:823–6.

41 Pillai M. Allegations of abuse: the need for responsible practice. *Med Sci Law* 2002;**42**:149–60.

42 Strong PM. *The ceremonial order of the clinic: parents, doctors and medical bureaucracies*. London: Routledge and Kegan Paul, 1979.

43 RE: B (Children) [1999] EWCA Civ 1772 (5th July, 1999) http://www2.bailii.org/cgi-bin/markup.cgi?doc=/ew/cases/EWCA/Civ/1999. (accessed 11 March 2003).

44 P, C and S v *The United Kingdom* [2002] Appl. no. 56547/00, Judgment 16/07/02 Strasbourg. http://hudoc.echr.coe.int/hudoc/ (accessed 10 March 2003)

45 Fisher G, Mitchell I. Is Munchausen syndrome by proxy really a syndrome? *Arch Dis Child* 1995;**72**:530–4.

46 Donald T, Jureidini J. Munchausen syndrome by proxy: child abuse in the medical system. *Arch Pediatr Adolesc Med* 1996;**150**:753–8.

47 Morley CJ. Practical concerns about the diagnosis of Munchausen syndrome by proxy. *Arch Dis Child* 1995;**72**:528–9.

48 Goldman LH, Yorker BC. Mommie Dearest? Prosecuting Cases of Munchausen Syndrome by Proxy. *Criminal Justice* 1999;**13**:26–33.

49 Ingleby D. Professionals as socializers: The "psy complex". *Research in law, deviance and social control*, 7. London: JAI Press, 1985.

50 Wall N. Judicial attitudes to expert evidence in children's cases. *Arch Dis Child* 1997;**76**:185–9.
51 Frank AW. "How can they act like that?": Clinicians and patients as characters in each other's stories. *Hastings Center Report* 2002;**32**:14–22.
52 Latour B. *Science in action: how to follow scientists and engineers through society.* Cambridge, MA: Harvard University Press, 1987.
53 Jureidini JN, Shafer AT, Donald TG. "Munchausen by proxy syndrome": not only pathological parenting but also problematic doctoring? *Med J Aust* 2003;**178**:130–2.
54 Brody H. Narrative ethics and institutional impact. In: Charon R, Montello M, eds. *Stories matter: the role of narrative in medical ethics.* New York: Routledge, 2002.

13: Confounding the experts: the vindication of parental testimony in shaken baby syndrome

JAMES LE FANU

Shaken baby syndrome (SBS) invokes a powerful and persuasive image of child abuse where a parent violently shaking their child by the shoulders causes a rapid to-and-fro movement of the head generating shearing forces that tear the veins in the subdural space – the space between the lining of the brain and the brain itself – and the veins in the retina. The trauma to the veins causes severe bleeding resulting in the "characteristic" features of SBS: a brain scan shows a blood clot under the surface of the skull (a subdural haematoma or SDH), while visual inspection of the retina through an ophthalmoscope reveals the presence of flare-shaped retinal haemorrhages (RH). For 15 years the presence of SDH and RH in a child with a head injury has been considered virtually cast iron proof of SBS resulting in hundreds of parents (and others involved in the care of small children) being accused and convicted of attempting to murder their children – with predictably serious consequences for all concerned. Then two scientific papers, published in 2001, challenged the clinical and neuropathological basis of SBS with necessarily profound implications for the soundness of those earlier convictions.[1,2]

This chapter seeks to do two things. First it clarifies how doctors in particular (but also the police and social workers) have been able to present so convincing a narrative of SBS as being diagnostic of this particular pattern of head injury as to invalidate parental protestations of their innocence. But secondly it demonstrates how the "denied" pattern of events as described by parents can now be seen to offer a much better explanation than SBS for several patterns of head injury in children. Put another way, the parental description of events would now appear to be more accurate than the experts' interpretation that the child's injuries could only have been brought about by shaking. It is, of course, well recognised that doctors will make diagnostic errors that might have been avoided if they had paid closer attention to the patient's story. But this situation is quite different as it involves a systematic denial of the authenticity of parental testimony in favour of a preconceived series of events that would have had to have occurred to account for the child's injuries.

It would be impossible in a single chapter to expound and explore the full implications of the "unmasking" of SBS over the past two years. I have chosen rather to present several narrative "snapshots" based on discussions and interviews with parents and other interested parties. My initial involvement with SBS followed a request for assistance from a family accused of having shaken their child and this subsequently led into a wider investigation of the issues. Though medically qualified (and a part-time general practitioner), my expertise is as a medical writer and commentator for the *Telegraph* newspapers to which I have contributed a twice-weekly column over the past 12 years.

Finally, it is necessary to recall that the events described below were taking place against the background of increasing concerns about the impartiality, and reliability, of medical expert opinion in other fields – Munchausen syndrome by proxy, "recovered" memories and, most dramatically, the acquittal of Sally Clark, Trupti Patel and Angela Cannings of the charge of having murdered their children. This might suggest we are witnessing a more generalised phenomenon involving the confounding of experts in which narrative research could, by highlighting the significance of parental testimony, play a central role.

We start with "a parental narrative" from October 2000 in which eight-month-old Jack Bennett tumbles off the parental bed resulting in his mother, Sarah, being convicted of attempted child murder in the Family Court nine months later.

A parent's narrative

Sarah and James Bennett live in inner-city London with their two young children. They belong to the cultural/alternative end of the middle class spectrum and are intelligent, witty, and popular people, with many friends. The story begins in the parental bedroom one October evening. Three-year-old Zoe is hanging around while Sarah has just positioned eight-month-old Jack on the bed and turned round to find a book. This is her account of the events that followed:

Suddenly there was this terrific crash. I spun round and there was Jack whimpering on the floor. He screamed, went stiff, then floppy then became semi-conscious. It took about five minutes for the ambulance to arrive and another twenty minutes to reach the hospital ... when the doctors were examining him his legs started twitching as if he were having a fit and soon after they told me his left pupil had begun to dilate and that he needed an urgent scan. [The scan showed a large subdural requiring a three and a half hour operation.] The waiting was terrible. The time seemed to pass so slowly until at one o'clock in the morning we learned that "all had gone well" and Jack would be staying in the intensive care unit.

Sarah and James' distress during their bedside vigil over the next few days was further compounded when Jack's bandaged head rapidly increased in size (for which the neurosurgeon could give no clear explanation), making him appear even more damaged and vulnerable. The only other significant (in retrospect) event was a visit from the ophthalmology senior registrar who, after examining Jack's eyes, added to the anxiety by telling them he had noticed "retinal haemorrhages". He replied to their questions as to whether this would affect his sight with the enigmatic comment "I will have to speak to my superiors to consider the significance of all this". Then, four days after Jack's operation, Sarah and James were summoned to a side room to see the consultant (whom they had not yet met).

We were both alarmed as we thought we were about to hear bad news about Jack's latest scan. The consultant introduced herself, looked briefly through the notes and dropped the bombshell. She told us she had no doubt that Jack's injuries were far too severe to have been caused by simply falling off a bed, rather he must have been "shaken with considerable force for a prolonged period of time". He had, we learned, sustained two separate injuries – a blow to the head, resulting in the subdural followed by the violent shaking that had resulted in the retinal haemorrhages. We were, of course, appalled to think that anybody could have done this to him – and it took a few seconds for me to realise I was the only suspect. The police and social services, we were told, had been informed and had already started their investigations. From that moment we would be kept in the dark about everything. We were never told the result of Jack's investigations or how he was doing. We had to pull every bit of information out of them – it was like getting blood out of a stone.

The next day it was the turn of the social workers who started off by saying the police were very worried about the seriousness of Jack's injuries which required him to have been shaken for at least two minutes. It did not occur to me at the time, but it is actually very difficult to shake anything – let alone an eight-month-old baby boy – for two minutes – you should try it. They told us the only safe option for Jack would be for him to be taken into foster care and had already applied for a court order to be heard on Monday morning. It was by now 6 pm on Friday evening so we had just the weekend to try and find a solicitor.

Come Monday they were able "with great difficulty" to reach the compromise solution where Jack would, after leaving hospital, go to live with a neighbour while Sarah would only be allowed to visit if there was another adult present. This, Sarah believes, was their most important victory because "if we had lost him [into foster care] we would never have got him back."

There followed several gruelling and stressful months during which they were arrested "at home" by the police and endured almost daily meetings with solicitors, social workers, the guardian *ad litem*, and other interested parties. Despite their ordeal they were in a considerably better position than most as at least they "spoke the language" of the professionals they had to deal with and were not overly intimidated by them. They did not, of course, speak the language of technical medical jargon, in which the accusation against Sarah of attempted infanticide was couched and which is the concern of the next section.

The author's narrative: interrogating the diagnosis of SBS

In May 2001, after hearing of the misfortune that had befallen the Bennetts, it was suggested I could perhaps help them make sense of the medical evidence as submitted by the various experts prior to the court hearing due in a couple of months. I readily agreed but confessed to knowing very little about SBS at the time. The combination of my both being in medical practice and writing a twice-weekly medical column requires that I know at least something about most of the important issues in medicine – so my "not knowing" much about SBS was, I subsequently realised, significant in itself, reflecting the lack of controversy about the diagnosis. The perception of the diagnosis as being effectively unchallengeable ("everyone knows that subdural and retinal haemorrhage equal SBS") makes it virtually impossible for parents to mount a defence and though, of course, they have the right to seek an independent opinion, this frequently turns out (given the overwhelming consensus about SBS) to be supportive of the prosecution's case.

My ignorance was also significant for a further reason as it reflected the secrecy that surrounded the family court proceedings – so neither I, nor indeed the parents in similar situations to the Bennetts, were aware that this "sort of thing" was going on the whole time (there are no official figures but the few UK pathologists in this field report there are one or two cases a week which would suggest roughly a hundred a year). Put another way, it would be easier to suspect there was something amiss if it were more generally known that hundreds of apparently respectable parents over the previous few years had similarly been accused by doctors of attempting to murder their children.

Two days spent in the library at the Royal Society of Medicine reading up the medical literature (which is vast, but the reader is referred to Duhaime *et al*[3] for a comprehensive review) confirmed the apparently uniform consensus of the significance of subdural and retinal haemorrhages as being characteristic of SBS.[3] (It would have been useful to have known – which I could not because it would not be published for a further two years – that an "evidence-based" interpretation of the literature 1969–99 would find that consensus to be "unsustainable" because of "serious data gaps, flaws of logic, inconsistency of case definition and a serious lack of tests capable of discriminating Non-Accidental Injury (NAI) cases from natural injuries".[4]) I did, however, unearth three possible leads. First, the consensus on SBS was not quite as unanimous as it appeared. The doyen of British forensic pathologists, Professor Sir Bernard Knight, in a letter to the *British Medical Journal* in 1995 had expressed serious doubts about the validity of the diagnosis. Its precise mechanism of action, he claimed, was "not clearly defined", its potential for serious trauma was "not supported by existing experimental data", and the clinical findings were "not in themselves specific".[5] Second, I discovered that minor accidental incidents were sufficient by themselves to cause a large bleed into the subdural space and hence, as neurosurgeons at Atkinson Morley Hospital pointed out, "NAI is a less common cause of SDH than it is believed to be".[6] Thirdly, while the literature on the biomechanics of retinal haemorrhages was highly technical, clearly there were several other possible causes besides shaking, including a sudden rise in intracranial pressure causing obstruction of the venous return from the retina – which is known as Terson's syndrome.[7] Thus it was possible to see how Sarah's testimony offered a clear alternative aetiology to Jack's injuries – where his trivial fall resulted in a large SDH, while the sudden rise in intracranial pressure caused the retinal haemorrhages, as in Terson's.

It was, however, not obvious where next to turn, when fortuitously a letter in *The Lancet* that same week from a paediatrician, Marvin Miller, from Dayton, Ohio, appeared to confirm this pattern of events: "acute encephalopathy, cerebral oedema and retinal haemorrhages" he wrote, "all *result* from a subdural haematoma".[8] Clearly Dr Miller was fishing in the same waters and a telephone call confirmed he too had been dealing with a case very similar to Jack's. More importantly, though, he drew my attention to a paper published just one month previously from forensic pathologist John Plunkett with its self-explanatory and highly pertinent title "Fatal paediatric head injuries caused by short-distance falls".[1] Plunkett had trawled through 75,000 records of the National Electronic Injury Surveillance System (NEISS) and similar databases in the United States and retrieved 18 independently witnessed head injury fatalities in children from falls of less than 10 feet. "Four of the six children in whom fundoscopic examination was described in the medical records had bilateral retinal haemorrhages," he added. By definition these children had not been shaken so Jack's injuries could have occurred as Sarah had described – the only difference being that, unlike the children in Plunkett's series, he had survived. Now, Plunkett's article had only just been published so the expert witnesses for the prosecution in Sarah's case would be unaware of his findings. Would this persuade them to drop the case against her?

The expert's narrative: the court hearing

The court hearing lasted five days and took place "in camera" as required by law though the written evidence of the experts for the prosecution and defence convey some sense of the arguments deployed:

> While the findings of subdural and retinal haemorrhage in the absence of other signs of trauma is stated by many to be the result of non-accidental injury which is caused by shaking there is published evidence to support the belief that short household falls can result in [the same pattern of injury], usually when the child falls onto a hard surface.

But the experts for the prosecution – particularly Jack's consultant and a neurosurgeon – insisted on SBS as the sole possible explanation:

> The combination of acute subdural and retinal haemorrhages is extremely common in non-accidental shaking-impact syndrome and therefore overwhelmingly on the balance of probabilities, is likely to be the cause of the injuries.

The judge found the consultant to be "an impressive witness" and ruled that "the burden of proof necessary to substantiate the charge that the mother had caused the injuries had been established". She dealt with the small matter that Jack's elder sister Zoe had actually witnessed his fall by suggesting that Sarah had first shaken him in another room "in a moment of frustration" and then placed him on the bed in a position that he would then topple off and thus provide a plausible subsequent explanation for his injuries. The judge ruled that Jack be allowed to return home on condition that another family member moved in lest Sarah seek to harm him again. He also ruled that both parents would have to undergo psychiatric counselling to help them to come to terms with what had happened and provide assistance in overcoming their "denial".

A further parental narrative: the protean faces of SBS or "what's in a syndrome?"

Following Sarah Bennett's conviction, I had come to realise there must be something seriously amiss about the whole concept of SBS. Several doctors echoed Professor Sir Bernard Knight's trenchant criticisms – a neurologist described the lack of objectivity of SBS experts as "beyond belief", while a pathologist remarked he was "amazed" at the uncritical acceptance of "shoddy and unscientific studies". Then there was the experience of other parents, such as television producer Rioch Edwards-Brown, accused of shaking her six-month-old son Riordan and whose narrative revealed two further disquieting aspects about SBS. First, the diagnosis, it seemed, encompassed several different types of clinical presentation and pathological findings suggesting it was not so much a "syndrome" (with the specificity of causation that this implies) but rather a catch-all diagnosis for any "unexplained" head injury in children. Then, her testimony confirmed how these extraordinarily serious allegations were being made without the most elementary attempts to substantiate them with other circumstantial evidence of abuse or to rule out other more innocent explanations. Why should this be? This is her story as recounted during an extended interview:

Riordan was born a month and a half prematurely and at his six weeks check his GP, worried about a history of vomiting and, detecting a mild left-sided weakness, referred him back to the hospital for further investigations. Eventually a CT scan revealed a small intracranial bleed that the consultant told us was related to his prematurity and accounted for his symptoms. A week later, while in my arms, Riordan had what seemed to be an epileptic fit and he was readmitted as an emergency to hospital. The following day we were told the consultant wanted to see us together – and so we were expecting bad news. She told us that she had looked at the scan again and had changed her mind. Riordan had been "picked up by the ankles and hit against a hard surface and shaken". We were told that "as a matter of procedure" the social services had been contacted and meanwhile if we attempted to remove Riordan from the ward the police would be informed. Subsequently we were interviewed by social workers who told us we would have to come up with "a good explanation" for Riordan's injuries, but in the meantime an application had been made to the Courts to place him in foster care. It was 4:30 on a Friday afternoon, the hearing was the following Monday and we had just over an hour to find a solicitor before their offices closed for the weekend.

So far, so familiar.

We were standing in a call box just outside the ward, frantically ringing round to get legal representation when quite unexpectedly we were approached by a sympathetic nurse. Riordan's original notes had gone missing soon after his admission but here was this nurse, carrying them in her hand. She handed them over and drew our attention to the measurements of his head circumference soon after birth.

These showed his head had increased by nearly four centimetres in just ten days – for which the only possible reason, as everyone subsequently agreed, was that birth trauma must have caused the bleeding under the skull (bleeding which the doctors should have been alerted to by the rapidity in growth in head circumference in the immediate neonatal period). The hospital, though not the consultant, belatedly offered a grudging apology, and Ms Edwards-Brown, angered by the false charges against her, formed a support group for parents – which would play a significant role in the final "unmasking" of SBS.

The counter-expert's narrative: the scientific assault on SBS

So far we have noted the diagnosis of SBS has been invoked to account for two very different patterns of clinical events resulting in two different types of neuropathology both of which can be caused by mechanisms other than shaking – Jack's acute subdural with retinal haemorrhages and Riordan's birth trauma related chronic subdural. But there is also a third, whose "deconstruction" in an article "Neuropathology of inflicted head injury in children" by Dr Jennian Geddes published in *Brain* would, with Plunkett's paper on short distance falls, provide the momentum for the scientific assault on SBS.[2] This requires first a brief historical diversion for its significance to be properly appreciated.

The concept of Shaken Baby Syndrome was first proposed in the 1970s to account for a particular type of injury in severely battered babies. They had all the stigmata of fractures, bruises, and cigarette burns and almost invariably suffered bleeding within the brain but sometimes without direct evidence of injury to the skull. Perhaps it was suggested, the perpetrator had violently shaken the child and the to-and-fro agitation of the brain within the skull could have torn the delicate blood vessels on its surface.[9] Shaking could, in a similar way, it is claimed, account for the frequently observed haemorrhages in the back of the eye by tearing the blood vessels to the retina.[10] This explanation was hypothetical as, for obvious reasons, no one had ever directly observed the sort of severe shaking required to cause such injuries. But an American neurosurgeon, Ayub Ommaya, provided some confirmatory evidence in a series of experiments in which monkeys sitting in a truck were catapulted forward along a 20 foot track. Their unsupported heads jerked backwards so forcefully as to cause concussion and, sure enough, at autopsy there were multiple contusions in the substance of the brain and bleeding on its surface.[11] Further biomechanical studies suggested the infant would also have to have been flung against a surface such as a padded mattress to generate the necessary decelerations to account for the full range of pathological findings. Subsequently some authors have advocated using the term "shaking–impact syndrome" to describe what is commonly known as SBS.[12] Now, if shaking could account for this pattern of injury in a severely battered child then logically *any* child with brain and retinal haemorrhages could also have been shaken – even when there was no other blemish on their bodies to suggest that they had ever been abused: hence the prosecution case against Sarah Bennett and Rioch Edwards-Brown. This extrapolation would require, by necessity, that the same pattern of neuropathological injury be present in all cases – but, crucially, this was not the case. The subdurals in the original cases of SBS – in which there was other powerful circumstantial evidence of abuse – constituted only a thin, often scarcely detectable, layer of blood on the outer surface of the brain. Further, autopsy studies had shown Diffuse Axonal Injury (DAI) in the brain caused by the shearing forces generated by the violent movement of the baby's head.

Now, turning to Dr Geddes's paper in *Brain*, she had performed the first careful histochemical evaluation of the pattern of brain damage in 53 children who had died from presumed non-accidental (abusive) head injury – which had been independently confirmed in two-thirds either by confession of the perpetrator or because of the presence of some other unexplained extracranial injury typical of child abuse.[2] Dr Geddes noted the thin subdurals on the surface of the brain but found evidence of Diffuse Axonal Injury in just three out of the 53 brains from these indisputably "shaken" babies. In a personal interview, she subsequently clarified the importance of these surprising findings for the diagnosis of SBS.

My main interest is in morphology – looking at the pattern of brain damage in great detail and trying to work out what has been going on. My predecessor, Carl Scholtz, had identified evidence of DAI in the brains of babies who died from alleged SBS.[13] Everybody said "that's it", that's why these babies died: the shaking causes the DAI that kills them and SBS can be diagnosed from the presence of the subdurals on the surface of the brain and the retinal haemorrhages induced by shaking.

Then in the early 1990s our histochemical techniques became much better and we began to realise that scattered axonal damage was not specific to trauma: the brain could swell from hypoxic damage irrespective of the cause of death. So when I started looking at my brain samples I wondered whether the pattern of damage might be ischaemic rather than traumatic – and that is what the paper in Brain *shows. These babies rarely have DAI, their brain damage is due to hypoxia. Our most recent research suggests that hypoxia also accounts for the thin subdurals on the surface of the brain and the retinal haemorrhages due to disturbance of the microcirculation to the eye. Now, babies stop breathing for many reasons, one of which could be "shaking" by disrupting the respiratory centre at the level of the craniocervical junction. But equally a respiratory arrest for any reason could, by causing profound hypoxia and brain swelling, produce the thin subdurals and retinal haemorrhage "characteristic" of SBS. So there were these experts turning up in court arguing these babies have sustained very severe brain damage from repeated acceleration and deceleration forces caused by shaking – but it just is not true.*

In retrospect it now began to appear quite obvious how the SBS experts had got it wrong. They had been so convinced by the imagery of how violent shaking could disrupt blood vessels in the brain and eye they had not contemplated the possibility that some entirely different mechanism might be responsible – namely that hypoxia would both damage the vessels and cause the brain to swell with the result that blood leaks into the surrounding tissues to cause the "characteristic" subdural and retinal haemorrhages. Their false premise had then been further extended to encompass within the rubric of SBS all types of SDH and RH, irrespective of their aetiology.

It took some time for the implication of Dr Geddes' findings to sink in but by early 2003, with a group of dissident experts now constituting an unofficial opposition to the SBS juggernaut, the tide began to turn. In March an Edinburgh jury was persuaded that a childminder, Tina Macleod, had not, as the prosecution alleged, shaken a child in her care, Alexander Graham, to death; rather they accepted the pathological findings of brain and retinal haemorrhages were due to acute oxygen deprivation brought about by the disruption of the respiratory centre at the craniocervical junction by the sudden flexing of the neck as he fell from the sofa to the ground. One month later the prosecution – in a *volte face* that would have been inconceivable just a few months earlier – declined to pursue their case against another nanny, 23-year-old Michelle Petchey. The court had heard on the first day how, in the familiar litany of SBS allegations, the baby's injuries were so severe as to be equivalent to "falling from a first floor window or serious head injury caused from a road traffic accident". The following day the judge advised the jury to return a "not guilty" verdict after hearing the prosecution would present no further evidence. Over the following months the same pattern became evident in the family courts with solicitors reporting a sharp fall in the number of cases because SBS experts presumably had become more hesitant in making their allegations.

The parental testimony revisited

Thus, in just under a year, the unifying concept of SBS as a readily recognisable *syndrome* of child abuse had disintegrated into three distinct types of neuropathology. So, now, the long ignored parental testimony suddenly became scientifically important in clarifying the clinical events that might predispose to these different patterns of subdural and retinal haemorrhage. So what did the parents say had happened? Despite the thousands of parents worldwide who have been accused of SBS over the past two decades their account of events does not feature in the medical literature *at all* – other than disparaging references to its presumed falsity. Thus the late Robert Kirschner, pathologist at the University of Chicago, and a significant figure in the creation of the concept of SBS, observes "the parent may present his story with truthful details, but facts are inverted, shaded or omitted in an attempt to conceal the true circumstances of the injury". He even provides a "dirty dozen" of "common suspicious stories", including: "the history of an infant falling from a sofa to the floor is so common that we label these deadly items of furniture 'killer couches'".[14] The parental experience of being at the receiving end of this sort of sarcastic disbelief may have gone unrecorded in the medical literature but it does exist – in the letters and statements collected over the past seven years by Ms Edwards-Brown and kept in the archives of the support group she had set up.

First, the parents' letters. These need no explanatory gloss other than to note their tone of authenticity. They are the letters of ordinary, decent but unsophisticated people caught up in a crisis over which they have no control:

* *Please, if there is any way you could help with our situation, by yourself or anyone you know, could you please get in touch. We can honestly say, hand on heart, we haven't done anything to hurt our baby. We are now been [sic] assessed and we got told [sic] that when we go to the finding of facts hearing and we still insist that we haven't done anything, our twins will probably go up for adoption.*

- *Throughout this we have cooperated with the authorities completely but the threat hangs over us from the social services like the sword of Damocles that should we fail to comply with their instructions, then they will move swiftly to remove S from our care. They have acted like preverbial [sic] storm troopers throughout this entire episode. Our allocated social worker threatened and deceived my family from day one, telling us to keep open minds when hers is completely closed around the notion that the injury has been inflicted by either (or even both?!) parents, initially assuring us that her sole object was to 'get the baby back home' (to win our confidence I guess) when she now openly admits that she will not allow baby back home unless one of her parents admits to causing injury, or the baby is "older and stronger" and her parents have some form of therapy.*

- *I have recently been reading an article about parents being wrongly accused of hurting their babies and doctors' evidence wrecking people's lives. I am in that situation and it is almost killing me. I am really at the end of my tether cos we have done everything the local authority have asked and more but they always twist things and make us look bad. I really need help to keep my boys. Will you help me?*

- *When we read the story of baby Riordan we felt like we were not alone, someone else had felt the same fear and sorrow we too had felt. Though we had different circumstances, the accusations were the same and the pain equally as bad. We have been through absolute hell and still have lots of problems coming to terms with what happened but our son's disabilities are part of him and part of us, we love him no less, he is our beautiful baby boy.*

The second source of parental testimony are the "statements of events" recorded by Ms Edwards-Brown over the past seven years. The limitations of such volunteered testimony are self-evident, none the less if the pattern of clinical events described by parents correlated with the three distinct types of neuropathology outlined above, this would clearly be important. The following analysis is based on 98 "statements of events". The details provided by parents, quite contrary to Kirschner's assertion that it is vague and inconsistent, are *so* precise and consistent it is possible, virtually from the first sentence, to anticipate what the subsequent outcome will be. There was no difficulty in identifying three patterns of clinical events that were compatible with the patterns of neuropathology already outlined.

Minor trauma

The first group (37%) gave a history of minor trauma (such as a fall from a bed or sofa) with either immediate loss of consciousness or delayed presentation of the subdural bleed and retinal haemorrhages. This is in line with the Plunkett series from the United States of independently witnessed minor falls resulting in an acute intracranial bleed with the retinal haemorrhages being due to a sudden rise in retinal venous pressure.[1]

Chronic malaise

The clinical presentation in the second group (29%) is quite different. There is a period of variable length of non-specific symptoms, such as vomiting and lethargy warranting repeated medical consultations until a CT scan shows the presence of a chronic subdural. The most likely aetiology here is a subdural bleed at birth, which, though usually associated with prematurity or a difficult labour, can also follow a normal delivery.[15]

Respiratory arrest

The precipitating event in the third group (22%) is suggestive of respiratory arrest – often followed by attempts at resuscitation – that could result in the subdural and retinal haemorrhages characteristic of hypoxic encephalopathy as described by Geddes.[2]

A fourth type of presentation, epileptiform seizures (12%), is also discernible, presumably secondary to underlying intracranial pathology – and is thus uninformative about possible aetiology.

So each of these three patterns of clinical events correlate with a distinctive type of neuropathology – the acute subdural (as in Jack's case), the chronic subdural (as in Riordan's case), or the thin subdurals of hypoxic encephalopathy (as in Alexander Macleod's case).

Conclusion

It would, of course, be of great interest to hear from the experts themselves as to how they interpret the deconstruction of SBS by Plunkett, Geddes and others and to what extent they have changed the opinions which in the past they have expressed so forcefully in the witness box. Regrettably, despite my several requests for an interview, they have declined, perhaps understandably, to contribute such a closing narrative. It seems appropriate, therefore, in conclusion to interpret the conflicts between professional and parental narratives outlined above in the light of Clive Baldwin's four narrative tactics (see Chapter 12, pp 211–15).

Silencing and narrative constraint

The [parents'] accounts were silenced in a number of ways ... (Baldwin, p 211)

Here we note from the outset the professionals' intimidatory approach, "ambushing" the parents with the diagnosis of SBS without any prior warning, presenting it as a fact ("your son has been violently shaken for several minutes") without acknowledging the possibility of uncertainty or ambiguity. Next there is the further intimidatory tactic of denying the anxious parents information about the clinical progress of their very sick child, with its obvious implication that they don't deserve to know as they are responsible for the child's injuries. Then there is the doctor's early involvement of the police and social workers leading to yet more accusatory interrogations. The doctors, of course, are required to notify suspicions of child abuse but the police and social workers appear to proceed on the basis that the parents are likely to be guilty – because the doctors would not have made such serious allegations against them without first ruling out more innocent explanations for the child's injuries. These intimidatory tactics are more likely to be successful when (as happens) they succeed in driving a wedge between the parents, hence the "come on, one of you must have done it" gambit — so the mother, knowing it was not her, wonders whether it might have been the father after all.

This process of "softening up" is just a prelude to the yet more potent intimidatory weapon of technical obscurantism: the couching of the charge of SBS in a language in which the professionals are fluent, but the parents are not. This creates the bewildering and disorienting sense of "not knowing what they are talking about".

Recuperation

Recuperation is the process whereby one narrative interprets aspects of the other narrative as indicative of its own validity ... (Baldwin, p 212)

The phenomenon of recuperation is illustrated by the way parents are trapped in a situation of being "damned if they do, damned if they don't". Thus the central tenet of SBS requires that severe physical violence be necessary to cause its characteristic pattern of injury. The parents are then faced with the option of confessing to something they did not do (for which they may be offered the inducement "if you say you did it, we will let you see your child again") or insisting their child's injury was accidental, in which case their denial is proof they are lying – and thus further evidence for their guilt.

The process of recuperation can also be seen at a more abstract level in the tautologous nature of the diagnosis of SBS. The tactics outlined above almost guarantee that any parent accused of SBS will be convicted – thus swelling the statistics of the number of "proven" cases of SBS. This in turn leads to yet further convictions as "on the balance of probabilities" the presence of subdural and retinal haemorrhages is evidence of SBS etc.

Asymmetry

> ... there was a marked asymmetry between how professionals viewed the narratives of the mothers and the narratives of other professionals. (Baldwin, p 213)

This has already been noted in the attitudes of police and social workers who interpret the doctor's referral as presumptive evidence of guilt. It also applies to the judiciary, whose judgments consistently favour the prosecution experts (again, "they must know what they are talking about or they wouldn't have made such serious allegations"), while the opinions of witnesses for the defence can be dismissed as being those of apologists for child murder.

Character work

> ... the [parent] is highly dangerous because, contrary to her appearance as a loving mother ... the "reality" is that she is attempting to deceive the doctors ... (Baldwin, p 214)

The question of "character" lies at the heart of the falsehoods that sustain the diagnosis of SBS. The question is: do ordinary, decent parents without a blemish on their characters attempt to murder their children? Common sense, every day experience dictates the answer must be "no". To be sure children are abused and battered, but psychological profiles of their abusers consistently show them to be psychopaths, recidivists, drug addicts or alcoholics. This is not the profile of those accused of SBS. They *appear* as loving, concerned mothers and fathers, because presumably they *are* loving, concerned mothers and fathers.

So why do the experts not see this, or, to be specific, what is the source of their certainty that these parents have deliberately injured their children – despite the complete absence of other circumstantial evidence to support the accusation of NAI? There would seem to be three possibilities. In the first the doctors are acting in good faith, they see no reason to challenge the prevailing, and overwhelming, consensus. They are convinced by the SBS paradigm. The second possibility arises from the observation that a relatively small group of doctors appear to be responsible for a disproportionate number of allegations. They are sometimes referred to as the "hardliners" and given their frequent appearance as witnesses for the prosecution, they might be considered "professional witnesses" (for which they receive generous fees). The third, and very obvious, explanation is that they cannot admit they may be wrong (even if they have doubts) because to do so would necessarily mean acknowledging their responsibility for repeated miscarriages of justice in the past – with all the terrible consequences for those concerned.

References

1 Plunkett J. Fatal paediatric head injuries caused by short-distance falls. *Am J Forensic Med Pathol* 2001;**22**:1–12.
2 Geddes J, Hackshaw A, Vowles G, Nickols CD *et al.* Neuropathology of inflicted head injury in children. 1. Patterns of brain damage. *Brain* 2001;**124**:1290–8.
3 Duhaime A-C, Christian CW, Rorke LB, Zimmerman RA. Non-accidental head injury in infants: 'The Shaken Baby Syndrome'. *N Engl J Med* 1998;**338**:1822–9.
4 Donohoe M. Evidence-based medicine and shaken baby syndrome. Part 1. Literature Review 1966 to 1998. *Am J Forensic Med Pathol* 2003;**24**:239–42.
5 Knight B. The shaken infant syndrome: shaking alone may not be responsible for damage. *BMJ* 1995;**310**:1600.
6 Howard MA, Bell BA, Uttle YD. The pathophysiology of infant subdural haematomas. *J Neurosurg* 1993;**7**:355–65.
7 Medele RJ, Stummer W, Mueller AJ *et al.* Terson's syndrome in subarachnoid haemorrhage and severe brain injury accompanied by acutely raised intracranial pressure. *J Neurosurg* 1998;**88**:851–4.
8 Miller M. Shaken impact syndrome. *Lancet* 2001;**357**:1207.
9 Guthkelch AK. Infantile subdural haematoma and its relationship to whiplash injuries. *BMJ* 1971;**2**:430–1.
10 Caffey J. On the theory and practice of shaking infants. *Am J Dis Child* 1972;**124**:161–9.
11 Ommaya AK, Faas F, Yarnell P. Whiplash injury and brain damage: an experimental study. *JAMA* 1968;**204**:285–9.
12 Duhaime AC, Gennarelli TG, Thibault LE, Bruce TA *et al.* The shaken baby syndrome. A clinical, pathological and biomechanical study. *J Neurosurg* 1987;**66**:409–15.
13 Vowles GH, Scholtz CL, Cameron JM. Diffuse axonal injury in early infancy. *J Clin Pathol* 1987;**40**:185–9.
14 Kirschner RH, Wilson H. Pathology of fatal child abuse. In: Reece RM, Ludwig S, eds. *Medical Diagnosis and Management.* Philadelphia: Lippincott, Williams and Wilkins, 2001.
15 Towner D, Castro M, Eby Wilkins E. Effect of mode of delivery in nulliparous women on neo-natal intracranial injury. *N Engl J Med* 1999;**341**:1709–14.

14: Narratives of compound loss: parents' stories from the organ retention scandal

RUTH RICHARDSON

One mother thought the pathologist had understood, until the close of the interview, when he stood up, shook hands, and then slipped her child's heart into his pocket as he walked away. To him it was a specimen – to her it was the core of her dead child's being.[i]

Introduction

I am a historian. My work is focused on the death culture of the British Isles, particularly on the use of the dead to the living, and beliefs concerning the dead body.[1-7]

I became interested and involved in the aftermath of the furore surrounding the organ retention scandal as a speaker at seminars and as a historical consultant to a national parents' organisation.[ii,iii,iv] As a result, I have encountered many people affected by organ retention. Disjunctions between the stories some doctors tell, and tell each other on this issue, and those I have heard personally from parents and relatives suggest a clash of world views.

Good practice

Most medical professionals, and particularly the pathologists with whom I have had contact, regard it as imperative that the public be better educated concerning the needs of pathology. This certainly seems a positive suggestion, and it is to be hoped that government and medical organisations will take it seriously. It would be beneficial, it seems to me, if medical professionals for their part were to attain improved anthropological perspective on indigenous death cultures, and law and ethics in this field.

Shortcomings in post-bereavement practice have become recognised in the past when professionals have been persuaded to listen to the experiences of those for whom they care. In the last quarter of the twentieth century, following the work of some influential observers in this field, a number of pressure and support groups formed specifically to address the care of the bereaved.[8,9,10] It became recognised that bereavement is a profoundly idiosyncratic, and yet culturally embedded process, with its own associated pathology: that the bereaved should themselves be seen as proper recipients of care and concern.[v]

There followed a period during which bereavement (particularly after the death of children) received increased attention, and special consideration. The restorative value to bereaved families of making farewells appropriate to their own cultural norms became better understood. Routines in healthcare settings were looked at in a new light. Aspects of care that include the dead body (such as parents seeing and/or holding their stillborn babies, should they wish to) have since become elements of good practice.

The Bristol, Alder Hey, and *Marchioness* cases have shown, however, that bereaved families remain significantly disadvantaged when it comes to protecting the dead from unwanted physical interference.[vi]

The organ retention scandal

"Organ retention" is the term now used to describe the removal of organs from the bodies of the dead at post-mortem, their keeping, storage, use, destruction, and disposal. The revelation (made inadvertently by a witness before the inquiry into the deaths of children at Bristol Royal Infirmary) that unauthorised retention had been commonplace in medical institutions, was a profound shock both to those involved, and to the wider public.[13]

Human materials had for many years been taken at post-mortem and kept without informing relatives. The law did not stipulate the need for specific consent, requiring only "reasonable enquiry" to establish *no objection*, a requirement which professionals ducked in the interests, they thought, of science.[vii] Organs and body parts taken from the dead became "specimens", and thereby fell into what has been characterised as a mind-set suffused with professional folklore, which took advantage of what could be treated as a grey area of the law to exploit it by custom and practice.[viii]

These human body parts were erroneously regarded by pathologists as their own property, or the property of the institution for which they worked, or of whomsoever they chose to pass it on to. No administrative oversight existed, locally or nationally, concerning whereabouts of body parts after removal, and book-keeping was often defective or non-existent. Medical ethics did not seem to apply to specimens.

Secrecy concerning the provenance of human specimens and body parts for medical museums and teaching had been assiduously cultivated for many years, in fact ever since the days of bodysnatching and the passage of the Anatomy Act in the 1830s, as I have recounted elsewhere.[15] From what I have gleaned from conversations with bio-medical scientists, the revelations at Bristol (and later at Alder Hay), which drew back the curtain on such covert procedures, were exceedingly unwelcome. Long before the government ordered a national census, there seems to have been a great deal of alarm behind closed doors inside NHS hospitals, and within the research institutions to which much of this human material had been passed. The notorious case of the artist Anthony-Noël Kelly – convicted and sent to prison for the theft of human body parts from the Royal College of Surgeons in 1998 – was fresh in many memories.[16,17]

The organ retention revelations at Bristol, Alder Hey, and elsewhere were met with a range of medical reactions. A few professionals perceived organ retention as ethically indefensible, and argued that it was time to move on.[18] Others disputed allegations of illegality or ethical questionability, believing doctors retain organs in good faith, and for good reason, portraying relatives as making a fuss about nothing, regarding them merely as doctor-bashers, or media attention-seekers (see, for example, Bennett[19]).

Such imputations seem so much at odds with the personal stories I have heard from relatives affected by organ retention, that I believe it historically important to analyse and explain the predicament in which they found themselves. My hope is that anyone experiencing bewilderment concerning the furore surrounding organ retention might find here some resolution to their incomprehension.

This chapter offers a composite impression of the stories I have personally heard from people affected by the retention of organs. I took no notes when people told me their stories. At the time, I had no intention at all of writing about the experience. Our meetings were on staircases, in tea-rooms, in lobbies, in ladies' toilets, on station platforms, in the street: informal settings where talking and weeping, and comforting take place after official business is over.[x] I was not being a historian in these encounters. I was being a witness to suffering.

Parents and children: no "ordinary" deaths

Many of those who told me their stories were affected by organ retention at Bristol and Liverpool, specialist hospitals there being initially at the eye of the storm. Others have come from country villages or inner-city districts in various parts of the country. The institutions responsible for quarrying their children's bodies were generally teaching hospitals with high reputations, and high levels of local loyalty: they include famous London hospitals such as Guy's and Great Ormond Street.

More recently, as the scale of the scandal emerged to include families in every part of the country, and, as members of the public realised that the problem was not confined to infants, more and more people have found themselves involved.

Most of those whose stories are mentioned here were part of the first wave of discovery. Their children had died from a variety of causes. In each case, all medical help had failed. None of the parents I've met blamed doctors for the death at the time. Their trust in the profession had initially been absolute. They thought everything that could have been done to save their child, had been done.

Organ retention was so widespread that outsiders discussing it sometimes lapse into generalities and statistics. But it is important to be aware that in every case, the dead person was an individual, as is each of their survivors. Every relative who spoke to me spoke of their dead with love, as a named individual, with a personality and a presence that was cherished. Many parents carried photographs. All referred to their child by name, and as a person. So although objectively these were "ordinary" deaths, each had lost someone who to them was an extraordinary and special person.

Those whose stories I have been privileged to hear have suffered not only the loss of a child, but, as I shall explain, the extra trauma of compounded loss. Yet parents are generally dignified and restrained in their grief. Their desire to tell their stories is strong, and derives, I believe, from a deep sense of having been intimately maltreated by strangers.

Narrative pattern

Their narratives share many features, most of which relate to the chronology of death, hospital and post-mortem procedures, funerary observances, and subsequent discovery. Their time-frames and speed of discovery vary considerably. Some of the deaths took place twenty or more years ago, others more recently. In some cases deaths were swift, in others, long-anticipated.[ix]

The death itself was something with which relatives knew they had to come to terms, and in the natural course of things, many had done so. But the subsequent discovery of the treatment of their dead, and of themselves, left them aghast, profoundly shocked.[13]

As we shall see, discovery of the fact of retention could be protracted, and fraught with obstacles. In many cases, bereavement was felt as only the first (and because inevitable, sometimes the least) in a series of blows, which have left many of these parents with a sense of being subject to a process of victimisation which began at the hospital, very soon after the loss of their child.

Consent

At the time these parents lost their children, post-mortem examinations (autopsies) in the UK were either coroner's or hospital post-mortems. If a death was unexplained, or if the patient had not been seen by a doctor within 14 days of death, it could become a coroner's case, and families had no legal right of objection to post-mortem examination. If, on the other hand, the death was expected, or occurred in hospital of a known cause, a post-mortem could be requested for reasons of medical understanding, and parents' permission was necessary.[20]

Most of the children discussed had died in hospital, and although several parents had wanted to be with their child after death, they quickly grasped that lack of hospital facilities precluded such togetherness. Some were mindful of the need for a post-mortem examination to ascertain cause of death, though many do not recollect having signed a consent form. None received a copy of the consent form.

When shown these documents later as proof, some could not recall the act of signing, though they recognised their own signature. In a daze of grief, some had hardly known what they were doing, or in the great chasm of loss in which they had become engulfed, memory of such administrative details had somehow bleached away. Others thought they had no option. A few now believe their signatures were forged.

None of the parents who have spoken to me was aware at the time, nor were they informed, that they could appoint a representative to attend the post mortem, or that they might involve an undertaker immediately, or that parents might take their child home and conduct the funeral from there. Parents believed themselves powerless, entirely at the hands of medical officials.

Shock following loss can induce temporary impotence or paralysis of will. In many cultures, customary death rituals work to relieve the bereaved of responsibility immediately after a death. Relieving the bereaved of unwanted responsibility is part of their support and care. Here, however, this helpful aspect of institutional rituals and routines served simultaneously to beguile the bereaved into a false sense of safety. Official procedures ensured they unknowingly relinquished control over the body of their dead.

This is a pivotal moment in many of the stories related to me. It is invariably a focus of profound regret on the part of parents, regret sometimes aggravated by anger and intertwined with self-blame, because it was at this juncture (parents now perceive) that substantial later suffering could have been prevented. Instead, ushered away, they were irrevocably separated from their child: trusting their precious child to people they believed benign. Parents' sense of maltreatment invariably begins here, at the inception of the process of deception, in which they were unwittingly cast in the role they believe they still sustain: that of *dupe*.

Conflicts of interest and of perception are pivotal here, too. To parents, the body of a dead child remains that child. In the wider culture, the dead body is the focus of a multiplicity of cultural beliefs and observances. To medicine, the body is a specimen, a source of information, both about the death of that particular child, about human pathology and physiology in general, and beyond, a rich resource for teaching, experimentation, and research. This conflict is of long standing.[6,21,22]

Ignorance and the post-mortem process

When parents signed a piece of paper to permit a post-mortem examination, they assented to the need for medical understanding of the death of their child, and perhaps to the possibility that the knowledge gained might benefit others with the same condition. Damage to their child was not contemplated in that gesture.

For most non-medical people, the autopsy process is not a pleasant matter to contemplate, and this is particularly the case for the newly bereaved. Until this scandal began to unfold, post-mortems were not much talked about. This was a silence that suited all parties, until it became clear that what parents had taken as a silence of consideration was more manipulative. Most parents knew only that their child's body would soon be ready for burial. Almost all were ignorant of the details.

Perhaps naively, those who were aware that there would be a post-mortem, thought that because their child died (for example) of heart or kidney failure, only their heart or kidneys would be looked at. They had no notion of a standardised process, which involves removing, examining, and often slicing and sampling all internal organs, including the brain, in the search for pathological signs that might illuminate cause of death.

Parents were completely unaware that body parts belonging to their child might be taken and kept without asking. A number of them had no real notion of the research value or the possibility of therapeutic re-use of their dead child's organs. Some parents however agreed to donate tissue, or a single organ (usually their child's heart) for medical research. Several parents mentioned that they actually offered their child's organs up for transplantation, only to be told they would be of no use.

These parents were not hostile to medical progress, they wanted to assist it, but it was only later that they discovered that the term "tissue" had been used to mean entire organs, entire organ systems. In some cases the whole contents of a child's bodily cavities, and more, were not just removed for examination, but kept, preserved and stored, without parental consent. Whether this was done for teaching or research is not always clear: many parents now suspect the likelihood of commercial exploitation.

Funeral directors

In most cases, when the body was "released for burial", a funeral director collected the dead child from the mortuary, and was responsible for preparing it for the family to visit at the company's chapel-of-rest or "funeral home".

The laying out of a dead body discloses its past history to those who do the work of undertaking, especially in regions of Britain, like Merseyside, where embalming is fairly common. Undertakers are used to dealing with bodies that have undergone post-mortems. They cannot have been entirely without suspicion when children's eyes or testicles were missing, when bodies whose long bones had been extracted flopped in a particular way, or when eviscerated bodies weighed less than might be anticipated.

In a few cases, after discussions about funeral arrangements with funeral directors, relatives accepted final disposal (burial or cremation) without seeing the body. Others chose to view. Several parents told me that they were allowed only to observe their child in its coffin: disallowed by the undertaker from touching or holding the body of their own child. It is, I think, a measure of their general deference to, or trust in, authority that parents should accept and observe these restrictions at such a time. Others might say they had been rendered powerless by officialdom.

There is perhaps a submerged professional narrative here, in which funeral directors (like many doctors) gain professional satisfaction from keeping their own counsel, perceiving their discretion as protecting the bereaved from unnecessary distress. Though it may be protective, such silence is also an arrogation of power: it robs the bereaved of agency. Some parents now distrust undertakers, perceiving them as part of a conspiracy of silence which operated to keep them in ignorance of what had happened to their child.

Doubts and suspicions

There is often a hiatus in parent narratives at this point. Funeral rituals and burial or cremation, messages of condolence, flowers, grave-visiting, erecting of monuments, or other forms of commemoration – the normal social processes of bereavement and coming to terms with loss – intervened. Time passed, and bereft families tried to get on with their lives.

It seems generally at some later stage that something happened to raise the suspicion to consciousness that all was not well.

Several parents have said that a sense of doubt first emerged at the funeral home, when they had an intuitive sense of a lack, a curious sense which none could name. This was something beyond the simple passing of a spirit, a sense that something other than death had occurred. Viewing the dead can serve as a confirmation of the fact of death, helping prevent denial. In these cases, the sense of lack was not a simple recognition of a passing, but seems to signify a lack of satisfaction with the presence of their dead child. Something about the body struck them as wrong. A few of the phrases parents used have stuck in my memory:

- "There was something missing."
- "She wasn't *there*."
- "She wasn't in that grave, I just knew she wasn't."
- Their child looked "not quite right".
- The coffin seemed, unaccountably, "very light".

Nebulous doubts such as these were repressed or laid aside at this stage, only to emerge again later. Several parents mentioned some niggling doubt or unanswered question, which kept posing itself: sometimes in dreams.

News gets out

In all the stories told to me, parents suffered these doubts in silence for a considerable period, not knowing quite what to do with them. Individuals were isolated, their concerns were nebulous, they doubted their own intuitions. Many felt haunted by their own misgivings. Some look back on this period as one of mental agony. Some felt if they voiced their suspicions, they would be regarded as mentally ill. A few have described to me their intense relief when they discovered that what they had feared was revealed to be true, because they had doubted their own sanity. A few have said that, with hindsight, they now wish they had not verified their own fears, as the process of uncovering the truth has caused them distress.

In the case of the Bristol mother whose doubts led to the original disclosure in 1996, the discovery (from a note on the post-mortem report, which most parents never get to see) that her daughter's heart had been retained occurred four years after her child's death. Having no idea what retention meant, she started asking questions. Being a persistent kind of person, and having a lawyer to advise her, meant she was able to obtain answers that eventually lifted the lid on the entire affair during evidence to the Bristol Inquiry. As the story of the Bristol heart operations unfolded, the retention of her daughter's organs became part of the story reported in the media, and other parents began to ponder whether retention might have happened to their child, too.

As parents made enquiries for themselves, and began to verify the truth of their own intuitions, they began communicating with one another, and hitherto isolated individuals became a critical mass.

No one knows how many parents have yet to reach the stage of making an enquiry. At first, in most of the stories told to me, concern or distrust seems often to have been tempered with doubt and distancing, people thinking initially that this could never have happened to them. The interval between wondering and doing something to find out was often interrupted or delayed by sometimes lengthy and repeated periods of pondering, oscillating with denial. It was over a year before one man expressed his fears to his own wife, who then admitted to him that she had been wondering, too. Those who have so far come forward to claim their child's parts, or to protest at what has been done, have passed through this stage to make enquiries. How many are still vacillating is not known.

Disorganisation or lack of candour?

The interval between enquiry and discovery was often very difficult for these parents: wanting news, yet apprehensive of what it might mean for them. Parent after parent has told me how they had girded themselves up to telephone or write to the hospital concerned to ask whether any parts of their child had been kept, only to undergo sometimes months of suspense, awaiting a reply.

Despite the currency of the news stories to which parents were reacting, many hospitals seem not to have acted promptly to establish proper channels through which parents might seek and receive information. Their enquiries were apparently unexpected.

Hospital personnel deputed to deal with these matters seem largely to have lacked much of a notion of the pain their call might cause, or indeed, that a parent might deserve the opportunity to decide when and how they might wish to receive information. Answers could come at inconvenient or inappropriate times, with no emotional preparation, delivered by staff who themselves had apparently received no training in the telephone manner needed to convey such information. For one mother, the news came on the anniversary of her child's death. Another answered the phone and was told the news in the middle of her surviving child's birthday party.

Discovery often did not put an end to the matter, because it transpired later, that many parents had been given answers only to those questions they knew how to formulate. A parent who, suspecting their child's heart had been taken, asked about the heart, might be informed some time afterwards that, yes, the heart had been retained.

But few hospitals revealed the real extent of retention without a lengthy process of further probing, reassurances subsequently revealed to be false, and yet further probing: a process which for some parents was shocking, repugnant, demeaning, and agonising, revelatory not only of what had been done to their child, but of their own naivety and powerlessness, past and present. They felt collateral victims in a damage-limitation exercise.

In many places disorganisation was the order of the day, and this sometimes gave the appearance of deception. Parents felt entangled in a complicated choreography of pursuit and evasion, in which it became apparent that the original deception was being further compounded by a lack of candour.

Mutual help

Eventually, the parents who have spoken to me had discovered others in the same predicament, which evidently brought some sense of relief: the pooling of experiences, sharing of grievance, mutual support, strength, and better strategic understanding.

Parents have staffed helplines, co-ordinated meetings, run newsletters, liaised with pathologists and with government. Some, despite what has happened to them, have even helped defend the need for paediatric pathology.

For many, though, the entire process has been not simply one of painful discovery – but of *disillusion*, because they now no longer know who or what to believe. One grandparent told me bitterly that even if the Chief Medical Officer was to state his name, he would not believe him. It is clear that for some of those affected, the entire medical world has forfeited trust.

Scale of retention

Over time, it has emerged that there was no standard for pathological practice in the UK. Procedures varied from place to place, according to the professional training, or standards, or indeed, the idiosyncrasy of the pathologist. The only consistent element in all affected institutions seems to have been disregard of informed consent. Some institutions retained only one or two affected organs per child, but elsewhere the scale of unauthorised retention was much more extensive.

The case of a little boy, Michael Robinson, who died in Liverpool, illustrates the scale of the retention process. Ten years after her boy's death, his mother discovered that before releasing his body to her for burial, the hospital pathologists had taken Michael's heart, brain, liver, lungs, kidneys, spleen, intestine, trachea, oesophagus, diaphragm, stomach, bladder, and connecting tissues, including muscle, ligaments, and bone. Michael's case is one among thousands.[x]

Other children's eyes, tongues, testes, and ovaries have been taken, all without parents' knowledge or consent.

None of the parents I have met had any inkling why the bodies of so many children should have been ransacked in this way. A sense of sinister acquisition and injustice pervades their conversation. Medically trained readers may perceive this naivety as suspect, but it might be worth recollecting that in our culture, integral burial was for centuries believed to be fundamental to spiritual peace and crucial to resurrection, while evisceration was regarded by the state as a punishment for enemies and the worst of criminals: reserved for murderers and traitors sentenced to be drawn and quartered.

Secondary burial

Confirmation of organ retention brought parents shock, disbelief, and sometimes anger, but later, acceptance, and then a craving to mend the damage in some way. For some this has involved reclaiming their child's lost parts, and setting in train novel disposal rituals. A number of self-help organisations have been established by families, the one in the Liverpool area is named PITY II – Parents who Inter Their Young Twice – after this striking and unusual necessity. Some children have now had more than two funerals, because other lost parts were located after a second funeral had already taken place.

It was this state of chaos that induced the government to call a moratorium on the whole process of request and discovery, to allow institutions breathing space to prepare for and deal appropriately with enquiries.

There is wide public sympathy for these families, reflected in media coverage. A disjunction between so-called "scientific" and "lay" (that is, non-medical) perceptions of the human body pervades this entire debate. Yet it is clear that "science" is not the real issue. Some doctors appreciate and understand the enormity of what has happened, indeed some have criticised in print professional colleagues who continue to propound the need for taking specimens without asking, or who disparage families hoping to reunite their lost child's remains.[18] I have personally witnessed other doctors react defensively by asserting the scientific necessity of pathological research and shroud-waving its demise, or who find refuge in derision, particularly towards families' emotional attachment to fragments of tissue. To some medical professionals the process by which these families recover tissue blocks and slides, containing microscopic amounts of tissue, seems incomprehensible, even farcical.

But to parents wishing to make some restitution to their dead child, whose body has been to their mind mutilated after death, or whose entire bodily contents have apparently disappeared, a tissue slide may seem infinitely precious. Tissue blocks and slides are regarded as valuable by medical professionals, too, the valuation having a different basis. Neither view is illegitimate, but legally and morally, parents have the primary claim. Revised DOH guidelines (which required no change in law to become operational)[23] currently require firm evidence of informed consent from next-of-kin prior to the removal or retention of organs or body parts from the dead.[xi]

Organ retrieval

Of course, parents are often at a loss to know what to do about the organs of their child, whose body has been buried or cremated years before. For many, retrieval is best done by an undertaker. But for some the need not to involve "professional" outsiders again has meant returning to the hospital in which their child died, meeting the pathologist, and witnessing for themselves what has been kept.

For two such mothers, visiting a pathology lab for the first time and meeting the person responsible for quarrying their child was both illuminating and distressing. Those they had thought ogres turned out to be human – people who tried to commiserate and to offer plausible explanations for what had happened. But both mothers ultimately found themselves unable to empathise with pathologists, mainly because they were unable to trust them.

One mother thought the pathologist had understood, until the close of the interview, when he stood up, shook hands, and then slipped her child's heart into his pocket as he walked away. To him it was a specimen – to her it was the core of her dead child's being.

"Clinical waste"

In quite a number of instances, information, when it at last emerged, provoked not only disbelief, but shocked incomprehension when emotionally battered parents learned that only one or two parts of their child could now be located, because the remainder had been disposed of as "clinical waste".

The ability to regard human body parts as "clinical waste" seems to be unique to those who have undergone medical or paramedical training. Most parents who have told me their stories regard all the parts of the body of their child as special, still a focus of love and concern because they are inherent with the identity of their child. In scientific terms this view is impeccable: even a sliver of tissue has sufficient DNA to establish identity.[xii]

Not knowing the fate of the constituent parts of their child is, for some people, heartbreaking. That someone else might possess unrestrained power to classify and dispose of parts of their *own child* along with soiled dressings as "hospital waste" is to them a scandalous and malignant wrong.

That the designation "clinical waste" might have been used as a cover for other nefarious uses is, of course, suspected by many. There is a thriving international market in human materials taken with or without authorisation.[25]

Compounded loss

The narratives whose telling I have witnessed reveal that substantial imaginative and emotional injury has been wrought upon the bereaved parents by the unconsented post-mortem evisceration of family members. Lack of openness has compounded these bereavements with fresh pain from other losses:

- Loss of self-respect, for being hoodwinked (sometimes repeatedly).
- Loss of trust in the National Health Service, which allowed a process parents perceive as plunder to take place on thousands of occasions, by subterfuge, over many years.
- Loss of the opportunity to donate organs to another person, or to research, which might have provided some positive mitigation to the death. Donation could have given some of these parents real comfort, could have brought something positive to the tragedy of their bereavement. Deception denied this possibility. Whatever positive purpose or meaning their bereavement might have allowed, has thus been taken from them too.
- Loss of innocence. This loss means that natural reactions to many things are tarnished, people and things can no longer be taken at face value. For example, suspicions arise where before trust was freely given. Some parents have described to me their distress every spring, when love-hearts are everywhere for Valentine's Day. For them the symbolism of the heart no longer stands for love, but for loss, damage, and hurt. At such times parents are aware that they have lost something of profound significance, and their sense of exclusion from the rest of humanity is painful.
- Loss of respect for professionals, whom parents regard as having no consideration towards ordinary people. To them, most doctors are trained to be two-faced: saying one thing (which sounds caring) and doing another (which is damaging).
- Loss of trust in the law and its machinery, by which an artist was sent to prison for theft of body parts from a medical institution, but nothing at all has been done to address what parents perceive as medical assault and theft from the bodies of their children.
- Perhaps, above all, the most painful loss is the loss of undamaged recollection of their own child. Many parents and relatives have effectively been robbed of imaginative or recollected images of their child, which had previously given comfort. Now their memories are irrevocably overlain with bitterly distressing images of mutilation and damage.
- For some, the experience has meant a profound loss of spiritual or existential comfort.

From what I have said it will be understood why many of these bereavements have become harrowing. For some, the difficulty of achieving closure by any ordinary means has become frustrated into exacerbated irresolvability.

Rituals to heal the lacerated imaginative memory of a child lost not only by death, but by evisceration and abstraction of the remains, do not (and perhaps cannot) exist. I have been told of suicides among the bereaved.

Nevertheless, these parents advise and support each other, and some have been resourceful and imaginative in designing rituals appropriate to their predicament, as in this example:[xiii]

From your Mum

My Precious Son. Stephen, Robert Smith

1966–1999

They never let me hold you, the night you went away,

There was so much I wanted to tell, I couldn't say.

I have all the lovely memorys of you at your work bench. The tree you planted in our Garden, your dog Sheena, she missed you so much, and fretted for you, we had to take her to Christy's, to let her see where you were so she could get well. Stephen you are still and always will be a part of me. I trusted those Doctors to get you well again, and I really do think they tried, but it was not ment to be.

What I have never been able to get over Stephen, was I had a Gut instinct, that things were not right, and I told my parents and family, and my minister, but know one believed me, they said such a terrible thing, could never happen. But I knew different. It was a mothers instinct. I knew that one day the truth would come out, and I thank God it has. I have waited 33 years for this my Son and never for one day have I forgot you, and never could because I had right on my side. God was with me. Now I can say Goodbye my child. If only the people would look around them, and know what they are doing (the Evil that they are doing) and the hurt and upset they are causing to all these Parents. They say in the name of Research. It was wrong, Stephen. Every child is so very precious, and we did not want it to happen, but could not do anything about [it]. But at last the truth is out, and one day we will be together. I have your organs Stephen and your little Casket, so when my life is finnished you will go in with me, and we will never be apart again. We shall be in heaven together. I know you are waiting Stephen, it wont be long now. Daddy sends his love. We shall

soon be altogether, never to part again, and one day when these Butchers
meet there maker, they will hang there heads in shame, and will have to
attone for what they did. I still carnt forgive them, after all these years.
But now Ive said goodby to you, perhaps I will heal my heart.

Many parents regard themselves, as well as their dead, as victims of profound abuse. They are very concerned, too, about the damaging impact of imaginative dismemberment/damage to the dead child's siblings, cousins, friends, and children elsewhere who witness upsetting headlines. Most are deeply angry, although in meetings few actually articulate this anger – the generality of these parents are in fact surprisingly restrained in their public utterances. Some have decided to seek redress in the courts, so as to achieve some proper public recognition of the damage they feel has been inflicted on them.[26] They believe this may be the only way the medical profession can be made to comprehend the nature of the assault that has been inflicted on their dead, and on themselves. Others, despite what has occurred, remain fiercely loyal to the National Health Service, and have decided against such a course. Parents' organisations pursuing compensation have lost members over this issue.

Government has been helpful in recognising the wrong done to these parents. Rules concerning the cremation and the burial of body parts have been changed in these cases, a national census of organs and body parts has been conducted to assess the scale of the problem, and to assist reunification if sought for; institutions concerned have been asked to foot secondary and further funeral bills provided they are modest; and the Retained Organs Commission has been appointed to reassure the public, and to propose legislative change.[27,28]

'The rights of the dead.'

The organ retention scandal has revealed a profound culture clash between medical and public perceptions concerning the decent treatment of the dead, and definitions of consent, assault, and theft.[29] Fundamental issues surrounding the rights of the dead, the rights of the bereaved, the development of ethical routes for bodily donation for medical research, demand proper attention and oversight. Clarity concerning access to and ownership of patients' bodies and body parts (including genetic material) are urgently in need of acceptable resolution. Illicit, deceptive, and unethical behaviours towards human bodies and their parts should be recognised as such, and consigned to the past.

Most of the parents who have told me their stories are not hostile to scientific enquiry. Indeed, had they been asked to assist by donation, a good proportion would have done so. Parents object emphatically to the violation of consent resulting from arrogant medical behaviours, which appear to them predatory and mendacious.[29]

By general agreement, human body parts should be transferable only by free gift from next of kin, never taken without asking.[xiv] Effective legislation assigning penalties for unconsented removal and retention is in their view the only possible positive outcome of their distress.

Endnotes

i   The epigraph derives from an observation made in this chapter.

ii   For the various possible meanings of "retention" see *The Bristol Royal Infirmary Inquiry*. London: The Stationery Office, 2000; II: Evidence, para. B.46. The document is available on the Web at: http://www.bristol-inquiry.org.uk/interim_report/report2b.htm.

iii   Although most cases discussed involved children, a wide variety of relationships are represented among those involved in organ retention. For "parents" in this chapter please understand "families", and for "child", "relative".

iv   Speaking engagements include: 1999: Institute of Biomedical Sciences Congress, Birmingham; Albert Norman Lecture, "The fate of the body and its parts at the hands of medical science". 2001: "Purloined parts and the public interest", University College, London; "Who owns the body?", Imperial College Medical School, London; "The history of bodily donation", Guy's Hospital Medical School, Royal Free Hospital Medical School, London; 2002: "Understanding the organ retention furore", British Medical Association, London; "Organ retention: what can history teach us?", Retained Organs Commission, London; 2003: "The impact of thefts of the body and body parts on communities in America and Britain", 72nd Anglo-American Conference of Historians, London; "Taking and giving", National Institutes of Health, Washington, USA.

v   Influential works include John Hinton, *Dying*,[8] Colin Murray Parkes, *Bereavement*,[9] and above all, Lily Pincus, *Life and death: coming to terms with death in the family*.[10] Charities formed subsequently include: Child Bereavement Trust, Cot Death Society, CRUSE, and SANDS.

vi   At Bristol, a series of fatal paediatric heart operations was investigated after a combination of whistleblowing from within the institution and parental pressure from without. The findings of the Bristol Infirmary Inquiry under Professor Ian Kennedy, were published in 2000 (see note ii above). The inquiry into events at Alder Hey Hospital, Liverpool resulted from revelatory evidence given at the Bristol inquiry, concerning an unauthorised collection of children's hearts, and wholesale eviscerations by Dr Van Velsen, who fled the country. The furore was subsequently investigated by Sir Michael Redfern, and reported upon.[12] The *Marchioness* case involved a riverboat disaster on the River Thames in 1989. The bodies of the dead had their hands amputated by mortuary staff, who failed to seek consent from next of kin. The amputations were done apparently to allow identification, under the authorisation of the Westminster Coroner, who seems to have exceeded his powers. Outraged next of kin demanded his resignation, and he was relieved of his responsibilities in this case. See: http://www.geocities.com/jndenio/ChronTable.htm.

vii   An outline of the current law is provided by the Department of Health,[13] see pp 30–35.

viii   The point about professional folklore is from the *Bristol Royal Infirmary Inquiry interim report*.[14]

ix The Chief Medical Officer's Census of retained organs and body parts covered the period 1970–2000, and suggested that "54 000 organs body parts, still-born children or foetuses retained from post-mortems since 1970 were still held by pathology services in England".[13] Retention after operations and post-mortems dates from long before 1970.[4]

x Michael's mother has kindly permitted me to mention his name, and details of his case.

xi Even the Royal College of Pathologists now recognises this primacy. Draft guidelines issued by the RCP in 2000 stated: "relatives have as much right to preserved organs as they do to the body, and it is possible ... that they may be held to own them."[24]

xii The meshing of traditional and scientific notions of identity are well illustrated by a portrait of Sir John Sulston, a scientist involved in the Human Genome Project, recently commissioned by the National Portrait Gallery, London. The artist, Marc Quinn, chose to feature Sulston's DNA profile rather than his face.

xiii The text here is a transcript of a message left by the mother of Stephen Smith at an art exhibition by the artist Denise Green at Bolton Art Gallery, in 2002. The artist, herself a mother whose son's organs were retained without consent, created an extraordinary and positive event titled "Never Again" which allowed parents affected by organ retention the opportunity to use art as a form of public expression/comfort/farewell. Stephen's mother is happy for her letter to appear here. I understand Stephen died as a child in 1966. The interval until his organs were located was one of great existential uncertainty for both of them. The text is as Stephen's mother wrote it, with the exception of one word omitted by mistake. I include the letter here, as it seems the finest way the real voice of a parent could be conveyed directly. Copyright of the letter remains with Mrs Smith.

xiv In this parents agree with the whole-body donors surveyed in Richardson and Hurwitz.[29]

xv The case came to court while this book was in press. See Dyer, C. Organ scandal parents win case. *The Guardian*, 27.3.2004.

xvi The Retained Organs Commission published its Valedictory Report while this book was in press. See http.www.dh.gov.uk/roc 31.3.2004. The new Human Tisssue Bill is due to be discussed in Parliament this summer (2004). It contains provision for a three year jail sentence for keeping organs without consent.

References

1 Richardson R. *Death, Dissection and the Destitute*. Routledge UK/Methuen USA, 1988; Penguin Books, 1989; 2nd edn, Chicago: Chicago University Press, 2000.

2 Richardson R. Hurwitz BS. Donors' attitudes towards body donation for dissection. *Lancet* 1995;**346**:2779.

3 Richardson R. Transplanting teeth: reflections on a cartoon by Thomas Rowlandson. *Lancet* 1999;**354**:1740.

4 Richardson R. A potted history of specimen-taking. *Lancet* 2000;**355**:935–6.

5 Richardson R. Bodysnatchers; Burke and Hare; The corpse; Funeral practices. Sections in: Blakemore C, ed. *Oxford Companion to the Body*. Oxford: Oxford University Press, 2001.

6 Richardson R. From the medical museum: Pennant's serpent. *Lancet* 2001;**357**:966.

7 Richardson R. Coroner Wakley: two remarkable eyewitness accounts. *Lancet* 2001;**358**:2150–4.

8 Hinton J. *Dying*. Harmondsworth: Penguin, 1967.

9 Murray Parkes C. *Bereavement*. Harmondsworth: Penguin, 1978.

10 Pincus L. *Life and death: coming to terms with death in the family*. London: Abacus, 1978.

11 Lovell A. A Bereavement with a diference: A study of late miscarriage, stillbirth and perinatal death, 1983. London; Polytechnic of the South Bank, p 29–34.

12 Redfern M, Keeling JW, Powell E. *The Royal Liverpool Children's Inquiry Report.* London: The Stationery Office, 2001.
13 Department of Health. *Human Bodies, Human Choices.* London: Department of Health Publications, 2002, p 3.
14 *Bristol Royal Infirmary Inquiry interim report: removal and retention of human material.* London: The Stationery Office, 2000, p 18.
15 Richardson R. *Death, Dissection and the Destitute.* Chicago: Chicago University Press, 2000, pp 239–64.
16 Wildgoose J. Catalogue essay for A-N Kelly's exhibition *Birthdays.* London, 1999.
17 Wildgoose J. An acceptable body of work? *Daily Telegraph*, Arts & Books section, 9 May 1998, p A7.
18 Burton JL, Wells M. The Alder Hey affair: implications for pathology practice. *J Clin Pathol* 2001;**54**:820–6.
19 Bennett JR. The organ retention furore: the need for consent. *Clin Med (J R Coll Phys Lond)* 2001;**1**(3):167–71.
20 Department of Health. *Human Bodies, Human Choices.* London: Department of Health Publications, 2002, pp 5–6.
21 Richardson R. The corpse and popular culture. In: Richardson R. *Death, Dissection and the Destitute*, 2nd edn. Chicago: Chicago University Press, 2000.
22 Richardson R. The corpse as an anatomical object. In: Richardson R. *Death, Dissection and the Destitute,* 2nd edn, Chicago: Chicago University Press, 2000.
23 Department of Health. *Human Bodies, Human Choices.* Department of Health Publications, 2002;**4**:22–35.
24 Royal College of Pathologists. *Tissue retention: draft guidelines.* London: RCP, 2000, para. 6.4.
25 Hedges SJ, Gaines W. Donor bodies milled into growing profits: little-regulated industry thrives on unsuspecting families. *Chicago Tribune*, Tribune Investigative Report: The body parts business, 21 May 2000, section 1:1–2.
26 Department of Health. *Human Bodies, Human Choices.* Department of Health Publications, 2002, p 5.
27 Brazier M. Organ retention and return: problems of consent. *J Med Ethics* 2003;**29**:30–3.
28 Dyer C. Doctors' arrogance blamed for retention of children's organs. *BMJ* 2000;**320**:1359.
29 Richardson R, Hurwitz BS. Donors' attitudes towards body donation for dissection. *Lancet* 1995;**346**:277–9.

15: The power of stories over statistics: lessons from neonatal jaundice and infant airplane safety

THOMAS B NEWMAN

I have always been a person more comfortable with numbers than with narrative, demanding data rather than accepting anecdotes. Recently, however, I have been increasingly impressed with the power of stories over statistics. As a general paediatrician, epidemiologist, and father of two, I have recently encountered this power in two areas: neonatal jaundice and infant airplane safety. These seemingly disparate areas provide stories I think illustrate some common themes that I hope to clarify, at least for myself, by retelling.

The jaundice story is one of me trying to practise and help write guidelines for treating jaundice in newborn infants according to the best evidence. Ironically, the more of an expert on the evidence I have become, the more difficulty I have practising according to that evidence. This is because becoming a "jaundice expert" means that one is consulted on medico-legal cases, and then becomes very familiar with rare but tragic stories. These stories are so powerful that it is hard to keep them from overriding evidence in determining practice.

To understand the jaundice story, a little medical background is necessary. Jaundice is a yellow colouring of skin and the whites of eyes caused by the build-up of bilirubin, a yellow pigment that comes from haem, the oxygen-carrying part of haemoglobin. Although in adults jaundice may be visible at lower levels, jaundice in newborns becomes visible when plasma bilirubin concentrations rise above about 6 mg/dl.[1]

Newborn babies tend to become jaundiced just after birth because their liver is not yet efficient at excreting bilirubin; during intrauterine life the mother's liver has been doing that task. So most newborns become a little jaundiced, then their liver kicks in, they start excreting bilirubin, and the jaundice goes away.

Rarely, however, as a result of increased breakdown of haemoglobin or an immature or diseased liver, bilirubin in the blood can build up to toxic levels that can cause a kind of permanent brain damage called kernicterus.[i] Kernicterus can be prevented by monitoring the baby for jaundice – visually and through undertaking serial blood tests – and by using treatments to keep plasma bilirubin from rising to dangerous levels. Two such treatments are currently available: phototherapy (shining light on the baby's skin) and, if this fails to work fast enough, exchange transfusion, a more drastic treatment which replaces the baby's blood a little at a time with donor blood.[ii]

The difficult question for clinicians and parents concerning neonatal jaundice is: what is a reasonable approach to preventing rare but devastating cases of kernicterus? Obviously, key questions are what bilirubin levels should trigger phototherapy and exchange transfusion. But monitoring and follow-up questions are perhaps even more difficult.[2] For example, do all newborns need to have their bilirubin measured, or only those noted to be jaundiced? How soon should the bilirubin be checked again if it is high? How low is low enough that we can stop worrying about it?

The neonatal jaundice story starts for me in 1980–83, when I was a resident in paediatrics at the University of California at San Francisco. At that time, we treated babies with phototherapy if their bilirubin rose above a concentration of 14 mg/dl (239 micromol/l), and we did exchange transfusions for bilirubin levels exceeding 20 mg/dl (342 micromol/l). In fact, as a resident I did several exchange transfusions for jaundice in otherwise well babies. Unfortunately, it turned out that 1980–83 was not a good time to be transfusing blood in San Francisco. Although we did not know it at the time, the blood supply was contaminated with human immunodeficiency virus (HIV). We also did not know at the time that most of the exchange transfusions we undertook then were unnecessary.

In 1983, in an article entitled "Bilirubin 20 mg/dl = vigintiphobia,"[3] Watchko and Oski questioned the "fear of twenty" that led to exchange transfusions for jaundice in healthy babies. Subsequently my colleagues and I reviewed[4] and re-analysed[5] existing studies and came to the same conclusion: that jaundice in healthy newborns was being overtreated. We recommended a "kinder, gentler" approach,[6] which was largely adopted for a 1994 practice guideline of the American Academy of Pediatrics.[7] Since then there has been a dramatic shift towards less treatment of neonatal jaundice.[8] That's the good news.

The bad news is that beginning in the mid 1990s, there has been concern that kernicterus may be "coming back."[9,10,11] This "return"[iii] of kernicterus has mostly been blamed on very early discharge of mothers and babies after delivery, with inadequate follow-up. (These so-called "drive-through deliveries" peaked in the US in the mid-1990s, just before federal legislation required insurers to cover at least a 48-hour stay post partum.) But some of these cases also seem to have occurred because of lack of clinician concern about the dangers of neonatal jaundice. This is something for which I may have some responsibility, since my colleague Jeffrey Maisels and I have been among the main proponents of the view that the dangers of neonatal jaundice are almost certainly less than previously thought.

The extent to which kernicterus is coming back remains a key question. How many cases are there, and is the number really increasing?[iv] The answer is that we don't know. For the past 7 years I have been doing research on neonatal jaundice in the Northern California Kaiser Permanente Medical Care Program (NC-KPMCP), a managed care organisation that covers about 3 million people, with about 28 000 births per year. My colleagues and I have been systematically searching for cases of kernicterus in this population. We have examined records of all infants with very high bilirubin levels among the 111 000 births between 1995 and 1998,[12] and all children with cerebral palsy among the 239 000 births from 1991 to 1998, and did not find any cases.[v] We do not know how this compares to other settings, but we do know that kernicterus is rare. My best guess is that the annual incidence is somewhere between 2 and 4 per million. This makes kernicterus about 200 to 500 times less common than other causes of cerebral palsy and sudden infant death syndrome.

Meanwhile, in the 1990s I began to get calls from lawyers who wanted me to serve as an expert witness in medical liability cases involving children with alleged kernicterus. This typically involves the lawyers sending me a stack of medical records, which I examine and offer my opinion on. Sometimes it ends there – my opinion is not what the lawyers are looking for and the case settles quickly or they try to find someone more sympathetic. But on other occasions I am named as an expert, and then start reading depositions (interviews by attorneys of people involved in the cases), and occasionally I am asked to provide a deposition myself.

When that happens, I become quite familiar with various claimants' narratives concerning the development of kernicterus. Parents' stories are uniformly poignant and heartbreaking. Attorneys trying to establish damages will go over in great detail what the affected child can and cannot do, including its care requirements. For example, I might be informed about a typical day, perhaps what it is like getting the child dressed, fed, and into his or her wheelchair for one of various therapy sessions, and how frustrating it is for the child to be unable to move, speak, or feed himself. Some of these children get a lot of pain at times from muscle stiffness, and I feel so sorry for the parents, when I imagine what it must be like to watch one's child suffer in that way. Most seem to have sleep problems, and although this is not covered in detail in most depositions, it is clear that the parents' stress and exhaustion from having such a child places great strains on marriages, many of which do not survive.

One of the cases with which I became quite familiar is that of Cal Sheridan. In addition to Cal, who suffers from kernicterus, Cal's father Patrick was also a victim of a medical error. Patrick had a spinal tumour that the couple were initially led to believe was benign. But when it recurred and was found to be a sarcoma, Susan and Patrick examined his medical record and found that the original pathology report had, in fact, concluded that the tumour was a sarcoma. Somehow, this report had been filed away in error and not been brought to the attention of the treating physicians. Patrick has since died from this tumour.

These experiences have resulted in Cal's mother, Susan Sheridan, becoming an extremely articulate and capable spokesperson for improvements in patient safety.[vi] After an article about herself and Cal appeared in *USA Today*,[13] other parents of children with kernicterus contacted her, and together they formed a parents group, "Parents of Infants and Children with Kernicterus" (PICK).

I have been amazed at how big a difference this parents group has made to the public's awareness of kernicterus, despite the small number of babies affected. As a result of efforts by PICK, the Centers for Disease Control issued a report in the *Morbidity and Mortality Weekly Report* about kernicterus,[14] the Joint Commission on Accreditation of Hospital Organizations issued a "Sentinel Event Alert" for kernicterus,[15] and the Agency for Healthcare Research and Quality awarded a contract for an evidence report on neonatal jaundice.

Unfortunately, in spite of all of these efforts, other than knowing that the condition is rare, we remain little better informed about the risk of developing kernicterus. Without this basic sort of information, it is hard to come up with evidence-based guidelines to address the detection and monitoring of neonatal jaundice. But the stories (and storytellers) are powerful.

I notice this power in the deliberations of the American Academy of Pediatrics (AAP) committee in charge of developing guidelines for management of jaundice in newborns, on which I serve. I have now met many of the women in PICK, and know that they want the AAP to recommend that all newborns have a bilirubin level measured before they leave hospital. I like and admire these women, who are unselfishly spending so much of their time and energy trying to keep what happened to their infants from happening to others and it would be nice to be on their side, heroically fighting to prevent an awful disease. On the other hand, I teach and am a strong proponent of "evidence-based medicine" and would hate to endorse a new screening recommendation that is not based on good evidence. In this case, the "evidence" is only the poignant stories of the kernicterus cases, many of which, when closely scrutinised, do not clearly support pre-discharge bilirubin testing as a preventive strategy. In order to justify screening, estimates of how many newborns would need to be screened to prevent one case of kernicterus are required as well as information on the cost and accuracy of the test, and knowledge of what to do with the results.[vii]

I feel the strength of the stories also in my own practice caring for newborns. I remember one particular episode when I was covering the normal newborn nursery on a Friday night. My wife and I were watching a video we had rented when I received a call from Valerie, one of the home health nurses, about a baby whom I had discharged from the nursery a few days earlier. We had started Baby V on home phototherapy the day before for a bilirubin level of 19·5 mg/dl. Valerie reported that the breast milk had come in and the baby was nursing better and had gained weight, so she had elected to continue the home phototherapy even though the bilirubin level was 20·5 mg/dl. She just wanted to make sure that was OK with me.

Now this report and plan were totally reasonable. In fact, I knew at the time that in the Northern California Kaiser Permanente Medical Care Program in 1995–6, during which time there was not a single case of kernicterus, only about half of all babies with documented bilirubin levels of 20–25 mg/dl were treated with phototherapy.[17,viii] None the less, I was very uncomfortable with the idea of a baby at home with a bilirubin level of more than 20 mg/dl. I kept envisioning this child developing kernicterus and my having to face the baby's mother, having let her down. I envisioned her attorney asking me why, when I had been on the AAP committee that wrote the guideline, I had not followed it.

I did not in fact call the home health nurse back to advise her to admit the baby to hospital; and of course the baby did just fine. But that evening all these thoughts were intrusive on me to the point that I could not enjoy the movie (much to my wife's annoyance!). And I remember thinking, "Who needs this? Next time I'll just follow the guidelines and admit such kids to the hospital, so I don't have to worry and can enjoy my movie."

So my experience dealing with neonatal jaundice has been a powerful indication to me of the power of stories over statistics.

Unlike the situation with neonatal jaundice, recommendations regarding infant airplane safety are only a recent interest of mine. In fact, I had not given this issue a second thought until late in 2001, when I noticed that the American Academy of Pediatrics (AAP) publicly supported a federal regulation requiring children under two years of age to ride in infant safety seats on airplanes.[18] This would require their parents to buy a ticket when previously the children had travelled free of charge if carried in a parent's lap. This AAP statement was a particular disappointment to me because for some time I had been trying to get the AAP to make its position statements more evidence-based[ix] and its Committee on Injury and Poison Prevention – which authored the statement on infant airplane safety – had presented virtually no evidence to support the position adopted.

Drs Brian Johnston and David Grossman (of the Harborview Injury Prevention Center in Seattle, Washington) and I decided to look further into the issue of infant airplane safety. The issue had first been raised by the US National Transportation Safety Board (NTSB) after the 1989 crash of United Airlines Flight 232 outside of Sioux City, Iowa, in which an unrestrained infant had died. The NTSB recommended a rule to the US Federal Aviation Administration (FAA), requiring universal infant restraint, but the FAA dragged its feet. In 1994, another "lap child" died in a potentially survivable crash, and the NTSB again asked the FAA to take action. This time the FAA agreed to study the issue, and in 1995, presented a report to Congress.[x]

The FAA estimated that only about five airplane crash deaths could be prevented over 10 years by adopting the rule of universal infant restraint on airplanes.[20] On the other hand, because the additional cost of an airplane ticket for a child is likely to lead some families to drive rather than to fly, the FAA estimated the regulation would cause an increase of about 87 deaths over 10 years, due to road deaths resulting from diversion to car travel. Thus the FAA estimated that the overall effect of adopting the policy would be 82 excess deaths over 10 years.

The FAA analysis was not accepted by the NTSB and received a hostile reception at a Congressional Hearing. A major point of dispute was the FAA's estimate that 20% of families with children under 2 years old would choose to drive rather than fly if they needed to buy a ticket for their young child. In the excerpt below, Congressman Peter De Fazio questions Louise Maillett, Acting Assistant Administrator for Policy, Planning, and International Aviation for the FAA about this estimate:

Mr DEFAZIO: How many people were surveyed in conducting this study? ... What was the size of the sample?...

Ms MAILLETT: There were no passengers surveyed for this report to Congress.

Mr DEFAZIO: No passengers were surveyed? So we know how they're going to perform, but we didn't ask any of them?

Ms MAILLETT: We looked at a wide range of research that has already been performed.

Mr DEFAZIO: You looked at research, which is econometric data which has to do with estimated price elasticity of ticketing, which has nothing to do with parents and their care for their children or any of that. You didn't survey anybody. Why didn't you do a survey? ... I studied economics. There is no reliability to any of this. This is a lot of gobbledegook. That's what it is.

Brian, David, and I did some analyses ourselves, to test the sensitivity of the results of the FAA to various assumptions about things like the proportions of families choosing to drive rather than to fly, the distance of the trips and the safety of the drivers.[21] We came up with about the same number of possible children's lives that could be saved from reducing airplane crash fatalities. This is a number we can estimate with some confidence, because there are good data on the number of fatalities in survivable crashes per 100 million enplanements. These numbers are very small, so UAL flight 232 notwithstanding, there just is not much room for improvement.

To avoid the contentious issue of how best to estimate the proportion of families that would choose to drive, rather than fly (since even responses on a survey might not reflect what people would actually do), we instead left that variable as an unknown, and simply estimated numbers of deaths that might be saved or caused as a function of this unknown proportion (Figure 15.1). We took into account the probable age distribution of drivers (few teenagers or elderly), their low likelihood of alcohol use, and their probable higher proportion of travel on the interstate highway system, all factors associated with lower than average fatality rates per hundred million vehicle miles travelled. Even with this estimate, however, if more than about 5–10% of families chose to drive, the policy would lead to a net increase in fatalities.

Perhaps the most striking feature of our analysis was the cost per death prevented by adopting a universal restraint policy for children under two. Even ignoring the possible deaths from diversion to car travel, the estimated cost per death prevented was about $6·4 million for each $1 cost of the round-trip airplane ticket for the child, or $1·3 billion if the ticket cost $200.

The issue of cost effectiveness of requiring child safety seats was raised in Congress:

CONGRESSMAN GEREN: ... five million enplanements. Say it only costs $20. That's $100 million ... If we gave you $100 million and you were entrusted with saving lives, where would you apply it, top priority?

Barry Sweedler, Director, Office of Safety Recommendations of the NTSB – the agency that is, in fact, entrusted with saving lives – initially

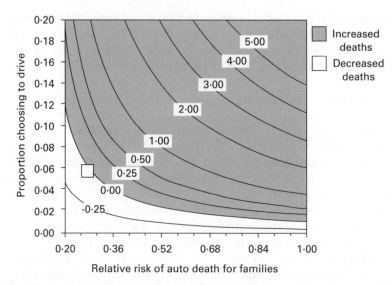

Figure 15.1 Estimated numbers of deaths in the USA that could be caused or prevented by a regulation requiring safety seats on commercial airplanes for children < 2 years old, as a function of the proportion of families choosing to drive and their relative risk of death (per 100 million vehicle miles traveled) compared with the US national average. The yellow square indicates the base case estimate, in which the relative risk is about 0.3, and the policy will lead to a net increase in deaths if more than about 6% of families choose to drive. From BMJ 2003;**327**:1424–27 20 December. Available electronically bmj.bmjjournals.com/cgi/content/full/327/7429/1424?maxtoshow=&eaf

parried the question, but Congressman Geren persisted. Finally, he received the following answer:

> *MR SWEEDLER: There is a long list of safety issues that need addressing, and I think it's probably best for us to try to lay out what the issues are and try not to prioritize which safety issue is more important than other safety issues ... this seems to be one of those areas where it just seems to make common sense to go ahead and take that extra step.*

Unlike the case with neonatal jaundice and kernicterus, here is a case where we have excellent data. However, as in the case with jaundice, the stories are very much more powerful than the statistics. In this case, Jan Brown-Lohr, a flight attendant from UAL Flight 232, told a particularly compelling story:[22]

> *Ms BROWN-LOHR: My name is Jan Brown-Lohr. I have been a flight attendant with United Airlines and a member of the Association of Flight*

Attendants for 20 years. Thank you, Mr Chairman and members of the committee, for allowing me to speak about my personal experience.

I was the chief flight attendant in the Sioux City, Iowa, DC-10 accident on July 19, 1989. A flight attendant's primary responsibility is passenger safety, and on that day I came to the full realization that passenger safety only applies to those over the age of 2 years old.

It was a golden July day when disaster struck. The number two engine exploded, severing all hydraulic lines and leaving the pilots with only the number one and number three wing engines to maneuver the airplane. I have never known such terror.

We had 40 minutes to clear the snack service, secure the cabin, and then, according to procedures, we prepared the passengers for the emergency landing.

As we waited for the brace signal from the cockpit, I mentally reviewed if everything had been covered and remembered that we had several lap children. I picked up the microphone again and instructed those parents to place their children on the floor, which would give some advance time to brace themselves, as well as their children.

What I had been taught in flight attendant emergency training class now became senseless in reality. I could hardly believe I was giving these absurd instructions, but that was all we had.

What followed has been viewed countless times – an unbelievable impact that mere words could never adequately describe – the plane breaking into three sections, being engulfed in a flash fire, and my section finally stopping upside down in a corn field.

I was finally forced to leave the wreckage due to prohibitive and deadly smoke. The first person I encountered was a mother of a 22-month-old boy – the same mother I had comforted and reassured right after the engine exploded. She was trying to return to the burning wreckage to find him, and I blocked her path, telling her she could not return. And when she insisted, I told her that helpers would find him.

Sylvia Tsao then looked up at me and said, "You told me to put my baby on the floor, and I did, and he's gone." My first thought was, "I'll have to live with this for the rest of my life." I then replied, "That was the best thing to do." That was all we had. Evan was killed ..."[xi]

I ask all of you members of the audience, take a moment today and try to bend down and hold an object on the floor at your feet. Feel the anxiety, tension, and fear in the airplane cabin. Imagine you looking down at your most precious possession, your child, who is at the mercy of whatever lies ahead, and you are frantically praying for safety.

What baby body count will force safety for vulnerable little people? Which parents will make the sacrifice of their infant's injury or death? And which official who opposes child restraints will explain to that grieving parent statistics on cost and highway hazards?

I will not allow Evan to be forgotten, nor his message that small children deserve the same measure of safety which every other passenger enjoys. We flight attendants will be relentless in the pursuit of infant safety on airplanes.

Thank you very much for the opportunity to appear before you today.

When I read this testimony on the internet I found it extremely compelling. (I am sure that in person it must have been even more so.) I began to wonder whether to continue writing my scientific paper on the costs and benefits of the proposed regulation. And I understood how rational people could favour the regulation – no flight attendant and no family should have to go through what was described in the testimony.

I did complete and submit the article about infant safety seats on airplanes, just as I had left Baby V at home on phototherapy. But I was impressed enough with the power of stories in both of these areas that (being on sabbatical and therefore feeling entitled to branch out into a new area) I decided to look into the area further,[xii] in hopes of gaining a better understanding on how best to understand and harness this particular power.

What makes these stories so powerful? First, the brains of human beings appear built to process stories better than other forms of input. Psychologist Robin Dawes[23] suggests changing a quotation by evolutionary biologist Stephen Jay Gould "Humans are the primates who tell stories" to "Humans are primates whose cognitive capacity shuts down in the absence of a story".

Second, the storytellers themselves are important. It is not just that these awful things happened, it is that they happened to the person telling the story. This enables a connection with the listener or reader beyond what would be possible if the story were recounted by a dispassionate observer, and it infuses the storyteller with a passion to tell the story over and over again, thus multiplying its influence. As someone who has looked at the numbers and data to project consequences of both hyperbilirubinaemia and unrestrained infants on airplanes, I like to present and publish my results, but the fact is, for me this is just a small part of my job. I cannot bring the same level of passion and sustained commitment to telling the story of my results that a Sue Sheridan or Jan Brown-Lohr can for stories of events that have happened to them.

Third, the powerful effect of these stories relates to the way people estimate probabilities. If we are trying to estimate the risk of kernicterus, one method we use is to base the estimate on how readily we can recall or imagine a case, and in what level of detail. This technique, referred to by Kahneman and Tversky as the "availability heuristic"[24] leads us to overestimate probabilities of events that we can easily and vividly imagine. It presents a real challenge to subspecialists in general, but particularly to experts in rare diseases, who, if they write guidelines, are likely to write them with a distorted sense of probabilities.[25] This is the problem I was encountering while trying to watch that video with my wife – recollections of children with kernicterus were just too vivid and available.

Finally, these stories are compelling because they describe particularly tragic outcomes and because they appear to offer a solution – a way to extract some meaning and redemption from tragedy, by preventing its reoccurrence.[xiii] There are at least 100 children with idiopathic cerebral palsy for each one with kernicterus, but because there isn't a clear way in which their disabilities could have been avoided, they do not make as compelling a story. John Adams, a risk researcher I was lucky enough to get to know while in London (and his colleague Michael Thompson) put it this way:[26]

> Rather than understanding policy-makers as problem-solvers who apply objective, scientific, and value-free methods to cure society's ills … think of policy-makers as performers who seek to persuade an audience …

> A policy argument, in consequence, tells a story: it provides a setting, points to the heroes and villains, follows a plot, suggests a solution, and, most importantly, is guided by a moral.

The trouble with these compelling stories, however, is that their apparent simplicity and focus can lead to suboptimal decisions in a complex world. As HL Mencken said, "For every complex problem, there is a solution that is simple, neat, and wrong." Poignant stories may focus our attention on a particular salient event that happened to a particular person, to the neglect of complicated considerations like what else we might do with our resources, and how we should make these decisions.

An example of this is screening mammography, particularly for women younger than 50 years, which is costly and not very effective. As David Eddy wrote on that topic:[27]

> The essential purpose of a cost-effectiveness analysis is to calculate the net benefit or harm to a population if resources are put into one activity rather

than another. *But that question does not even arise if you do not look past one activity that interests you ... From this narrowed perspective, the results of cost-effectiveness analysis are not only moot, they are an irritant* [emphasis added]. The scope of concern of a specialty society, an advocacy organisation, or a disease-oriented charity might be narrowed in this way. Conversely, if one's scope is broader, encompassing other patients and other diseases, and if one understands the implications to real people of limited resources and misplaced priorities, then the results of cost-effectiveness analyses are critically important.

Those of us who do try to have a broader scope run into problems, however. One is that it is harder for us to find compelling stories and storytellers. We may know that more lives could be saved by course of action A than B, but if the specific people benefiting from course of action A are harder (or impossible) to identify, we cannot tell their stories. This relates to a well-known paradox in how people perceive risk and value risk reductions: we tend to over-value relative risk reductions, at the expense of absolute risk reductions.[28,29,30] Thus, an intervention that could reduce the number of cases of kernicterus by 50% (preventing perhaps 8 cases per year) might be valued more than one that could reduce the risk of cerebral palsy in general by 1% (preventing about 80 cases per year) – these 1% being perceived as a "drop in the bucket".

When we cannot identify the specific people who would benefit or be harmed by a specific course of action, we are reduced to impersonal numbers and calculations that are often viewed with distrust. As Congressman Jim Lightfoot of Iowa, whose district includes the site of the Flight 232 crash, put it during the congressional hearing at which the FAA presented its report:

The question, I think, Mr Chairman, comes down to how many more children must die, how many more have to be hurt before we reach the threshold of FAA's ghoulish cost/benefit ratio?

What can be done about the power of stories over statistics, and how can it be more appropriately harnessed? I am new to this field, but based on my experiences, I have a few suggestions.

First, we should be careful about having experts in particular diseases write guidelines for preventing those diseases. It is fine to have experts write guidelines about how to *treat* the diseases (provided treatments are not too costly) but particularly when it comes to prevention, for which the number of interventions that might be recommended is potentially limitless, a widened perspective that includes some awareness of other ways the resources could be spent seems important. This is the approach taken by the US Preventive Health Services Task Force, with the result that their recommendations have greater credibility than those of specific disease – advocacy groups or subspecialty societies (whose recommendations tend to be self-serving).

Second, raise awareness of this problem – teach writers of treatment guidelines about problems like the availability heuristic, and the power of stories and storytellers. The first step to overcoming these biases is knowing how and why they occur.

Third, I have started to collect my own stories. In this effort, it helps that I continue to see patients myself. For example, here is a story that I've told to illustrate the need for more thoughtful allocation of health resources:[xiv]

One thing I do about four weeks a year is act as the attending physician for children in the hospital at UCSF with general pediatrics problems. The last time I did that I took care of a six-year-old girl named Alice, who was having trouble breathing because of her asthma. I wanted to talk to her primary care provider to let her know that Alice had been admitted. So, as is my custom, I took a stack of charts over to the phone, so I could write some notes in case I got put on hold while waiting to talk to the doctor. In fact, I got through all of the charts, and I was still on hold waiting to speak to a live person. Anyway, I finally spoke to the doctor, who said she hadn't seen Alice for a while, but agreed with what we were doing.

When I next saw Alice's mother, I asked if she had had any trouble getting through to her pediatrician. She became very sad, and said, almost crying, "Doctor, it's very hard for me to make an appointment for Alice to see her doctor, because my breaks at work are only 15 minutes."

When I tell this story, I point out that we all need to realise, when we order $2000 magnetic resonance imaging scans, that the cost of one scan is enough to hire someone to answer the phone in the paediatric clinic for nearly a month.

Finally, I think it is helpful to try to discuss *how* decisions should be made separately from particular decisions. I tried this in an informal conversation with several of the original PICK mothers at a meeting of the Pediatric Academic Societies a couple of years ago. I explained that when I am attending in the nursery I typically have 10 or 20 families to see, in addition to circumcisions, teaching rounds, and other parts of my job. It is unusual for me not to feel at least a little rushed. I posed the question: how should I decide how many minutes to allocate to different prevention issues? How do I choose between the dangers of jaundice, and, for example, those of guns in the household or passive smoking? When we are writing up our information for parents of newborns, how should we decide how much space to allocate to each problem, knowing that the fatter the packet gets the less likely it is to be read? My goal was to achieve some consensus that one part of the calculation *had* to be some estimate of how common the problem was, and how much difference talking or writing about it might make. Was I successful? I don't know. At least I think we parted on friendly, mutually respectful terms. But the answer I got to the question about how I should allocate my minutes talking to families was perhaps not surprising. It went something like this: "That's your problem. Our problem is preventing kernicterus!"

Endnotes

i   This used to occur most often when a baby had a blood type incompatible with the mother's, and antibodies from the mother crossed into the baby's circulation, causing destruction of red blood cells (haemolysis) resulting in haem being converted to bilirubin at a much faster rate than the liver could handle. But this sort of haemolysis most of the time can now be prevented, so it has become rare.

ii An alternative type of treatment, haem analogues that are given to inhibit the enzyme that catalyses the first step in the production of bilirubin from haem, is currently under investigation.

iii I put "coming back" and "return" in quotes because there is no good data that kernicterus had disappeared in the 1980s, as some have claimed.[10] Reviewing some of the cases does suggest a relationship with early discharge or inadequate treatment. But for others, particularly those related to infections or an inherited deficiency of the enzyme glucose-6-phosphate dehydrogenase, it is hard to understand why such cases would not have occurred at a steady, low level during the 1970s and 1980s.

iv The kernicterus alarm was sounded primarily by Drs Lois Johnson and Audrey Brown, both of whom were from a generation of paediatricians who trained when kernicterus was quite prevalent, in stark contrast to me; I still have never seen a case of neonatal kernicterus. In presentations and reports[9,10] they showed a graph that makes it appear that the number of kernicterus cases had been rising dramatically, but such a conclusion from this graph would be unwarranted, because the graph showed only cases that have come to their attention, and they only started asking people to tell them about cases around 1995–6.

v   Drs Johnson and Brown, joined by Dr Vinod Bhutani, reported on 90 cases from a kernicterus registry in 2002 (Journal of Pediatrics 2002;**140**:396–403), but their report does not help much with estimating the number of new cases annually as it includes no reference to a defined population base over a defined period of time and the registry's inclusion criteria for the diagnosis of kernicterus were not specified.

vi Recently she has also begun to address high contingency fees charged by plaintiff's attorneys, with which she has had considerable experience by now.

vii A particular problem is the difficulty of knowing what to do with the result. Because the test is far from perfect, proponents suggest that in order to avoid missing any cases of subsequent hyperbilirubinaemia, results of the pre-discharge bilirubin level need to be considered abnormal and repeated in about 60% of newborns,[16] and then in many cases repeated several more times, potentially leading to a lot of unnecessary trips to the doctor's office, laboratory tests and worry.

viii I also knew that the number 20 mg/dl was not based on particularly good data. Those of us on the guideline development committee realised that jaundice had previously been over-treated, so we added an arbitrary 5 mg/dl to previous treatment thresholds.

ix   This is a mission I have been pursuing since 1992, when the AAP Committee on Nutrition recommended screening many children for high blood cholesterol.[19]

x   The entire hearing, which makes fascinating reading, is available online at: http://commdocs.house.gov/committees/Trans/hpw104-63-000/hpw104-63_0-htm.

xi   Jan Lohr-Brown's testimony also included this further story: "Six years ago, when I addressed this subcommittee on the same issue, Lori Michaelson also testified. Lori, her husband, Mark, their 11-month-old daughter, Sabrina, and their two older sons were aboard that flight 232 in July 1989. In her testimony, Lori recalled her distress when one of my colleagues told her to place Sabrina on the floor for our emergency preparation. She said, 'I can still remember the look in that flight attendant's eyes as we both knew this baby had a slim chance of surviving a crash landing. Picture me, a person only five feet, three inches tall, trying to bend over to reach the floor to hold on to my baby' – a task that was almost physically impossible. ... On impact, Sabrina flew through the cabin, landed in an overhead storage bin, and was rescued by a heroic passenger who re-entered the fiery wreckage when he heard her tiny cries."

xii   I agreed to prepare a lecture on the topic for the International Centre for Health and Society at University College, London (where I was doing my sabbatical). Trisha and Brian heard that lecture, which is what led to this chapter.

xiii   Thanks to Brian Hurwitz for pointing this out in a letter to me following my lecture.

xiv   From: "Healing American Healthcare", originally a sermon given at multiple Unitarian Universalist congregations in the San Francisco Bay Area, also a talk at the David Rogers Health Policy Colloquium at the Cornell University School of Medicine, December 12, 2002. For full text, see http://itsa.ucsf.edu/~newman/ Healing_American_Healthcare_10Nov02.htm.

References

1   Davidson L, Merritt K, Weech A. Hyperbilirubinemia in the newborn. *Am J Dis Child* 1941;**61**:958–80.

2   Maisels M, Newman T. Jaundice in full-term and near-term babies who leave the hospital within 36 hours: The pediatrician's nemesis. In: Brittion J, ed. *Clinics in Perinatology*, vol 25. Philadelphia: WB Saunders, 1998, pp 295–302.

3   Watchko J, Oski F. Bilirubin 20 mg/dl = vigintiphobia. *Pediatrics* 1983;**71**:660–3.

4   Newman TB, Maisels MJ. Does hyperbilirubinemia damage the brain of healthy full-term infants? *Clin Perinatol* 1990;**17**(2):331–58.

5   Newman TB, Klebanoff MA. Neonatal hyperbilirubinemia and long-term outcome: another look at the Collaborative Perinatal Project. *Pediatrics* 1993;**92**(5):651–7.

6   Newman TB, Maisels MJ. Evaluation and treatment of jaundice in the term newborn: a kinder, gentler approach. *Pediatrics* 1992;**89**:809–18.

7   American Academy of Pediatrics. Provisional Committee for Quality Improvement and Subcommittee on Hyperbilirubinemia. Practice parameter: management of hyperbilirubinemia in the healthy term newborn. *Pediatrics* 1994;**94**(4 Pt 1):558–65.

8   Seidman DS, Paz I, Armon Y, Ergaz Z, Stevenson DK, Gale R. Effect of publication of the "Practice Parameter for the management of hyperbilirubinemia" on treatment of neonatal jaundice. *Acta Paediatr* 2001;**90**(3):292–5.

9   Brown A, Johnson L. Early discharge and reemergence of kernicterus in term infants. Presented at the 1995 Annual Meeting, American Academy of Pediatrics, Section on Perinatology, San Francisco, CA. 1995.

10   Brown AK, Johnson L. Loss of concern about jaundice and the reemergence of kernicterus in full term infants in the era of managed care. In: Fanaroff A, Klaus M, eds. *Yearbook of Neonatal and Perinatal Medicine*. St Louis: Mosby Yearbook, 1996, pp xvii–xxviii.

11   Ebbesen F. Recurrence of kernicterus in term and near-term infants in Denmark. *Acta Paediatr* 2000;**89**(10):121–37.

12   Newman T, Liljestrand P, Escobar G. Infants with bilirubin levels of 30 mg/dl or more in a large managed care organization. *Pediatrics* 2003;**111**(6):1303–11.

13 Appleby J, Davis R. Was it medical negligence, or bad luck? Judge, jury differ on boy's disability. *USA Today* 2000;October 11:1.

14 From the Centers for Disease Control and Prevention. Kernicterus in full-term infants – United States, 1994–1998. *JAMA* 2001;**286**(3):299–300.

15 Joint Commission on Accreditation of Hospital Organizations. Kernicterus threatens healthy newborns. *Sentinel Event Alert*, Issue 13, April 2001.

16 Bhutani VK, Johnson L, Sivieri EM. Predictive ability of a predischarge hour-specific serum bilirubin for subsequent significant hyperbilirubinemia in healthy term and near-term newborns. *Pediatrics* 1999;**103**(1):61–4.

17 Atkinson L, Escobar G, Takayama J, Newman T. Phototherapy use in jaundiced newborns in a large managed care organization: Do physicians adhere to the guideline? *Pediatrics* 2003;**111**:e555–61.

18 American Academy of Pediatrics. Restraint use on aircraft. Committee on Injury and Poison Prevention. *Pediatrics* 2001;**108**(5):1218–22.

19 American Academy of Pediatrics Committee on Nutrition. Statement on cholesterol. *Pediatrics* 1992;**90**(3):469–73.

20 Federal Aviation Administration. Report to Congress: Child Restraint Systems. Report of the Secretary of Transportation to the United States Congress pursuant to Section 522 of the Federal Aviation Administration Authorization Act of 1994, P.L. 1033–05. Washington, DC: US Department of Transportation, 1995.

21 Newman T, Johnston B, Grossman D. Effects and costs of requiring child restraint systems for young children traveling on commercial airplanes. *Arch Pediatrics Adolesc Med* 2003;**157**:969–74.

22 Brown-Lohr J. Testimony before the US House of Representatives, Subcommittee on Aviation. Hearing on H.R. 1309: Child safety restraint systems requirement on commercial aircraft. 1996: vol 2003.

23 Dawes R. A message from psychologists to economists: mere predictability doesn't matter like it should (without a good story appended to it). *J Economic Behav Org* 1999;**39**:29–40.

24 Tversky A, Kahneman D. Judgment under uncertainty: heuristics and biases. *Science* 1974;**185**:1124–31.

25 Newman TB, Maisels MJ. Less aggressive treatment of neonatal jaundice and reports of kernicterus: lessons about practice guidelines. *Pediatrics* 2000;**105**(1 Pt 3):24–5.

26 Adams J. *Taking account of societal concerns about risk: Framing the problem.* A report for the Health and Safety Executive. London: HSE, 2002.

27 Eddy D. Breast cancer screening in women younger than 50 years of age: what's next? *Ann Intern Med* 1997;**127**:1035–6.

28 Smith V, Desvousges W. An empirical analysis of the economic value of risk changes. *J Political Economy* 1987;**95**:89–114.

29 Featherstonhaugh D, Slovic P, Johnson S, Friedrich J. Insensitivity to the value of human life: a study of psychophysical numbing. *J Risk Uncertainty* 1997;**14**: 283–300.

30 Gyrd-Hansen D, Kristiansen IS, Nexoe J, Nielsen JB. Effects of baseline risk information on social and individual choices. *Med Decis Making* 2002;**22**(1):71–5.

Commentary

BRIAN BALMER

Why would people place more faith in stories than statistics? While the academic literature does not provide any definitive answer, recent research on the public understanding of science provides us with pointers. Although the public is far from homogeneous, there is strong evidence from qualitative studies that, contrary to the so-called "deficit model" where the public is construed as totally ignorant, people do not wilfully ignore scientific and technical expertise.[1] Instead, they sometimes make sense of complex issues, such as statistics, risk or genetics, by relating abstract information to specific contexts and even develop their own "lay expertise".[2]

Such lay expertise can sometimes be technical knowledge, for example certain AIDS activists have studied the science of their disease and used this knowledge to negotiate how clinical trials are carried out.[3] More usually, lay expertise is different in kind to the generalising tendencies of statistics and science, focusing on local and experientially gained knowledge. So, an expert paediatrician, Thomas Newman, still learns things in court from parents who have become expert in managing their children's disability. The flight attendant quoted in the chapter has unenviable expertise gained first-hand in an airline disaster.

Sometimes lay expertise directly challenges expert assumptions about how society operates. In the 1970s, British agricultural workers had their claims about the harmful effects of the pesticide 2,4,5-T dismissed as anecdotal and were repeatedly told that scientific evidence contradicted their stories.[4] The pesticide was safe, claimed government scientific advisers, so long as the manufacturer's instructions were followed. This contention was challenged, not because of the science *per se*, but because "following the safety instructions" involved taking such impracticable measures that it would have meant the workers could not do their jobs. One worker compared the situation with working in a laundry and being told to avoid the steam. In this case, local knowledge about the practicalities of day-to-day spraying was incompatible with the implicit and impoverished assumptions about working practices adopted by scientists in the laboratory test environment. In another example, predictions of the effects of the Chernobyl explosion on British livestock were challenged by farmers because scientists generalised findings from clay soils to acid peats. But, as Wynne has shown, radioactive caesium behaves very differently in the peats found in upland areas.[5]

Lay expertise does not always contradict technical expertise. This point is exemplified in interviews with people diagnosed with inherited familial hypercholesterolaemia, where higher cholesterol levels raise the chances of a heart attack, but also where there are no symptoms that individuals can detect. These patients:

> accept the diagnosis they are given and follow medical advice, but most of them only do so to the extent that it can be accommodated relatively easily into their daily lives ... The "scientific fact" of above-average personal risk is consciously weighed against the implications for a restrictive existence [and a compromise is reached]. People are not ignorant of, nor do they fail to understand, the technical assessment ... [instead they] evaluate its implications for action with regard to the quality of their whole lives.[6]

All of these observations about lay expertise suggest that any tension between expert statistics and lay narratives should not be construed as a straightforward confrontation between truth and fiction. Narratives may capture contested values that technical information masks. Sociologist Dorothy Nelkin gives a hypothetical example of an experiment involving vivisection.[7] Pharmaceutical manufacturers and anti-vivisectionists might (hypothetically) agree on the soundness of the empirical data obtained. Indeed, they all might concede that the experiment will lead to new drugs, and that the animals will suffer. But the response to the question "is it worth it" is likely to provoke different answers, each related to competing sets of values. Likewise, with our United Airlines flight attendant, her narrative allows her to articulate that, for her, the seat belt question is less about costs and more about equity: "that small children deserve the same measure of safety which every other passenger enjoys". If this point needs further clarification, try a thought experiment in which you react to the same calculations and debates, but in this imaginary society at issue is the extra burden of introducing seat-belts for women or ethnic minorities who, unlike the rest, travel in separate seats without safety restraints.

Of course, the vivisection example is simplistic in its division between irrefutable facts and contestable values. Regulatory science is rife with disagreements over the interpretation of data and, more philosophically problematic, what will even count as acceptable evidence.[8,9] Moreover, aggregated, generalised information such as statistics, smooths over assumptions and local variations.[10,11] Calculation of the trade-off between extra costs of flights and lives saved inevitably makes assumptions about such matters as: whether and how costs are passed on to consumers; that risk is best measured by accidents per miles travelled (rather than per journeys taken, or time spent travelling); whether one ignores the safety of the drive to and from the airport; or that people will not take the train or even stay at home (and do something else more or less risky). Now, although these may all be perfectly defensible assumptions, they remain implicit and not necessarily grounded in systematic empirical evidence. My aim in raising this point is not to denigrate or ignore the statistics, rather to say that even the most robust statistics will rest on assumptions – stories, if you like – about how the world works. Furthermore, once the statistics have been compiled, a narrative still needs to be told about what the statistics mean.

What this suggests is that the epistemological polarisation between statistics and narrative, that their power arises from totally different sources, is overstated. This, in turn, challenges the conclusion that decisions based on numbers are (or ought to be) inevitably superior to other ways of thinking about problems that are more narrative and contextually based. Instead, on closer examination, statistics may show themselves not to be wholly different from, but instead rather special forms of, narrative.

References

1 Gregory J, Miller S. *Science in Public: Communication, Culture and Credibility.* New York: Plenum, 1998.
2 Kerr A. The New Genetics and Health: Mobilizing Lay Expertise. *Public Understanding of Science* 1998;7:41–60.
3 Epstein S. *Impure Science: AIDS Activism and the Politics of Knowledge.* Berkeley, CA: University of California Press, 1996.
4 Wynne B. Frameworks of Rationality in Risk Management: Towards the Testing of Naive Sociology. In: Brown J, ed. *Environmental Threats: Perception Analysis and Management.* London and New York: Belhaven Press, 1989.
5 Wynne B. Misunderstood misunderstandings: social identities and public uptake of science. In: Irwin A, Wynne B. *Misunderstanding Science? The Public Reconstruction of Science and Technology.* Cambridge: Cambridge University Press, 1996, pp 19–46.
6 Lambert H, Rose H. Disembodied knowledge? Making sense of medical science. In: Irwin A, Wynne B. *Misunderstanding Science? The Public Reconstruction of Science and Technology.* Cambridge: Cambridge University Press, 1996, pp 63–83.
7 Nelkin D. Science, Technology and Political Conflict: Analysing the Issues. In: Nelkin D, ed. *Controversy: The Politics of Technical Decisions.* London: Sage, 1992.
8 Jasanoff S. Contested Boundaries in Policy-Relevant Science. *Soc Stud Sci* 1987;17:195–230.
9 Gillespie B *et al.* Risk Assessment in the United States and Great Britain: The Case of Aldrin/Dieldrin. In: Barnes B, Edge D, eds. *Science in Context: Readings in the Sociology of Science.* Milton Keynes: Open University Press, 1982.
10 Scott JC. *Seeing Like A State: How Certain Schemes to Improve the Human Condition Have Failed.* New Haven, CT: Yale University Press, 1998.
11 Porter T. *Trust in Numbers: The Pursuit of Objectivity in Science and Public Life.* Princeton, NJ: Princeton University Press, 1995.

Section 3:
Meta-narratives

16: Narratives of health inequality: interpreting the determinants of health

GARETH WILLIAMS

> Ah fuck it man stories, stories, life's full of stories, they're there to help ye out, when ye're in trouble, deep shit, they come to the rescue, and one thing ye learn in life is stories. Sammy's head was fucking full of them.
>
> (U Kelman, 1994)[1]

Introduction

Narrative analysis in medical sociology focuses upon individuals' experiences of ill health as expressed in the stories they tell or the accounts they give. Telling "a story" and providing "an account" each has very different, multiple connotations of course, but both can be said to produce "narratives" in some broad sense. Whether self-authored or co-authored, narratives are seemingly authentic representations of the ontology of experience. In other words, if life is lived as a narrative, then the representation of that life in narrative terms will contain sharp truths about the life of the person.

If narratives were only opportunities for self-examination their importance to the social sciences would be limited. However, "life's full of stories", James Kelman's fictional anti-hero tells us,[1] filling the cultural maps of our everyday lives, and for this reason narratives are important also for what they tell us about society. Narratives are small windows opening onto the gritty realities of social structure and social change from a particular position and point of view. In this sense, they provide not only truth about personal experience but also material through which we can understand more fully the dynamics of a time and a place.

For much of the time human lives are routine, mundane, and unproblematic, if not hassle-free. However, there are times when crises occur, taken-for-granted roles and relationships are disrupted, and everyday categories of explanation and understanding are challenged.[2] When you are in deep trouble, you need stories to help you out, to "come to the rescue", to use the quote from Kelman again. This process of "narrative reconstruction" is one through which people "reconstitute and repair ruptures between body, self and world by linking and interpreting different aspects of biography in order to realign present and past and self and society".[3] It is a way of understanding the relationship between agency and structure within the frame of personal experience. Although not often perceived as such within the sight lines of medical sociology, it is a process that draws on an imagery of hope and despair that has deep cultural roots.[4]

Taking the idea of narratives as a window upon society as my starting point, I want to explore the use of narratives to inform our understanding of the dynamics of health inequalities. The existence of health inequalities in Britain and other late-modern, capitalist societies is incontrovertible. In recent years explanations for these inequalities have focused upon the impact of social class and other inequalities in wealth, power and social position; emphasising that this is not just a question of there being poor people in society, but rather that there is a gradient marking the distribution of inequality throughout society. The ways in which these inequalities work to create differential patterns of morbidity and mortality in populations are complex. However, in recent years it has been recognised that the startling mortality and morbidity differentials in adult populations are the product of cumulative lifetime exposures to a range of social and physical hazards, clustering in the intense, multidimensional experience of social exclusion in particular places.

Much of the debate about health inequalities has quite properly taken place in relation to statistical evidence, focusing on the size, proportion, and distribution of health inequalities. However, it has increasingly been argued that if we are to understand the causal processes whereby social conditions shape health, we need to examine how social conditions are experienced, perceived and handled, and how they constrain the freedom of people to act in such a way that those conditions could be transformed, adapted or avoided in different ways. Narratives and narrative reconstruction offer a micro-realist perspective on the possibilities of health promotion and community health development, providing a "contextual" understanding of health inequalities. In this chapter I discuss the theoretical arguments pointing to the need for narrative approaches to developing fuller understanding of health inequalities, and go on to use a narrative approach to qualitative data about how people make sense of the social forces that shape their experiences of health and ill health. I argue that this approach complements epidemiological research on health inequalities by illuminating "the hidden injuries of class" rooted in history and social conditions.[5]

Place and time

During the 1980s the debate about health inequalities, in the UK at least, was shaped by the publication of the Black Report[6] and the cold reception it received in the emerging neo-liberal environment of Thatcherite economic and social policy. The Black Report's emphasis on structural change and economic equality implied redistributive policies that were out of kilter with the emerging *zeitgeist* of possessive individualism. For many years after that, the ideological conflict of the times sharpened and polarised the debate about health inequalities. There was an either/or quality to the discussion of Black's four explanations: materialist/structuralist; cultural/behavioural; artefact; and natural or social selection. As Macintyre, looking back, later concluded, the distinctions between these categories were in danger of becoming "false antitheses".[7]

In subsequent years a number of longitudinal data sets became available for analysis of the relationships between health and social factors over time. This allowed for a much more subtle and sophisticated understanding of the forces shaping individual lives, and the complex ways in which socioeconomic, cultural, and psychosocial factors interact to produce population health differences. Among those who continued to regard class inequality in material resources and structural conditions as the prime mover of health inequalities, it nevertheless became clear that our understanding of these relationships had to become more subtle and fine-grained:

> "social class", at any given point is but a very partial indicator of a whole sequence, a "probabilistic cascade" of events which need to be seen in combination if the effects of social environment on health are to be understood.[8]

The concept of a probabilistic cascade is an alluring one, expressing the way in which things can build up over time, exposing people to different kinds of risks and benefits at different points in the cycle or course of life – the way in which: "advantages and disadvantages tend to cluster cross-sectionally and accumulate longitudinally".[9] It implies a "causal narrative"[10] unfolding from the start of life, with numerous points of stress and strain, shaped by local circumstances that are themselves dependent upon national policies and global economic and social change.[11] Within this overwhelmingly determinist picture, there are also times of choice and situations of opportunity, but these too are unequally distributed in the population.[12]

Much of the sociological literature on health inequalities has struggled to move beyond a "social factors" approach that mimics epidemiology and brackets out any broader reflection on either social structures or the meanings that people give to the situations of inequality they experience. However, a constructive dialogue is now emerging between social epidemiology and more interpretative forms of social science.[13] The developments arising out of this dialogue emphasise the gains to be made from exploring lay perceptions of, and narratives about, health inequalities[14] in order to help explain why individuals and groups behave the way they do in relation to wider social structures – to link agency and structure to use the sociological language – through a detailed examination of contexts.

A deeper understanding of the complex relationships between an individual's capacity to act and the wider social structures/ relationships of power and control in which he or she operates is central to our understanding of the processes that generate and sustain inequalities in health experience across modern societies. Reconceptualising the notion of places or contexts to allow us to explore the way in which structures work themselves through into the dynamics of everyday life is central to this endeavour. Places can be conceptualised as the locations for "structuration" – the interrelationship of the conscious intentions and actions of individuals and groups and the "environment" of cultural, social, and economic forces in which people exist. Alongside this, there is recognition of the need for a deeper understanding of the role of the "subjective" – and its narrative articulation in the form of lay knowledge – in mediating these interrelationships.

Places have histories and people have biographies that they articulate through stories or narratives. The history of sociology is replete with attempts to theorise this macro–micro link, to look at the intersection of history and biography, but the theoretical directions suggested by this work have rarely been taken up in empirical research on inequalities in health. Attention to the meanings people attach to their experience of places and how this shapes social action could provide a missing link in our understanding of the causes of inequalities in health. In particular, the articulation of these meanings – this lay knowledge – in narrative form could provide invaluable insights into the dynamic relationships between human agency and the wider structures of power and control that underpin inequalities in health. Inside the occasionally convoluted theorising of the late Pierre Bourdieu is a simple message: "The social world is accumulated history",[15] and the stories about the "weight of the world"[16] hammer home the point that structure can be very heavy indeed, undermining individual and collective capacities and capabilities.

The weight of the world

What people know is not simply datum for epidemiological or sociological extraction. It co-constitutes the world as it is, and helps social scientists to understand how structures determine health and well-being through where people live and what they do. In some of the work that colleagues and I have undertaken over a number of years we explore "lay knowledge" as a way into theorising the structure–agency problem. We have done this by looking at the recursive relationships, to use the jargon, between people's "knowledgeable narratives"[17] and the places or locales in which they live. These narratives have been collected through in-depth unstructured/ semi-structured interviews, in which people talk about their lives at length in response to an interviewer's questions or comments. However, narrative analysis depends not on the reproduction of lengthy verbatim quotation – though it can take this form – but upon the identification of key meaning-points in the story being told. Narrative analysis may therefore be performed upon small fragments of data.

In one study in inner city Salford in the north-west of England undertaken in the mid-1990s, for example, we looked at people's perceptions and understandings of "health risks".[18] The interviews ranged across personal and social realities in an attempt to explore where the risks fall:

> *I think the biggest health risk is mentally ... 'cause it's a lot of pressure and there's nothing really for you to do ... you're sort of segregated all the time.*

In this powerful statement a middle-aged man is thinking about the position in which he finds himself and the forces that shape his experience of ill health. He resists the pressure to see everything as either his fault, or the fault of someone else, and begins to develop a sociological analysis. Within this fragment of a story he identifies the ways in which the world weighs upon him, drawing us into an understanding of what in our work-stress culture is an almost counterintuitive argument that the pressures which may lead to mental ill health are produced by the absence rather than the excess of activity. The startling use of "segregated" also invites pause for thought. Here is a white man living in an economically highly developed "free society", close to the heart of one of Britain's major cities, using a word more commonly associated with apartheid South Africa, or the deep south of the United States before the civil rights movement.

What does this narrative fragment tell us? This extract itself cannot be described as a story. It is something said in an interview that draws our attention to an analysis based on this man's biographical experiences. We could talk about his socioeconomic circumstances in more objective detail: the amount that he gets in benefits, the kind of housing he lives in, the accessibility of shops and public services, the quality of his friendships; all of which would be very important. But within this small fragment of the long story told in the interview, we are able to see "first order" lay concepts being used to generate an understanding that could not be delivered by "social facts" alone. It tells us something about the social organisation of everyday life in an inner-city locality. It begins to describe some of the effects of this on personal experience, and it offers certain concepts – pressure, segregation – with which we can better understand the way in which the determinants of health and inequalities in health play out in the relationship between this man and the place in which he lives. It thickens our understanding of social scientific concepts like "social exclusion" and "inequality".

The fragment tells us something about the life of this man. But we wouldn't want to stop at that point. It also offers us a window onto certain aspects of the society in which he lives. He is offering an interpretation of the multivariate economic, social, and cultural factors affecting him within the compressed or condensed form of his own life. It is precisely because the story is personal that it is able to offer a sociological interpretation that draws structure, context, behaviour, and ill health into a single frame. In this way, fragments of the narratives people develop for making sense of the trouble they are in can be highly political. Another respondent from the same study told us:

Smoking and drinking and drug taking, I put it down to one thing ... until money is spent on these areas ... there doesn't seem to be much point in trying to stop people smoking and what else. As long as the environment is going down the pan the people will go down with it.

Risk factor epidemiology tends to assume a freedom to make healthy choices that is out of line with what many lay people experience as real possibilities in their everyday lives. Knowledgeable narratives illustrate the need to contextualise risk factors – smoking, diet, alcohol, lack of exercise – by reference to the wider material and environmental conditions in which the risks are embedded. The respondents in this study understood the behavioural risk factors that made ill health more likely and for which they were, in a limited sense, responsible, but they were also aware that the risks they faced were part of social conditions that they could do little to change. For these working class residents of a declining inner city the "way of life" –in this case unemployment, poor housing, low income, stressful and sometimes violent lives – provided a context for "making sense" of smoking, drinking and drug taking, and other "behaviours". These narrative fragments, elements of stories, are complex bodies of contextualised rationality that are central to our understanding of social structure and its impact.[19]

Here we see, therefore, a reflexive understanding of "collective lifestyles"[20] and an analysis that recognises the limited purchase that practices and capabilities can have on change in the more deprived areas of economically developed societies. In a more recent analysis of data from a large study of people's perceptions of health inequalities the intense limitations on people's capacities to deploy "causal powers" were clearly articulated.[21] One single mother living on a housing estate with a "reputation" told us:

> *The doctor put me on Prozac a few months back, for living here, because it's depressing. You get up, you look around, and all you see is junkies ... I know one day I will come off, I will get off here. I mean I started drinking a hell of a lot more since I've been on here. I drink every night. I have a drink every night just to get to sleep. I smoke more as well. There's a lot of things ...*

In these quotations from research interviews, words and phrases like "segregated all the time", "the people will go down with it" and "there's a lot of things ..." carry a heavy semantic load that it is difficult to unpack with any certainty or finality. There are many different interpretations that could be made of what these people are saying, interpretations that they themselves might contest. The point is that their stories *are* interpretative. They are not merely descriptions waiting for social scientists to interpret them, and they invite us to acknowledge the ability of people to turn routine, taken-for-granted knowledge into discourse or narrative, and the need to find ways of interpreting the relationship between structure, context, and experience through a reading of people's own stories.

Exploration of the links between individual biographies and life courses is a new and important dimension of research on the links between social structure and health. This does not imply that material circumstances are not crucial, but rather that one of the routes through which material disadvantage affects behaviour and health is through people's ability to construct a sense of identity and purpose under very difficult social and economic conditions. In turn, their ability or capability to do this may be linked to the relationship between the critical periods and pathways of their own life courses and the places in which they are living.

Knowledgeable narratives and social action

Narratives provide a link between experience and structure, and in so doing they provide some understanding of what to do in difficult situations. Indeed, they are often revealed in situations in which difficulties or crises threaten to overwhelm and something must be done. Somers has recently developed a set of concepts that bring into the foreground the concept of identity and the role of narratives in an attempt to bring a new perspective to some of the problems contained in social theories of action. She argues that recent research is revealing the substance of narratives as central to our understanding of social action:

> that social life is storied and that narrative is an ontological condition of social life ... showing us that stories guide action; that people construct identities (however multiple and changing) by locating themselves or being located within a repertoire of emplotted stories; that "experience" is constituted through narratives; that people make sense of what has happened and is happening to them by attempting to assemble or in some way to integrate these happenings within one or more narratives; and that people are guided to act in certain ways and not others on the basis of the projections, expectations and memories derived from a multiplicity but ultimately limited repertoire of available social, public and cultural narratives.[22]

Knowledgeable narratives connect experience to structure in terms of a personal understanding of episodes rather than an abstract conceptualisation of events. The integrative act counters the disintegrating effects of difficult personal troubles. Somers identifies four dimensions of narrative: ontological, public, conceptual, and "meta". Ontological narratives, she argues, are used to define who we are and provide the basis for knowing what to do. It is through these that apparently disconnected sets of events are turned into meaningful episodes, as seen in the examples quoted from research interviews. Public narratives are those attached to cultural or institutional formations, such as families or workplaces, often by the mass media that transcend the individual. They often provide the legitimating context for ontological narratives. Meta-narratives are "master" narratives of progress, decline, crisis, which transcend the immediate context and are often used politically to construct a particular ideological position. Conceptual narratives are those which researchers construct, using concepts that lie outside both ontological and public narratives, drawing on them both but introducing concepts such as social class, behaviour change, mortality rate, and so on which might not be found in either ontological or public narratives.

From a theoretical point of view, Somers argues that the analytical challenge is to develop concepts that will allow us to capture the narrativity through which agency is negotiated, identities are constructed and social action mediated. She suggests that two central components here are narrative identity and relational settings – the latter being relations between people, narratives, and institutions. These notions, she suggests, provide a conceptual bridge to (re)-introduce time, space, relationships, and cultural practices into the process whereby people are categorised in research.

In relation to the determinants of health, personal narratives are characteristically linked to wider sets of changes. In situations such as the recent widespread announcements of the closure of steelworks in

South Wales, to take one example (there are numerous others in the global economy), we can see the notion of ontological narratives of health and illness explicitly bound up with public narratives of identity, work, and family life, and metanarratives of decline, injustice, and the end of history.

Following a major strategic review in February 2001 Corus plc announced that they were going to restructure their enterprise and activities in Wales. The company had 64 900 employees at the end of 2000, with approximately 33 000 of those employed in the UK, almost 11 000 of them working in Wales. The expectation was that the number of Welsh employees would be reduced to about 7000 by 2002, with well-founded anxiety that further jobs would go in the near future. In response to the restructuring, I was part of a team that undertook a major review of the likely impact and implications of the Corus decision. One small part of this involved interviewing a number of people working in the towns and villages within Blaenau Gwent close to the Ebbw Vale steelworks – health professionals, church ministers, welfare officers, and other "key informants", asking them about what they thought was going to happen in the area.[23] In addition to the effects of the direct loss of jobs on individuals and their families, many people with deep ties to the area were only too well aware that the direct loss of jobs in steel was only part of the story. In such circumstances, not only do individual workers feel the harshness of redundancy, the community as a whole is undermined.

One health visitor working in the area said:

People talk not only about the effect on individuals; it's the effect on the borough – everybody, regardless of whether they are employed by Corus or not. I think that there is a huge concern [...] that in an area that appeared to be going downhill anyway this is the final nail in the coffin.

Blaenau Gwent is a massively deprived area, all of whose electoral wards are ranked within the 40 per cent most deprived wards in Wales. It has amongst the lowest levels of earnings in Britain, a large percentage of the population with no qualifications, and high levels of long-term ill health. Moreover, with low car ownership and limited access to public transport the prospects of commuting to work are limited.

The nature of the work – in coal and steel – and its dominant relationship to the community generated powerful social solidarity. The withdrawal of the major industries from Blaenau Gwent changed the social and physical landscape. The same health visitor said:

Abertillery breaks my heart because it just was not like it looks now, it's just a dump.

Many respondents talked about the way in which the running down of the steelworks, as well as the mines, affected the way in which local people interacted with each other. Solidarity extended beyond the work into the "social capital" of the local community. An educational welfare officer told us:

The changes in the area over the past thirty years have been tremendous. It had a feeling all of its own thirty years ago, a very strong community of miners and steelworkers [...] and now that's gone.

A district nurse who had always worked in the area spoke in similar terms, drawing attention to the impact of these changes on structures of feeling:

That sort of comradeship has all gone. You knew who you could trust and everyone would help you, but that is disappearing, that sort of feeling is disappearing.

The nature of the work defined the kind of relationships that emerged: the communities, the politics, and the aesthetics. The sights, sounds, and smells associated with the steelworks imprinted themselves on the social and physical character of the surrounding towns. We see in these excerpts from interviews an understanding of the interweaving of personal narratives and social history. The sense of loss and decline is simultaneously expressed, in Somers' terms, in ontological, public, and metanarratives. Whereas in the past solidarity provided the basis for union and political action, the decline over thirty years and more has created a situation in which the resources for hope and resistance are depleted.

Not only are the people of the area poorer because of the loss of work, the historical evidence of what the place was and what the people did has been taken away. In Christopher Meredith's novel about a declining steel town, one of the main characters contemplates the last slab to come out of the mill:

Odourless invisible history would blow them all apart and they would hurtle away from each other through space and never really understand what had shifted them. Except blowing apart was the wrong idea because it was a continuing process, evolving and breaking slowly and then occasionally twitching like this. And it included everything.[24]

The decision to close the steelworks in Ebbw Vale can be seen as the last twitch of a long process of breaking down. The personal consequences of the historical process of "breaking slowly" and "twitching" can be seen in a fragment from an interview with a church minister:

In the space of six months about two years ago I buried five drug-related [deaths]. The youngest was 18 [years of age] and the oldest was a 27-year-old mother who lived in one of the streets up here. And I knew her parents fairly well, and she left a three-year-old boy for her parents to look after. It's a very, very, very real problem.

Poverty, inequality, social exclusion – however we describe the distribution of resources and opportunities – have direct consequences for individual lives: educational failure, crime, heart disease, drugs, and alcohol. Things – relationships, roles, jobs, thoughts, actions – are fractured and fragmented, no longer making sense in terms of what people understand from past experience. What our respondents spoke about were people hurtling away from each other, a process of fragmentation that is the condition underlying many of the problems people face. These narrative fragments were framed within an historical analysis of decline, providing a rich context for our understanding of the way in which ill health is determined by social forces and people's responses to it.

Conclusion

In thinking about developments in the analysis of social structure and health there is a widespread acceptance of the need for a deeper and more fine-grained understanding of the relationship between the individual and his or her social context. In some ways poverty, economic inequality, and the social conditions associated with them remain "explanation enough" of excess mortality and morbidity in particular populations and places. However, thinking about the "weight of the world", Bourdieu argued:

> using material poverty as the sole measure of all suffering keeps us from seeing and understanding a whole side of the suffering characteristic of the social order which, although it has undoubtedly reduced poverty overall (though less than often claimed) has also multiplied the social spaces (specialized fields and subfields) and set up the conditions for an unprecedented development of all kinds of ordinary suffering.[25]

In turning events into episodes, narratives provide an analytic opportunity for exploring the links between structure and experience and between explanation and action. Through exploration of the words people use in making sense of their circumstances we see the way in which the spaces of "ordinary suffering" have multiplied. Stories about these spaces are often very personal, but they are woven into interpretations about what is going on in the social worlds in which people live and work, or lose their work. In the case of the people living in Blaenau Gwent, in particular, people who were not themselves directly employed in the steel industry, we can see the way in which the experiences of individual people are explicitly linked to public narratives about workplaces and households and to metanarratives about progress and decline. These kinds of accounts are important, therefore, not only for what they tell us about individual lives, but also as windows upon the structures of society and the impact of these on experience.

References

1 Kelman J. *How Late It Was, How Late.* London: Minerva, 1994.
2 Bury M. Chronic illness as biographical disruption. *Sociol Health Illness* 1982;**4**:167–82.
3 Williams GH. The genesis of chronic illness: narrative reconstruction. *Sociol Health Illness* 1984;**6**:175–200.
4 Stachniewski J. *The Persecutory Imagination: English Puritanism and the Literature of Religious Despair.* Oxford: Oxford University Press, 1991.
5 Sennett R, Cobb J. *The Hidden Injuries of Class.* New York: Vintage Books, 1973.
6 Department of Health and Social Security. *Inequalities in Health: the Report of a Working Group (the Black Report).* London: HMSO, 1980.
7 Macintyre S. The Black Report and beyond: what are the issues? *Soc Sci Med* 1997;**44**:723–45.
8 Bartley M, Blane D, Davey Smith G. *The Sociology of Health Inequalities.* Oxford: Blackwell, 1998.
9 Blane D. The life course, the social gradient and health. In: Marmot M, Wilkinson R, eds. *Social Determinants of Health.* Oxford: Oxford University Press, 1999.
10 Prandy K. Class, stratification, and inequalities in health: a comparison of the Registrar General's Social Classes and the Cambridge Scale. *Sociol Health Illness* 1999;**21**:466–84.
11 Graham H. Building an interdisciplinary science of health inequalities: the example of lifecourse research. *Soc Sci Med* 2002;**55**:2005–16.
12 Williams GH. The determinants of health: structure, context and agency. *Sociol Health Illness* 2003;**25**:131–54.
13 Graham H. *Understanding Health Inequalities* Buckingham: Open University Press, 2001.
14 Popay J, Williams GH, Thomas C, Gatrell A. Theorising inequalities in health: the place of lay knowledge. In: Bartley M, Blane D, Davey Smith G, eds. *The Sociology of Health Inequalities.* Oxford: Blackwell, 1998.
15 Bourdieu P. Forms of capital. In: Richardson JG, eds. *Handbook of Theory and Research in the Sociology of Education* 1986 Westport, CT: Greenwood publishing group p 241
16 Bourdieu P, Ferguson PP, Emanuel S et al. *The Weight of the World: Social Suffering in Contemporary Society.* Cambridge: Polity, 1999.
17 Williams GH. Knowledgeable narratives. *Anthropol Med* 2000;**7**:135–40.
18 Williams GH, Popay J, Bissell P. Public health risks in the material world: barriers to social movements in health. In: Gabe J, ed. *Medicine, Health and Risk.* Oxford: Blackwell, 1995.
19 Good BJ. *Medicine, Rationality and Experience: an Anthropological Perspective.* Cambridge: Cambridge University Press, 1994.
20 Frohlich KL, Potvin L, Chabot P, Corin E. A theoretical and empirical analysis of context: neighbourhoods, youth and smoking. *Soc Sci Med* 2002;**54**:1401–17.
21 Popay J, Thomas C, Williams GH, Bennett S, Gatrell A, Bostock L. A proper place to live: health inequalities, agency, and the normative dimensions of space. *Soc Sci Med* 2003;**57**:155–69.

22 Somers M. The narrative constitution of identity: a relational and network approach. *Theory and Society* 1994;**23**:605–649.
23 Fairbrother P, Morgan KJ *et al*. *Steel Communities Study*. Cardiff University: Regeneration Institute, 2001.
24 Meredith C. *Shifts*. Bridgend: Seren, 1988, p 211.
25 Bourdieu P, Ferguson PP, Emanuel S *et al*. *The Weight of the World: Social Suffering in Contemporary Society*. Cambridge: Polity, 1999, p 4.

17: Narratives of displacement and identity

VIEDA SKULTANS

God's punishment contains its own reward, namely the ability to long for a paradise lost.

(E Wiesel, 1996)[1]

A man had three sons. Two were clever and the third went to England

(Arvids Sermulins, Bristol, March 2003)

Introduction

My chapter deals with narratives of displacement and exile from both an autobiographical and an anthropological perspective. There is a vast and complex socio-anthropological and psychiatric literature on these topics. The relationship between migration and mental health has been examined from Odegaard onwards. The term "culture shock" was first introduced to describe the impact of social and geographical displacement on psychological health.[2] It has been used extensively to understand the reactions of migrant communities, volunteer workers, and gap year students.[3] There is a growing literature on language problems as a barrier to communicating traumatic events to medical personnel.[4,5] However, with a few notable exceptions, there is relatively little on the actual experience of displacement.[6,7] Thus although readers may not need to be reminded of the potentially destabilising effects of exile and its accompanying susceptibility to psychological malaise and ill health, the actual experience of exile may be unfamiliar. Increasingly we have come to recognise the importance of acknowledging and interrogating the ethnographer's experience as a resource rather than an impediment. Judith Okely, author of a seminal work on autobiography and anthropology,[8] emphasises that the anthropologist can provide the academic community with unique insights into a particular cultural phenomenon by telling their own story: "The concern for an autobiographical element in anthropology is to work through the specificity of the anthropologist's self in order to contextualise and transcend it" (p 2). This is what I attempt to do in this chapter.

Narrative as a research tool has both been criticised on the grounds of giving an incomplete and unreliable version of the truth and, conversely extolled on the grounds of giving a more authentic "experience-near" version of the truth. My own position is closer to that of Rorty, who states that we have a duty to listen to narrative simply because the narrator is a human being. And if the told story diverges from the lived story it may well be that the told story tells us more about the values and aspirations of the narrator than might the lived story.

Hard facts on the incidence of psychiatric breakdown among Latvian exiles in post-war Britain are difficult to come by. In part because the documentation was never systematically gathered and in part because there was so much shame attached the perceived loss of control associated with mental illness. But anecdotal evidence suggests that the incidence of psychiatric hospitalisation and illness was high. My mother recollects doing Sunday tours of the psychiatric hospitals of southern England with the Lutheran pastor to visit Latvian patients who spoke no English. My conversations with an elderly GP of Latvian origin, Dr Svene, conjure up a similar picture. I have a list of some seventy Latvian names and the psychiatric hospitals to which they were admitted from a librarian who worked for the Latvian Welfare Fund (sent by Laimonis Cerins). However, the thin sheets of paper bear no dates or ages, nor do they tell us how complete this listing by an anonymous author was. In a sense, these people were lucky to have reached England at all. Had they broken down sooner they would not have gained entry to Britain. Kathryn Hulme describes how displaced persons who broke down in transit were shipped back to Germany: "The mumbling phantoms our doctors led off those ships and escorted to a mental institution were not aware they had made a round trip"[9] (p 221). Studies of psychiatric breakdown were carried out on the much larger Polish community and they suggest that the process of exile might have been even more difficult for the much smaller Latvian community.[10]

My interest in anthropology as the study of other cultures no doubt has its roots in my own experience as a child in a refugee family, my early memories of serial and unpredictable movements in displaced persons camps in Germany, and my ultimate belonging to two European cultures which nevertheless have radically different mind-sets and traditions. As Gadamer has so insightfully reminded us, learning a second language is a radically different exercise from learning a first language.[11] So too socialisation into a birth culture is different from socialisation into an adopted culture. In the first instance everything is taken for granted, whereas in the second instance everything is subject to questioning and filtered through one's earlier knowledge of the first language and culture. The fusion of the personal and the academic is evident in this chapter, which draws both upon my autobiographical and anthropological knowledge and uses my personal account to illustrate more general concepts of displacement and identity.

I arrived in England as an infantile appendage of the European Volunteer Workers Movement: not able to speak English let alone to do much hard work. The labour shortage in post-war Britain meant that key industries could not function and that their collapse undermined the economy. An editorial in *The Times* ran: "Want of labour is hampering the progress of a number of industries vital to the national well-being. The case for selective immigration of up to 500 000 workers during the next few years is exceedingly strong and it is regrettable that neither the government nor the labour movement appear to have given much thought to it" (17 January 1947). The coalmines, textile industries, and hospitals were all short of workers. As a result of this movement, some 80 000 workers of East European origin were removed from the displaced persons (DP) camps in Germany. Among them were Serbs, Ukrainians, Estonians, Lithuanians, and some 18 000 Latvians. These East Europeans constituted the first major influx of immigrants after World War Two. England in the late 1940s was not prepared for the values of multiculturalism and the displaced persons were referred to as "vagabonds and thieves". Many workers experienced hostility and derision. My early months in school were difficult because I could not speak English. On my way home from school I was regularly ambushed by the boys in my class, trussed up with rope, and beaten. The East Europeans might have seen themselves as political refugees but their host country saw them as economic migrants. Hulme, who worked as a welfare officer in the DP camps in Germany describes "country after country reaching in for its pound of good muscular working flesh"[9] (p 159). Each country had its own requirements and set its own terms. None wanted the economically dependent, that is, the young, the old, and the frail. In our case this meant that my mother and I were allowed entry into England in the winter of 1948 but my grandmother was left behind and could only join us some three years later. Hulme describes this as a "macabre stock market that dealt with bodies rather than bonds"[9] (p 201). Refugees, no matter what their educational and professional background, were accepted if they contracted to do a minimum of two years' unskilled work.

As Gunther Grass writes in *Crabwalk*,[12] my own life story began several years before I was born. In June 1940 as the period of the first Soviet occupation of Latvia drew to a close my maternal grandfather was arrested, tortured, and killed. Notes on his arrest referred to the fact that he was a plutocrat and that he had bought his daughter, my mother, a Steinway piano. My mother was 19 at the time and since the family home in Riga had been expropriated by Soviet forces, she and my grandmother took refuge on their farm in Vidzeme. Here my mother met and two years later married my father, Andrejs. I was born a year later in April 1944. By the summer of 1944 my father had been conscripted into the 19th Division of the Latvian Legion of the occupying German army. He died sometime the following winter of massive chest injuries inflicted as a result of hand-to-hand fighting in Kurzeme. With the advance of Soviet forces in the autumn of 1944 it seemed clear that unless we escaped, our lives would be in danger. Thus began our peregrinations in Germany and eventual transfer to England.

A place called *trimda*

The word exile conveys many ambiguities. Dictionaries define it in terms of an unwanted separation from a place one is no longer able to inhabit. As well as physical separation, war and loss, desire and longing serve to construct exile as a moral space characterised by absence. Exile is both backward looking and forward looking: "The exile in his aestheticised aloneness poses no threat. He is exempted from discussions about immigrants in general, for it is hopefully believed that, unlike the immigrant, the exile forever hopes to and one day will return home".[13]

The Latvian word for exile is *trimda* and people in exile are termed *trimdinieki*. Latvian is a highly inflected language and *trimda* is commonly used in the locative *trimda* to indicate place. As a child this word described for me where I was living. I grew up in a place called *trimda*. Its boundaries spanned several countries: Germany, Holland, and England and its features changed too. *Trimda* in Germany was mostly to be found in the open and on the outside. My earliest memories are of being on the outside of houses, looking in through windows at families going about their domestic activities and thinking how impossibly lovely it would be to live in a house of one's own. Impossible, not only because for us home was floor space shared with many other families, but because the reality of post-war Germany showed huge areas of towns in ruins and rubble. Sebald[14] gives us the telling statistic that there were 31·1 cubic metres of rubble for every inhabitant of Cologne and 42·8 cubic metres of rubble for every inhabitant of Dresden (p 3). The destruction of Germany and the enormity of civilian deaths (600 000) have remained unspoken subjects: "There was a tacit agreement, equally binding on everyone, that the true state of material and moral ruin in which the country found itself was not to be described. The darkest acts of the final act of destruction, as experienced by the great majority of the German population, remained under a kind of taboo like a shameful family secret, a secret that perhaps could not even be privately acknowledged" (p 10).

In some way less ambitious but no less impossible were the walks I took with my mother in Nordschtemmen which had as their end point the Marienburg Schloss. Each walk started out with my hope that the *herzog* would invite us in for coffee and cakes. Although my mother never disillusioned me of my hopes, the invitation and the coffee and cakes never materialised. If for Bachelard the answer to the question as to the benefit of a house is the protection it provides for the dreamer and her daydreams,[15] for me those dreams were inspired precisely by the absence of a house.

In Holland *trimda* meant waiting on a dark quayside left in charge of a large trunk that contained all our possessions whilst my mother went to sort out the documentation that allowed us to board ship for Harwich. *Trimda* meant distrust of adults concerned for a small child who must have appeared to be on her own. It meant spread-eagling my 4-year-old body across the trunk to protect our possessions whenever a well-meaning adult attempted to approach me.

Trimda *in post-war Germany*

There were some two million of us refugees from the east in Germany. Perhaps because I was so very young my experience of *trimda* in post-war Germany is a good illustration of the way memory is reinforced by later re-narrations. Childhood memories and their retellings were shaped on the one hand by the experience of social dislocation and disconnection and on the other by an enforced and unaccustomed physical proximity. Memories are cast in the form of parables that speak of the dangers of straying away from others and the life-threatening consequences that may ensue. My childhood memories are impossible to separate from the later uses to which adults put them and re-interpreted them in the light of their own experience. These memories are intertwined with themes of belonging versus solitude and understanding versus incomprehensibility.

Some names are clearly later additions. I know that the name of the ship we boarded in Riga was the *Fritzschob*, but I am unlikely to remember. Similarly, I know that I spent my first winter in Bad Blankenburg in the Thueringer Wald, and my first birthday in Dittersdorf. We spent the winter of 1944 in the Gau Sportschule in Bad Blankenburg and this is where I had my first Christmas. But after two months, the Sportschule had to be vacated in order to accommodate wounded soldiers. We were offered a room in the nearby village of Dittersdorf by a family called Baeringer. Herr Baeringer was the village elder. I know that they lived in the last house on the right going uphill out of the village, although how I know this I am not sure. A photograph taken in the spring of 1945 shows me sitting in a large and somewhat battered pram looking trustingly towards the camera.

Towards the autumn of 1945 with the approach of Soviet troops, Dittersdorf was no longer a safe haven and we were offered a lorry ride to Coburg, which at that time was in the American zone. In Coburg a huge refugee camp awaited us. We were housed in what had been until very recently a stable. After two weeks there we moved to Wildflecken in the American zone (where Kathryn Hulme worked as an UNRRA officer) and from there to Hanau in the British zone. Hanau had been virtually razed to the ground and only a few chimneys were left. We were housed in an army camp along with about a 1000 other Latvians. I have a photograph of myself from the Hanau period standing on a dusty road wearing a knitted dress and knitted socks. My mother, during the idle days that were forced upon her, either knitted or went on long walks in the countryside. We stayed in Hanau for about a year and my memories here are of being one of a large group of straggling children. I remember in particular a little boy named Karlis. Karlis had a fiery temperament that brought him grief. I remember watching him in bewilderment, as time and again he would distance himself from the rest of us and howl tears of rage. I know his behaviour perplexed me not only because of the repeated intensity of his feelings but because he chose to cut himself off from the rest of us.

In the spring of 1947 we moved to Nordschtemmen near Hanover, again in the British zone. Here we moved into part of an empty house on Heyersumerstrasse. It was the last house on the right coming from the station. It was here that I started to assert my independence exploring the area around our house. Opposite the house were fields where peas were grown and here I learnt to make quick forays until one day in my eager rashness I ran under a British army lorry. This was my first unpromising encounter with the country that I would later adopt. The episode was dramatic but left no lasting physical legacy apart from a small scar high on my forehead. It did however serve as a morality lesson for my family whose view of me as a risk taker was consolidated by the event and who used its re-narration to impress upon me that striking out on my own would have tragic consequences.

In the autumn of 1948 we moved to Klausthal am Zellerfeld. We had a room in what had been an old-fashioned-style hotel set in the midst of parkland. Again I had considerable freedom here. I made friends with the park attendant, one of whose jobs was to sweep the leaves into his horse-drawn cart and take them to a compost site. He sat on the rim of the cart with his legs swinging over the edge and I occupied a less exciting position in the middle of the cart on top of the leaves. On one occasion as evening was drawing in, he decided to go home early leaving me in sole charge of the horse and cart. For me this was an opportunity to assume a more commanding position by sitting on the edge of the cart and swinging my legs in the way I had seen my friend doing. Needless to say, things ended badly. I fell between the shafts of the cart missing the horses' legs but falling into a pile of soot and ashes. The park had a steep-sided and deep lake and it was there that I planned to wash off the evidence of my misbehaviour. My mother caught me as I dodged from tree to tree on my way to the lake. Again the regular re-narration of this episode served to emphasise the dangers of solitariness. I have recounted these episodes not in order to make a point about my own adventurousness but rather to show the uses to which they were put in family memory and how their use illustrates one of the central dilemmas of refugees, namely overcoming solitude and achieving connectedness.

Trimda *in England*

Trimda acquired new connotations in England. *Trimda* spread itself thinly across London and established little pockets for itself in Golders Green, Child's Hill, Hendon, Finsbury Park, Westbourne Grove and Bayswater. My parents managed to scrape together a loan for a small and somewhat dilapidated Victorian semi-detached house in Child's Hill. Whereas these places are now all to a greater or lesser extent incorporated into fashionable and expensive London, in the 1950s they were, with perhaps the exception of Golders Green and Hendon, down at heel, working class areas. Childs Hill, though geographically close to Hampstead, was socially a million miles away. But living in *trimda* entailed laborious journeys across London. The Lutheran pastor was in Golders Green. The dentist was three bus rides away in Finsbury Park. My weekly visits to the piano teacher took place in Westbourne Park. Sunday School was in the Latvian community centre in Bayswater. And the dachshund Duksis, whose inability to learn the required house rules regarding toilet practice meant his eventual expulsion to a Latvian family living in Hendon, led to weekly visits there by my sister and myself.

Trimda also meant that everything of importance had happened elsewhere and earlier. Authentic time and experience belonged to the remembered past. Inauthentic routine time belonged to the present. *Trimda* meant living between two worlds. The world that had made my family and me who we were and whose dissolution resulted in our presence here in England had no reality to those around us. Our lives were part of a story whose beginnings were beyond the experience and comprehension of our neighbours and my schoolmates. If, as Kent writes, "communication occurs through a hermeneutical guessing game engendered through genre",[16] then our stories lay beyond familiar genres, could not be guessed at, and ultimately made communication impossible. Kirmayer[7] refers to this painfully uncomfortable situation as absence of a consensual reality in the refugee's experience (p 725). If Czarniawska is able to pin down the anthropologist's outsider status so deftly, it is perhaps because of her own dual ethnic identity. She writes of, "A feeling that there is no 'inside' where researchers can safely reside but merely a series of antechambers, where being inside one is outside of another"[18] (p 34). For me the metaphor of the antechamber captures my experience as a child refugee. We are all born into stories that are already well under way and that are not of our own making. But for the refugee child the earlier story is more of a mystery and has to be pieced together from the fragments told by others. Little evidence of the beginnings of my story could be seen in my new environment. Sontag writes of the way photographs invite a meditation on the passage of time.[19] But for me, our photograph albums conjured up a world frozen in time. The photograph of my mother aged three holding hands with her two boy cousins sits on the same page as the photograph of her striking a romantic pose in a white confirmation dress and holding a bunch of white lilies. The temporal mixing of these photographs conferred an independent existence on different periods of my mother's life and that of all the other family members. Indeed, it served to swell the overall size of our family with younger and older versions of the same person living alongside each other in my imagination. But I had never experienced the reality that the stories and photographs represented.

Gifts to memory

In 1956 my mother started working for a Polish company that sent gift parcels to Poland. Following an advertisement in an exile Latvian newspaper (*Londonas Avize*), she began sending gift parcels to Latvia. The process was complicated because each parcel needed a licence from the Soviet embassy, different amounts of duty had to be pre-paid for each item sent and rules regarding maximum quantities for different kinds of item had to be observed. Despite the complications, my mother found herself inundated with clients. In the early years she sent somewhere in the region of 200 parcels a week. Most of her clients were men in their mid to late thirties perhaps a few years older than my mother. They sent parcels every two months or so and they spent over £100 per parcel, spending more than half of what they earned on these gifts to memory. They came to her office in South Kensington from places like Bedford, Luton, Rugby, and Corby. During the school holidays and on Saturdays I would help her or occasionally stand in for her. Putting the parcel together was itself a prolonged act of performative memory. Headscarves could not be chosen without recalling a wife's or mother's hair colouring and eyes. Warm boots were chosen by measuring them against a piece of paper that had traced feet distorted by cold and rheumatism. Choosing underwear evoked lost moments of physical intimacy. Asked about a bra size two open hands with splayed fingers evoked a powerful corporeal memory of a wife's breasts. These were families who had already been separated for some 12 years. Wives who had been in early adulthood when war separated them were now approaching middle age. Mothers who had been in middle age were now old women. And children who had been babies were now approaching adolescence. Memory judged their size by the width of a past embrace. Dates and years left them confused and looking to advice from my mother or myself.

Performative memory came into play most powerfully at Christmas and Easter. Parcels took a long time to reach their destinations in Riga or some remote country farmhouse – perhaps two or three months. Clients knew this from past experience and yet on Christmas Eve there would be a telephone call for my mother saying that there were some dozen or so men wanting to send their families Christmas parcels. Inevitably, she would be late back home for our own Christmas celebrations having helped to ritualise and share each man's solitary grief. Like the youthful African novelist Achebe who describes a childhood journey sitting in the back of a truck,[20] these men could see where they were coming from but not where they were going. Among the gifts that were sent in these parcels were paisley headsquares and shawls made of a fine wool. Every now and then I have come across a woman wearing a headsquare that I instantly recognise as having been sent by my mother. Latvia is dotted with women wearing these headsquares and as my mother poignantly remarked of her life's work, whereas I have my writing to show for my work, all she has are fleeting glimpses of a headsquare.

Dialogues with the past

A central problem for refugees is communicating and sharing a credible past. The present is meaningless unless it can be seen as connected in some logical way with what precedes it. Present events need to be situated within the wider narrative structures to which they belong[18] (p 4). But the problem for refugees is that that past is often not credible to the host community. As Taylor reminds us,[21] human beings need to "situate themselves somewhere in ethical space" in order to have a sense of self. And that ethical space can only be constructed through dialogue. To their English hosts, much of Eastern Europe remained a grey area. Few had heard of the Baltic countries, often confusing them with the Balkans. Many of my schoolmates at All Saints Primary School thought I came from Lapland. Their ignorance served to accentuate my own image of Latvia as a remote, fairy-tale land. Moreover, the fact that Russia had won the war also conferred a certain legitimacy upon the Soviet regime. Few English people could understand why the Balts had fled their countries. The Nazi crimes loomed large in post-war imagination whereas Russia had been an ally and Communist crimes were not acknowledged. This meant that Latvians could not share their past in their new country of settlement. As Wyman notes, "The mood of this congregation of the homeless and dispossessed, fleeing territory torn by the clash of opposing armies, was in sharp contrast with the jubilation erupting elsewhere as word came of the end of the war".[22] Rasma remembers the lack of comprehension:

They didn't know anything about our countries. No they didn't know even though they were intelligent people. They just knew that we were foreigners. And explanation was also very difficult because we didn't have the language. And many of us didn't make any attempt to talk or explain. And we are Latvians so we are very shy and withdrawn and we don't make any attempts to speak if we're not asked. We are Latvians. We are prone to silence.[i]

On being asked what their English neighbours thought were the reasons for being in England, Rasma recalls:

They asked "How did you get here?" But no one ever asked "Why did you come here."

She gives a graphic example of this lack of interest in the past and what was important to her employer:

She had ladies come for morning coffee from the church committee and the Women's Institute and then she always took me into her drawing room and showed me to her ladies. And what Mrs Kettlewell liked very much was that I curtsied. And she loved that and so she took me straight from the kitchen to the drawing room and introduced me to the ladies. And I had to shake hands and, of course, I curtsied because that was normal for us because we always curtsied to adults and the ladies loved that. But none of the ladies ever asked me anything.

Rasma is important to the household because her traditional manners help to raise its social standing. Her story, however, is of no interest. A report for the United Nations entitled *The Refugee in the Post War World* describes England as "probably the most difficult of all countries in which to be a refugee".[23] Certainly many Latvians spoke of the difficulties they experienced in establishing close friendships with the indigenous population. They threw their energies into setting up committees of various sorts, Saturday schools, choirs, and theatre companies. Their activities confirm Summerfield's claims that what traumatised people need is not so much counselling as help in rebuilding social and cultural institutions.[24]

But the difficulties of integration also meant that the ethical space inhabited by Latvian selves was constructed in dialogue with the past. Kirmayer[7] explores the twin concepts of the transactional and the adamantine self in order to make sense of the refugee's experience (p 726). The transactional self is constructed through dialogue and social interaction. It is, in a sense, the true heir of William James' multiple selves. However, the dislocation of refugees means that there is an absence of shared experience which threatens the consensual basis of a transactional self. The adamantine self, by contrast, relates to "some inviolable essence of the person, a monological self, that has been hidden, silenced or suppressed by the lies and coercion of others, or more subtly, by the efforts of that same self to some false and misprisoning image or ideal of itself designed to please and placate others" (p 726). Kirmayer dismisses the adamantine self as "something of a fiction", suggesting instead that selves are transitory, constantly reshaped and lacking coherence outside of the consulting room (p 726). I would rather suggest that the adamantine self is in dialogue with the past. Difficulties with the English language, solitary occupations such as agricultural or factory work forced many of my mother's clients to retreat into an adamantine self. However, their self presentation might have appeared adamantine but it was not monologic. They were in constant dialogue with their memories and the ritual of putting together and sending parcels embodied these dialogues.

The broader picture

What was the broader picture in which these kinds of selves evolved? There were some 125 000 Latvians who sought refuge on allied territory in post-war Germany. They were initially placed in camps in Germany but, from 1946 onwards under the European Volunteer Workers Scheme, they were offered work under restricted conditions in other European countries. (For a history of this scheme see work by Tannahill[25] and Kay and Miles.[26]) Women from the Baltic states were recruited as trainee nurses to make up the shortages in British hospitals. From 1946 onwards, under a scheme entitled Baltic Cygnet, over 2000 Latvian women entered Britain. To qualify for the Baltic Cygnet scheme women had to be young (aged between 21 and 40), able-bodied, not pregnant, and without dependents. A memo of the time sent by a Ministry of Labour official describes the young women from the Baltic states in quasi eugenic language: "The women are of good appearance, are scrupulously clean in their person and habits and have a natural dignity in their bearing".[27] A second scheme called Westward Ho was set up in 1947 and recruited men and women to agricultural work, the textile industries and domestic service.

Altogether some 18 000 Latvians arrived in Britain as a result of the Soviet occupation of Latvia, but by the mid-1950s the numbers had shrunk to around 10 000 because of further emigration to Canada and the United States. The numbers were tiny compared, say, to the numbers of Polish refugees and demobilised soldiers, who numbered around 200 000, and they felt even tinier because the areas of settlement were scattered throughout Britain. I have heard Latvians frequently refer to themselves as being "scattered like salt and pepper" throughout the world. My own life in England owes its beginnings to Windleston Hall, a DP camp near Newcastle, where my new stepfather worked as an interpreter for some hundred Latvian agricultural workers and to the English family who gave my mother and me a windowless room in return for her domestic work.

What emerges from a wider perspective is the discrepancy between the host country's perception of the refugees and their own self-perception. Refugees are so often referred to in non-human terms using naturalistic metaphors such as waves, torrents, and streams or more catastrophically as landslides and avalanches. The other term for European refugees, DPs or displaced persons, conjures up Douglas' definition of dirt as "matter out of place".[28] The naturalisation and objectification of the refugees is consistent with ignorance or denial of their stories. Post-war Germany was "flooded" with refugees from Eastern Europe and for the British and the Americans their management posed administrative and economic problems with regard to their future. However, whereas the refugees must have had huge anxieties about their future their energies went into preserving their past. As Gattrell[29] writes: "Far from being dissolved, collective identities grew stronger as a result of the need to devote resources to the tasks of survival, cultural improvement, and reproduction" (p 201). In the Latvian camp in Hanau, a school theatre and choir were set up.

Timeless memories and disconnectedness

Collective cultural identities were more fragile in England because of the dispersion of Latvians around the country. Malkki observed from the study of Hutu refugees that isolated camps nurtured ideas of Hutuness whereas dispersal in towns undermined collective identities.[30] Refugee narratives tell the story of loneliness in the host community. For Kundera exile is "A tightrope high above the ground without the net afforded a person by the country where he has his family, colleagues and friends, and where he can easily say what he has to say in a language he has known from childhood".[31] Arvids remembers the difficulties he had with English at school and saying to himself "I'll never go to England because English is so difficult". As it turned out he finds himself in the position of the third simpleton son who does end up alone in England. Working on a farm in Derbyshire he is faced with the problem that no one can understand what he is trying to say apart from the farmer's two young children. Arvids had arrived in England in October 1947 having just turned 21. He left behind his mother and brothers and sisters. By that time he had already lost his father:

> *My father was poisoned by the Germans in 1942. He was in hospital. He had some sort of problem in the head. And the whole of that hospital was liquidated.*[ii]

Arvids was, as he says, "The only one who was left on this side." Contact between the two sides was confined to infrequent letters.

The farmer allowed Arvids to use his gun to shoot the odd rabbit for his supper. Arvids used the gun to take himself off to the fields and be by himself:

> *Often in the evening when I'd finished work I said to myself I'll take the gun and go and see if I can see a hare or a rabbit. I simply went to the edge of the field and had a cry. I had a feeling of loneliness. Well, I don't know, but something was missing. You could say it was a feeling of closeness.*

Arvids' wife, Rasma, arrived in England in February 1949 with her mother but she too describes intense feelings of loneliness. Their ship docked in Harwich and they proceeded to Liverpool Street station where they were met by an Immigration and Refugee Officer representative. They were given tea and iced buns, pocket money, and a ticket for Bristol. They were met at Temple Meads station by Mrs Ketwell and her chauffeur-driven car. From there they drove to East Harptree in North Somerset. Rasma's mother worked as a housekeeper for the elderly Ketwell couple, cooking and cleaning the house. Rasma was aged 14½. The headmistress of the local school said she was too old to go to school. Instead she polished the furniture while her mother cleaned the floors. Rasma appreciated her attic room, the clean bed, and the ordered household. She says: "I learned how to live properly". However, the ordered household did not assuage her feelings of loneliness:

> *As far as my youth was concerned there was loneliness everywhere. I was very lonely because I missed out on school, I missed not having any friends, I missed out on my childhood. I was very lonely.*

The loneliness is accentuated by a story of a lost intimacy frozen in memory. The familiar past becomes an imaginary past transfixed in a timeless zone. If for Levinas time is the other, then an imaginary other distorts the experience of time.[33] Arvids assigns a special place in memory to his family and his hometown of Cesis.

Now talking of memory. When you leave home as a young man you keep so many memories of what you've left behind in your thoughts and in your mind. So many memories register themselves in your mind and you keep a hold of them. I kept all the dates in my mind of my mother's birth and my father's and my brothers' and sisters' and everything. And the view as you go along the road towards Cesis and Cesis itself ... all that is inscribed inside. I can say that all my life I have lived with that view, living on my own in England. And as you said to me, Vieda, I couldn't speak the language.

In these accounts authentic time belongs to the imaginary past. Inauthentic routine time belongs to the experience of exile and the present. Rasma puts this as follows:

In some way or another we were dazed. We drove ourselves forward and lived life from day to day without questioning.

These stories tell of an unreal present and a real past. They challenge the distinction that some Latvian oral historians have made between Latvian life stories being told in a passive witnessing mode and exile life stories being more actively authored and infused with agency.[34]

The return of the native

Although Latvian identity has been articulated in terms of attachment to place and past, for many return has not been straightforward. As Beer points out "The return of the native has often been an occasion of confusion, bloodshed and dismay as of rejoicing".[35] Certainly, the breakdown of political boundaries has led to a questioning of interpersonal boundaries and identities. As Beer writes: "That the native can return seems plain enough but can she or he return as a native?"[35] The country from which one has been exiled is no longer inaccessible. And yet for many Latvians its very accessibility has made it emotionally inaccessible in a way that it was not before.

For example, Arvids has this to say about his return visit in 1992:

Vieda, I walked all through Cesis, trying to find something from my past. I found my old house, and I recognised my house. I found an outhouse and I recognised the outhouse. On one corner there had been a memorial to the schoolboy battalion (of the First World War) now there was a statue to Lenin. And wherever you go something new has been built. Nothing stays the same. Everything changes. But in your thoughts you are searching for the past.

The sense of strangeness extends to people as well:

Now you know that this is your brother and this is your sister. But in some way or another you're a stranger. Somehow, you can't get the closeness that you had years ago.

Rasma, on her return to her home town of Liepaja, has this to say:

It didn't feel as if I was going back to Liepaja. It was strange. Everything was strange. Even my relatives were strange. We had been girls together but now everything was strange. It was a strange feeling.

After a separation of nearly two years from my grandmother, I too had experienced that feeling of strangeness. When she arrived from Germany and we met her in Liverpool Street station I am reported as saying: "Omite [granny] feels foreign."

Just as the imaginary country was kept alive through the telling of stories, so too the present confusion and sense of estrangement finds expression in stories. However, these stories have a social life. Earlier stories spoke of a golden past a lonely and disconnected present and a future return to the homeland. Contemporary stories speak of a search for a missing past and a return to the safety and predictability of England. The site of authenticity has shifted from memory to everyday experience and with that exile has been transformed into diaspora.

In this chapter I have made an experimental attempt to combine the role of ethnographer, informant, and author. To do so I have revisited some of my early feelings and memories and tried to subject them to the same kind of intellectual interrogation that one would any other ethnographic information. I have asked how my memories might have been shaped by their subsequent retelling and the concerns and values of the refugee community to which I belonged. In an obvious sense Sontag[36] is right when she claims:

All memory is individual, unreproducible – it dies with each person. What is called collective memory is not a remembering but a stipulating: that this is important, and this is the story about how it happened, with the pictures that lock the story in our minds (p 76).

But that stipulation is a collective act that requires performance before an audience, real or imagined. Thus in the retelling of childhood memories and the emotion-laden business of putting together gift parcels individual memory is transformed into something shared and reproducible. The need for such transformation is an ongoing challenge for refugees throughout the world.

Endnotes

i My chapter is based on autobiographical experience as well as some sixty hours of tape recorded interviews with émigré Latvians living in the UK. However, I have chosen to use extracts from the stories of only two people. They are Rasma and Arvids Sermulins, whom I have known for more than 12 years. They have asked that their names should not be anonymised.

ii Arvids father was a patient at the psychiatric hospital of Strenci in north Vidzeme. All the patients were killed in the summer of 1942. The director of the hospital, Dr Cukurs, subsequently committed suicide. The killing of psychiatric patients in Germany has been documented by Burleigh[32] among others. The history of these events in the Baltic States has yet to be written.

Acknowledgements

I wish to thank Trish Greenhalgh and Judith Okely for their encouragement and suggestions in the writing of this chapter.

References

1 Wiesel E. Longing for home. In: Rouner LS, ed. *The Longing for Home.* Southbend, IN: University of Notre Dame Press, 1996, p 28.

2 Mumford DB. The measurement of culture shock. *Soc Psychiatry Psychiatr Epidemiol* 1998;**33**:149–54.

3 Oberg K. Cultural shock: adjustment to new cultural environments. *Practical Anthropol* 1960;**10**:49–56.

4 Clark M, Owen D, Szczepura A, Johnson M. *Assessment of the Costs to the NHS Arising from the Need for Interpreter and Translation Services.* CRER and CHESS: University of Warwick, 1998.

5 Bischoff A, Bovier PA, Rrustremi I, Garriazzo F, Eytan A, Loutan L. *Soc Sci Med* 2003;**57**(3):503–12.

6 Fadiman A. *The Spirit Catches You and You Fall Down. A Hmong Child, her American Doctors and the Collision of Two Cultures.* New York: Noonday Press, 1997.

7 Kirmayer L. The refugee's predicament. *Evolution Psychiatrique* 2002;**67**:24–42.

8 Okely J. Anthropology and autobiography: participatory experience and embodied knowledge. In: Okely J, Callaway H, eds. *Anthropology and Autobiography.* ASA Monograph 29. London and New York: Routledge, 1992.

9 Hulme K. *The Wild Place.* London: Frederick Muller, 1954.

10 Cochrane R. Mental illness in immigrants to England and Wales: an analysis of mental hospital admissions, 1971. *Soc Psychiatry* 1977;**12**:23–35.

11 Gadamer HG. *Truth and Method,* 2nd edn. London: Sheed and Ward, 1999, pp 441–2.

12 Grass G. *Crabwalk.* London: Faber, 2003, p 1.

13 Daniel EV. The refugee: a discourse on displacement. In: MacClancy J, ed. *Exotic No More: Anthropology on the Front Lines.* Chicago and London: University of Chicago Press, 2002, p 272.

14 Sebald WG. *On the Natural History of Destruction.* London: Hamish Hamilton, 2003.
15 Bachelard G. *The Poetics of Space* (trans M Jolas). Boston, MA: Beacon Press, 1969, p 6.
16 Kent T. Hermeneutics and genre. In: Hiley DR, Bohman JF, Shusterman R, eds. *The Interpretive Turn. Philosophy Science and Culture.* Ithaca, NY and London: Cornell University Press, 1991, p 284.
17 Kirmayer L. Landscapes of memory: trauma narrative and disassociation. In: Antze P, Lambek M, eds. *Tense Past Cultural Essays in Trauma and Memory.* London and New York: Routledge, 1996.
18 Czarniawska B. *A Narrative Approach to Organization Studies.* London and New Delhi: Sage, 1998.
19 Sontag S. *On Photography.* Harmondsworth: Penguin, 1979.
20 Achebe C. *Home and Exile.* Edinburgh: Canongate, 2001, p 2.
21 Taylor C. The dialogical self. In: Hiley DR, Bohman JF, Shusterman BR, eds. *The Interpretive Turn. Philosophy, Science, Culture.* Ithaca, NY and London: Cornell University Press, 1991, p 306.
22 Wyman M. *DPs: Europe's Displaced Persons.* Ithaca, NY and London: Cornell University Press, 1998, p 16.
23 United Nations Report. *The Refugee in the Post War World.* Geneva: UN, 1953.
24 Summerfield D. War and posttraumatic stress disorder: the question of social context. *J Nerv Ment Dis* 1993;**181**:522.
25 Tannahill JA. *European Volunteer Workers in Britain.* Manchester: Manchester University Press, 1958.
26 Kay D, Miles R. *Refugees or Migrant Workers? European Volunteer Workers in Britain, 1946–1951.* London: Routledge, 1992.
27 BBC Radio 4. *The Archive Hour: European Volunteer Workers,* producer Mark Whittacker, 17 May 2003.
28 Douglas M. *Purity and Danger: An Analysis of Concepts of Pollution and Taboo.* London: Routledge and Kegan Paul, 1966, p 35.
29 Gattrell P. *A Whole Empire Walking. Refugees in Russia during World War 1.* Bloomington, IN: Indiana University Press, 1999.
30 Malkki L. *Purity and Exile: Violence, Memory and National Cosmology among Hutu Refugees in Tanzania.* Chicago: Chicago University Press, 1995, p 6.
31 Kundera M. *The Unbearable Lightness of Being* (trans MH Heim). New York: Harper and Row, 1984, p 75.
32 Burleigh M. *Death and Deliverance: 'Euthanasia' in Germany 1900–1945.* Cambridge and New York: Cambridge University Press, 1994.
33 Levinas E. *Time and the Other* (trans RA Cohen). Pittsburgh: Duquesne University, 1987.
34 Zirnite M, Hinkle M, eds. *Oral History Sources of Latvia: History, Culture and Society Through Life Stories.* Riga: Latvian Oral History Association, 2003.
35 Beer G. *Can the Native Return? The Hilda Hulme Memorial Lecture.* London: University of London Press, 1989, p 3.
36 Sontag S. *Regarding the Pain of Others.* Harmondsworth/New York: Penguin/Viking, 2003.

18: A thrice-told tale: new readings of an old story

CATHERINE KOHLER RIESSMAN

This chapter represents a re-working of my past work, distant and proximate. The illness narrative, developed in conversation with a man who had advanced multiple sclerosis (MS), was produced more than 20 years ago. Burt (a pseudonym) was an "accidental case" in my sample: his name appeared in the early 1980s in court records. In the book I published on gender and the divorcing process (based on many interviews), Burt did not appear; I folded his responses into broad gender comparisons.[1] But because of an interest in health and illness, I developed a case study drawing on narrative portions of the interview.[2] It was a reading, heavily influenced by Goffman,[3] that articulated how a severely disabled man whose wife had left him for another man, constructs positive identities through storytelling – he was a good husband, father, and worker. Burt claimed the status of hero, against all odds – a representation I now view as incomplete.

I returned to the interview with Burt as I was preparing a talk for the UK Narrative-based Medicine conference in 2001. As happens for many investigators, aspects of the life story continued to haunt me. In the intervening years, significant changes had occurred in the social world of disability, narrative theory, and in my perspective on the storied world of experience. Massive changes had undoubtedly occurred in Burt's world as well; given the severity of his illness, I imagine he had probably died. I could not go back and talk again with him, I could only re-read the text we had constructed together, in a long and memorable conversation. During the second reading I saw aspects of the man, and the social world contained in him, that I had not seen 20 years earlier. Developments in gender theory worked their way into my interpretation: I focused the lecture on Burt's performance of masculinity in the face of a disease that challenges capacities usually associated with masculinity.

During the discussion period, several members of the audience raised questions about my representation. Where was the disability rights movement? Was it ethical to return to data gathered in the past with new questions in mind? Where was I in the text that I had created from the life story? A physician in the audience later told me he felt I had "undressed" the man. I had positioned myself as the "fully dressed" distant observer. What about the undercurrent of sexuality (raised about Burt's interview, and even more so in the comparative case)? The issue of sexuality had come up every time I presented the material. Audiences, it seems, read the text differently than I did. So, back again I went to the interview.

The third reading of the illness narrative I develop here represents a response to these issues, and to my own re-thinking of the material. Going beyond previous readings, I examine my positioning in the research relationship and the historical times – contexts for development of the illness narrative. In sum, this is a thrice-told tale – a new case study, constructed from research materials I worked with one way many years ago, and another way a few years ago.[i]

Through the different readings, I hope to problematise meaning and representation in narrative accounts of illness – issues anthropologists have raised in other contexts. Literary critics add an additional dimension: When we read a text (a novel, biography, or the transcript of an interview), we enter it to actively construct its meanings. Readers can even imaginatively rewrite it.[5,6] But I am getting ahead of my story. First, some theoretical comments on the case study as a method, and the illness narrative as a genre.

The value of case studies

The case occupies a venerable place in the history of medicine, and case studies thrive in education, psychology, law, and other disciplines, but the concept is currently under siege. In evidence-based medicine, the individual case has been downgraded to the status of an "anecdote", but in teaching the case study thrives, for it is the best way to communicate practical knowledge to trainees. Through detailed examples clinicians come to understand what is involved in illness and treatment. In health research, case-centred methods are especially valuable, providing contextual knowledge that population-based and category-centred approaches do not.

A clinical case involves two social actors: the patient "presents" symptoms and makes claims about him or herself, and the clinician in turn "presents" his or her case to others in an expressive portrayal. A case study involves actions of a subject and actions of an investigator, who transforms a person into a "case". When done well, the investigator "recreate[s] the presentational features of the encounter in a way that replicates the experience of the investigation"[7] (p. 328). The reader or listener can then re-create the individual and setting in imagination, imagining him or herself in the social world of another.

For the field of narrative studies, these are congenial concepts, although studies of illness narrative have not always attended to them.[ii] A form of case study, the illness narrative emerged in response to biomedicine's focus on disease (rather than illness) and consequent neglect of patient experience. As Hyden[11] says, "patients' narratives give voice to suffering in a way that lies outside the domain of the biomedical voice" (p 49). But scholars conflate the study of illness narrative with patients' speech acts. Scant attention has been directed to the presentational features through which illness experiences are reflected – the "displays" of identity, illness, and health that can be observed, but are not always verbalised. Narrative research in general has assumed until recently the primacy of the spoken word over other forms of expression. Mishler says "we speak our identities",[12] but I would add that much remains unspoken, inferred, shown, and performed in gesture, association, and action. What narrators show, without language, is a way to make claims about the "self".

The investigator's actions in the production of an illness narrative also warrant closer investigation. Although the listener's role in co-construction during the interview itself has been well documented,[13-16] his or her analytic action – that is, the making of the case study – has received less attention (but there is some work in this area[17,18,19]). How, for example, do the investigator's social location, subjectivity, and frameworks of understanding enter into that investigator's analysis of another's narrative account of illness? More generally, how is the investigator positioned in the field of interpretation? These questions have received attention in anthropology for some time,[20-23] and more recently in sociology.[24,25,26] Investigator positioning is important because it shapes the production of knowledge. As Bell writes, "understanding the experience of illness involves more than 'simply' the experiences of others; it also involves the experiences of sociologists attempting to understand the experiences of others"[27].

As my "thrice-told tale" illustrates, investigators' understandings of interview texts can change over time. Cases in biomedicine are often subject to re-analysis as new theories of disease and laboratory methods develop (witness, for example, the re-interpretation of frozen tissue samples following identification of the HIV virus). It is rare in the social sciences for an investigator to return to previous case studies and re-interpret them in the light of theoretical "discoveries" and methodological advances. I begin to develop this terrain here.

Illness narrative as a genre

The past decade has seen a burgeoning literature on the illness narrative in the social sciences (see reviews[11,27,28,29]), a development that recognises subjectivity in adaptation to chronic illness: how disease is perceived, enacted and responded to by "self" and others.

The last decade has also seen a burgeoning literature on narrative identity: we "become" the stories through which we tell about our lives.[8,30,31,32] Illness narrative provides a way for sufferers[iii] to explain and contextualise their interrupted lives, and changing relationships with the social world.[33–37] The genre provides a way to view lives through the prism of illness, "the vantage point from which all other events are related"[11] (p 57), at least in the beginning of an illness. Gareth Williams[38] argues that "illness has become something of a trope upon which to hang all kinds of musings about the meaning of damaged bodies and damaged lives" (p 247). Aside from the potential healing function of stories (a discourse form that links past, present, and an imagined future), identity work is done – accomplished performatively.

Analysing illness narrative as performance builds on recent work in the UK and United States.[12,18,39,40] The general perspective originated, for me, in Erving Goffman's brilliant use of the dramaturgical metaphor:[3,41] social actors stage performances of desirable selves to preserve "face" in situations of difficulty, such as chronic illness. Goffman (cited[42]) continues: "what talkers undertake to do is not to provide information to a recipient but to present dramas to an audience. Indeed, it seems that we spend most of our time not engaged in giving information but in giving shows." To emphasise the performative element is not to suggest that identities are inauthentic (although such a reading is suggested by Goffman), but rather that identities are situated and accomplished with the audience in mind. To put it simply, one cannot be a "self" entirely by oneself, identities must be performed in "shows" that persuade. Expressive acts, they attempt to convince an audience – they are "performances-for-others"[43] (p 109). Hence the response of the listener (and ultimately the reader) is implicated in the art of narrative.[5,6,44]

Although not my focus here, narratives serve non-performative purposes as well – the world is not all a stage. Moving beyond Goffman, individuals work over universal human problems and moral questions in their life stories. As Silko remarks (quoted by Capps and Ochs[45]), "Stories … aren't just entertainment. Don't be fooled. They are all we have. They are who we are, and all we have to fight off illness and death" (p 152). So, too, there is a real world outside of narrative performance: social structures of inequality constrain lives and possibilities for narrating them. Narrators, however, do control the terms of storytelling where they occupy privileged positions.[46] Consequently, the performative approach emphasises narrative as action, an intentional project.[29] Analysis shifts from "the told" – the events to which language refers – to include "the telling",[47] specifically the narrator's strategic choices in illness narrative about positioning of characters, audience, and self. Investigators ask the following kinds of questions: Why was the tale told that way, and in that order? In what kinds of stories does the narrator place himself? When are stories inserted into an account of illness and what purposes do they serve? How does the narrator strategically make identity claims through a narrative performance, beyond the spoken word? What was the response of the audience/listener, how did she influence the development of the narrative, and interpretation of it? And, in my "thrice-told tale", how might the illness narrative be re-read with history and the research relationship in mind? To develop these angles of vision, I return to Burt.

Wanting a job and someone to love: an illness narrative

Forty-three years old when I met him, Burt was white, had a high school education, and advanced multiple sclerosis. After agreeing by phone to be interviewed (I had obtained his name from court records), I went to his home, and was surprised when an ageing man in a wheelchair answered the door. I wrote in my field notes, "He looked much older than 43 years." He asked for my help several times (he could not, for example, easily reach his urinal from the wheelchair), nevertheless I tried to conduct the pre-scripted interview. But Burt redirected the conversation at every opportunity to the topic most salient to him: how MS over the previous eight years had altered his life. Taking charge of the interview early on, he told story after story. Anatole Broyard, after his cancer, wrote about the process of storytelling: "[Ill] people bleed stories, and I've become a blood bank of them".[48] Burt bled stories, and I wanted to suture him. Perhaps asking the structured sequence of questions served to contain the flow. His resistance to the controlled format with extended storytelling reveals a man bleeding discontinuities – severed from the markers of masculinity in his life world.

Similar to other white working class men, the job had provided a secure masculine identity. Burt had been the breadwinner in a traditional marriage that lasted 21 years. As the disease advanced, his wife left him for another man. Burt had worked for a large, well-known company for 20 years. He recounted with pride how when he became ill, "they got me an electric wheelchair"; they also gave him a desk job. He continued to work until he "couldn't sit for too long in a wheelchair". Within the first five minutes of the interview he told me he was "planning on going back to work part time." Sitting across from him, it was hard to imagine. He said he had gone to see his boss several weeks earlier but had been told "things were kind of slow … there was nothing open right now … they would get in touch with [him]." I now wonder if they were putting him off. I learned after our conversation that the plant was downsizing; a year after we talked, another firm acquired the company, and the plant closed.

Returning to work meant returning to a familiar masculine identity, but I now also wonder if Burt wanted to return to work for human connection – an antidote to the isolated life he described. Looking back on my research materials with historical context in mind, I see Burt's extreme isolation in a time when the disability rights movement had not yet secured wheelchair access in communities – disability had not yet become politicised. Burt said that "being alone" was his greatest difficulty. A personal care attendant, who helps him with "hygiene … exercises … housecleaning … food shopping", is his "closest relationship". With the attendant's aid, he is able to get out of the house several times a month only, to play bingo or go to a movie. Otherwise, he watches TV alone.

When presenting an earlier version of this chapter in British Columbia, I witnessed the achievements of the disability rights movement in Vancouver, arguably the most wheelchair accessible community in North America – buses, museums, buildings, markets, and entertainment centres are all accessible, and I observed people in motorised wheelchairs in all of these locations. To be sure, the disability movement can accomplish much more, but as I think now about Burt's life story, I can imagine the life taking a different form. The illness narrative (and experience of MS) would be transformed in the context of current policies in some settings for wheelchair access.

Burt was not living in Canada, however; our conversation took place in the United States in the early 1980s, before disability rights entered policy debates. Like others with severe mobility problems, he was physically segregated at home, unable to leave without an attendant. He had very few social contacts. In our interview Burt longs for companionship and pines for his former wife: he continues to carry her picture in his wallet and shortly before we talked he had sent her a Mother's Day card, "but she has not responded".

Sometimes I watch a TV show that she liked to watch, "Love Boat" or something like that. She was always here Saturday night watching it with me. I sit here and I see these things and I feel depressed. Sometimes I hope that she would still be sitting here on the couch.

Other sources of companionship, tied to the marriage, have disappeared. Contacts with in-laws have "gone down the drain": "they don't call and they don't even write", and his adult son and daughter have moved out. It is unclear what led to estrangement, especially in relationships with children. Whatever the reasons, the limited possibilities for a public life, and the loneliness of the private sphere, are grimly apparent to me now as I re-examine the materials. I am reminded of Irv Zola's meditative narrative about his discovery – an American sociologist with polio – as he did ethnographic research in a village of the disabled in the Netherlands.[26] Extreme social isolation need not accompany polio or multiple sclerosis, except as social arrangements and physical barriers make it so.

Lacking fraternity and community, Burt is institutionalised at home. I now wonder whether he looked to the research relationship as a potential source of companionship. Subverting the interview format, he muses about how the younger generation has changed, reaching out to me – his audience – in a kind of plea for understanding. It was the first of his many attempts to position me as a friend:

Kids today are a lot different than they were in our time. I don't know – I am – I don't know how old you are. In your early forties, too? [I nod]. *We used to take the kids to the drive-in, something like that, but today – forget it, everything has changed. Now they have to go down to the Cape and spend the weekend down there. You are saying to yourself, "What is going on down there?"*

There is a hint of intimacy, even sexuality here – topics Burt returns to in our conversation. He describes "growing fond" of a nurse who took care of him during a recent hospitalisation:

I wish I could have some kind of real close relation with her, but she is married and has five children. That just about throws everything down the drain. I like the girl very much, she is more my age and I wish I could have some sort of relation with her. I feel something like that. That's what I need, a good woman companion.

He continues:

You know what I mean, you used to sleep with a woman for 21 years and now I'm sleeping in my own bed and there's no one beside me to keep warm, let's put it that way. Nights are cold – something like that. Somebody to hold on to, I miss that.

Burt wants "someone to talk to, you know, someone to love". Perhaps the research relationship offered a fleeting "woman companion", someone who listened, gave support, and expressed interest. Re-examining the transcript, I see how Burt repeatedly tries to position me (his audience) in a common world of meaning and connect me to his life world. He even created an opening in the fixed question/answer format designed to collect demographic information at the end of the interview – a dehumanised way to ask about religion (interestingly, we both subverted the structured format in this exchange):

CR: *How often do you attend religious services? Do you attend –* [I hand a card with frequency response categories].

315

> B: *Never.*
>
> CR: *Never? Not at all, not even on Easter Sunday?*
>
> B: *Not since I been sick. I watch it on Sunday at 10:30 on TV. When I can – when I can get somebody to get me up early enough to watch it. Are you Catholic?*
>
> CR: *I was raised as a Catholic.*
>
> B: *They have that passionate mass on Sunday at 10:30. Have you ever seen that? Channel 25 has it.*

I resisted religious positioning, as I resisted any promise of a continuing relationship.

As the long interview was ending, I asked another standardised demographic question, this time about income (again using the ghastly cards with fixed response categories). I learned Burt had no pension, and was living on meagre social security disability payments. Resisting the constraints once again of the structured format, he inserts a long story that recounts his last day at work several years previously – an association that suggests the huge significance of employment for him. In the story he positions himself as the central character in a heroic drama, with his boss and several doctors as supporting characters. He positions me, his audience, as witness to a moral tale depicting a man who wants to be a working man.

> *I had told my boss ahead of time that I was goin' to see him [the doctor].*   **Scene 1**
> *And he said, "Well, let us know, you know, as soon as you find out so we can get your wheelchair all, you know, charged up and fixed up and everything."*
> *So I had seen him [doctor] on a Friday*
> *and I'd called soon as I got back Friday told him [boss] I'd be in that following Monday.*
> *And he said, "Oh, it's goin' to be so good to have you back, you've been out of work so long."*

> *So I went in there [factory]*   **Scene 2**
> *[pause] and before I used to be able to stand up in the men's room you know, and urinate that way*
> *but this one time I took the urinal with me*
> *just in case I couldn't do it.*
> *So I got up, I get in there at 7 o'clock that morning*
> *and at about 9 o'clock I felt like I had to urinate.*
> *And I went over to where I usually go to try to stand up*
> *I couldn't stand up the leg wouldn't hold me.*
> *They have a handicapped stall.*
> *So I went into the handicapped stall to try and use the urinal.*
> *Couldn't use it.*

I had the urge that I had to go but nothing was coming out.
So back to my desk I went and I continued working.
And about fifteen or twenty minutes later I get the urge again.
So back to the men's room I go
back to the handicapped stall.
All day long this is happening.
I couldn't move my urine
everything just blocked up.

When I get home I figured well maybe it's because   **Scene 3**
I'm nervous coming back to work the first day on the job.
So I get home [pause] I still couldn't go.
So I called my doctor, Dr George
and he said, "Well, can you get up to [names hospital]?"
I said, "Well, I'm in my pyjamas."
He said, "Well, I'll send an ambulance"

So they sent an ambulance and brought me up there.   **Scene 4**
And he put a catheter on me
soon as he put that on I think I must have let out maybe two pints.
Everything just went shhhhh.
You know, I felt so relieved.
And he said, "Well, I'm goin' to keep you in," he says
"I want, I want this uh [pause] urinologist to take a look at you."
So it was Dr Lavini
I don't know if you know Dr Lavini he's one of the best around.
He looked at it and said, "We're going to have to operate."
Everything just blocked up.
They had to make the opening larger
so the urine would come out, you know, freely.
So I was in [names hospital] –

I had gone to work for that one *day ...*   **Coda**

This poignant, quintessential masculine narrative articulates a failure of the male body. It entangles us as readers emotionally in the bodily suffering of a man, and in his social suffering as he tries to return to work. A classic story in a formal sense,[49,50] it bleeds the pain of disability in social space.

But why does Burt insert this particular story here, as our interview was ending? When I have presented the text to other audiences, participants speak of "embarrassment" – the details are too intimate for strangers. Remember, Burt began the interview by talking about returning to work; so, too, does he end it. Stories about the job stand as bookends to the illness narrative, a testament to the crucial importance of paid work to the man's identity. But why, specifically, does he insert the story in response to a demographic question about income? Masculinity and income are linked in Western imagination – a man's worth is often tied to what he earns. Burt protects his masculinity, perhaps, by storying a day at the job. Perhaps, too, the insertion of an intimate detailed story about the masculine body sustains the intimacy Burt has been seeking all along – connection with a woman, with me.

There are other ways to read the text. It draws on the familiar Western cultural plot of contemporary biomedicine: a man struggles unsuccessfully against an invisible enemy, and is saved by doctors who can see into his body, and identify and correct a physical defect. Burt joins this well-known cultural narrative with his personal one about a particular illness event, located in a life context, not a disease localised in the body. The illness narrative includes the social suffering missing from the biomedical plot. It draws on the familiar – classic narrative devices: a setting, action, characters – set alongside the cultural narrative of biomedicine. Burt stages a dramatic representation: the action moves temporally through the fateful events that transpired on his last day at work. His representation includes discrete scenes: the Friday before (Scene 1), Monday, the beginning of the work week (Scene 2), that evening (Scene 3), and the final hospital scene. He creates characters, giving speaking roles to his boss, the two doctors, and himself. He positions himself in a moral story about what it means to be a virtuous man. In line with this interpretive reading, Burt chooses to perform his preferred self – responsible worker – as the long interview was ending, not other "selves" he has suggested earlier (lonely man wanting a woman to love). I leave it to the reader to ponder why the long story appears when it does – the function it serves in the illness narrative and research relationship.

As I muse about the closing narrative, I am reminded of another character and another scene – Willy Lowman, in Arthur Miller's *Death of a Salesman*, telling off his corporate employer when he is fired. A salesman for 34 years who was tired and ageing, he too wanted to be known as a working man. The employer, who extracted Willy's labour for 34 years, took work identity away. Burt's corporate employer is not portrayed so harshly, but he also used up the able-bodied man. Nor does Burt confront corporate power, as Willy did: "You can't eat the orange and throw away the peel ... A man isn't a piece of fruit." Thinking now about Burt's lack of a pension after 21 years with the same employer, learning about the downsizing and subsequent closure of the plant, I now see a vivid instance of how corporate capitalism and job loss have ravaged American workers. People in management and upper levels were given employment opportunities in the new corporation, and generous benefit packages. Line workers were not. The post-industrial wasteland in manufacturing in the entire north-eastern United States produced in the 1980s by acquisitions and mergers, capital flight, and the search for corporate profits, eclipsed the power of working men, bleeding masculinity embodied in factory labour.

Conclusion

What can we learn from the third reading of the illness narrative of a man severely disabled by MS? Although in earlier readings I positioned myself as the distanced observer, I did construct meaningful case studies to illustrate how the illness narrative, as a discursive form, allows a very ill man to connect strands of his existence: health, illness, gender identity, and the life worlds of marriage and job. The third reading I have developed here opens up my entanglement with the text, and the suffering of the man, avoided in earlier readings. Making visible the otherwise hidden feelings and bonds in the research relationship, as Rita Charon[51] does in her meditative account of her relationship with a patient, is my version of clinical reflection.

The shards of an illness narrative I have presented do not meet standard criteria of coherence, nor do they suggest a single authorised meaning. As we all do in our lives, Burt played out different identities, and there are gaps between them that I – audience/listener/reader – had to fill in, making connections through interpretation.

There are important differences between a literary narrative (a novel, for example) and a spoken/conversational one, but each involves interaction between text and reader. The constitutive activity of the reader supplies what is not in the text, bringing together text and imagination. It is the indeterminacy of the text itself that calls forth this aesthetic response, along with meaning-projection – inevitable because we can never experience another's illness experience. Like a work of literature, an interview transcript occupies a liminal space – a "peculiar halfway position between the external world of objects and the reader's own world of experience"[5] (p 8). The aesthetic response lies in the realisation accomplished by the reader. As Iser[5] (p 10) says, meaning is not concealed within the text itself: we "bring the text to life with our readings ... a [second] reading of a piece of literature often produces a different impression from the first ... [related to the] reader's change in circumstances" – her standpoint, feminist scholars would say. Burt's illness narrative is a "product of occasions of telling and reading"[17] (p 30) – several occasions of reading, each producing different meanings.

As a contemporary reader/interpreter of a narrative Burt and I developed 20 years ago, I tried to bring the text to life again by historicising it, placing the man's experience of disability in the context of historical and economic circumstances – realities we both took as given during our talk together. The literature of the time portrayed the disabled as "victims" – a discourse I certainly took for granted, and perhaps Burt did as well. "The reading process always involves viewing the text through a perspective that is continually on the move"[6] (p 285). Meanings, by nature, are shaped by their historical position "and cannot in principle be set apart from history"[6] (p 29). The third reading is profoundly influenced by history, specifically changes in my understanding of disability, learned from friends, colleagues, and social movements in the years since the interview. In the space between text and reader, "we learn not only about what we are reading but also about ourselves"[5] (p 29).

There are other lessons to be learned. First, cases matter in social research on health: examination and comparison of the smallest details of narrative accounts can reveal the social world hidden in "personal" stories, lending context to clinical case studies. Although Burt never acknowledged objective social conditions – he "naturalised" them – the life he represented is saturated with class and global politics – taken for granted inequalities inscribed in the consciousness of ordinary citizens: corporate pension plans (and their absence), the downsizing and migration in the United States of large industrial plans (benefiting executives, not workers), and restricted spaces for the disabled. Burt cannot move around his own community without a paid attendant because of structural conditions – social arrangements that are historically and class specific, and can be changed. The significance of the body's relationship to space is an often unperceived source of power: "The power over social space ... comes from possessing various kinds of capital ... The lack of capital intensifies the experience of finitude: it chains one to a place".[52] Working class men, like Burt, earn a living by bodily labour, a body that is "fit for work" displays health.[53] A strong work ethic runs through Burt's identity performance; his vigorous attempts to return to work (and to the topic in our interview) are efforts to minimise illness, embodying the value of a man in his economic world. In sum, detailed studies of cases can reveal how class, gender, and race/ethnicity – structures of inequality and power – work their way into what appears to be "simply" talk about a life affected by illness[54] – a sociological reading of the text that I develop elsewhere.[4]

Second, illness narrative encompasses more than the spoken word. I privileged the performative aspects of narrative – the "displays" of self and identity that are not only spoken but also enacted and embodied, actions that offer insight into an ill person's preferred way of being. As points of entry, I re-examined my field notes of observations and reactions, Burt's strategic placement of stories (when he inserted them into the fixed interview format) and aspects of their composition (choices about the positioning of characters, self, and audience) to look at what these actions accomplished performatively. How the protagonist presents himself as the central character in the illness narrative is suggested by associations, "asides", actions in the research relationship, and in the spaces he forges to introduce and expand upon particular topics. These "displays" and "doings" of identity go beyond speech acts, and the verbal in a strict semantic sense – what the text is "about" or what it "says". In addition, I used the performative view to interrogate myself – an active figure in the production of, and reaction to, the illness narrative. Similar to artistic performances, personal narratives that develop in interviews are alive and fluid, composed in the dynamic space between performer and audience, not composed solely by speakers and enacted similarly for different audiences.

Lastly, by looking back and reinterpreting past materials, I have made visible my role in constructing a case study. I included myself in the text as a vulnerable observer[55] in the past as a figure in the illness narrative (interviewer, audience, and composer of field notes), and in the present as a voice asking new questions. In all roles I am interpreter – active and positioned – as we all are when we listen to narratives, construct case presentations, or develop narrative studies of lives. Qualitative research in the modernist tradition has minimised and/or ignored the identities of the investigator and his or her relationship with the subject, assuming that scientific standards and ethics could produce unbiased generalisable findings. With the postmodern turn and the collapse of the knower/known distinction, investigator subjectivity and social location have entered the field of investigation,[27] for the investigator's positioning affects what he or she "sees" in the Other. The investigator is located at one level in the interview conversation, by virtue of social characteristics and commitments, and at another level between subject and audience, a translator. Acknowledging my shifting positions, I included myself as listener/hearer/knower/analyst/reader. Through the act of looking back, I emphasised different ways of seeing, interrogating my shifting identities and perspectives. Through my analytic process, my subject's shifting "selves" came into awareness. Different readings of the research materials could be accessed with these shifts in positioning.

I am not arguing that my third reading is "truer" than my first or second; they are, simply different. Although I think the thrice-told tale illuminates a layered complexity rather well, I am sure other readings from other historical and dispositional standpoints can illuminate the material in other ways. There is never a single authorised meaning, but interpretation cannot exclude from analysis the structure and patterns of the text itself[5] – reading is not unmitigated free association. Reading an illness narrative means engaging with a text and the relationship that produced it, entering imaginatively into its world. It involves discovery, "finding significance for oneself, and thus undergoing personal change through the experience of reading"[56] (p 838).

Re-examining data collected in the past – "accidental" cases that turn up when studying another topic – always raises issues, to which there are no easy solutions.[57,58] Returning to materials collected in the past opens up new insights for research in the future. I told this thrice-told tale as a positioned ethnographer; it is an example of the complicated ways researcher and reader are implicated in the production of knowledge about lives and cultures.

Acknowledgements

A somewhat different version of the case study, along with a comparative case, appeared in *Qualitative Research*, 2003;**3**(1):5–33. For comments on drafts, I thank Susan Bell, Gareth Williams, Elliot Mishler, Wendy Luttrell, and the Boston Colloquium on Qualitative Research in Health; for local knowledge, thanks to Ron Altimari. My deepest thanks go to Burt; may he rest in peace.

Endnotes

i   For another reading of the materials see Riessman.[4]
ii Several excellent collections of narrative studies in the social sciences include Brockmeier and Carbaugh,[8] Andrews *et al*,[9] and Hinchman and Hinchman.[10]
iii For a thoughtful discussion of the term "suffering" in illness research, including a critique, see Bell.[27]

References

1   Riessman CK. *Divorce talk: women and men make sense of personal relationships*. New Brunswick, NJ: Rutgers University Press, 1990.
2   Riessman CK. Strategic uses of narrative in the presentation of self and illness. *Soc Sci Med* 1990;**30**(11):1195–200.
3   Goffman E. *The Presentation of Self in Everyday Life*. New York: Penguin, 1969.
4   Riessman CK. Preforming identities in illness narrative: masculinity and multiple sclerosis. *Qualitative Res* 2003;**3**(1):5–33.
5   Iser W. *Prospecting: From Reader Response to Literary Anthropology*. Baltimore, MD: Johns Hopkins Press, 1989/1993.
6   Iser W. *The Act of Reading: A Theoretical Aesthetic Response*. Baltimore, MD: Johns Hopkins University Press, 1978.
7   Radley A, Chamberlain K. Health psychology and the study of the case: From method to analytic concern. *Soc Sci Med* 2001;**53**:321–32.
8   Brockmeier J, Carbaugh D, eds. *Narrative and Identity: Studies in Autobiography, Self, and Culture*. Amsterdam and Philadelphia: John Benjamins, 2001.
9   Andrews M, Sclater SD, Squire C, Treacher A, eds. *Lines of Narrative: Psychosocial Perspectives*. Routledge: New York, 2000.
10 Hinchman LP, Hinchman SK, eds. *Memory, Identity, Community: The Idea of Narrative in the Human Sciences*. Albany, NY: State University of New York Press, 1997.
11 Hyden LC. Illness and narrative. *Sociol Health Illness* 1997;**19**(1):48–69.
12 Mishler EG. *Storylines: Craftartists' Narratives of Identity*. Cambridge, MA: Harvard University Press, 1999, p 19.

13   Atkinson P. Medical discourse, evidentiality and the construction of professional responsibility. In: Sarangi S, Roberts C. Talk, work and institutional order. Berlin: Mouyton de Gruyter, 1999, pp 75–107.
14   Bell SE. Narratives and lives: Women's health politics and the diagnosis of cancer for DES daughters. *Narrative Inquiry* 1999;**9**(2):1–43.
15   Clark JA, Mishler EG. Attending to patients' stories: Reframing the clinical task. *Sociol Health Illness* 1992;**14**(3):344–70.
16   Mishler EG. *Research Interviewing: Context and Narrative*. Cambridge, MA: Harvard University Press, 1986.
17   Hall CJ. *Social Work as Narrative: Storytelling and Persuasion in Professional Texts*. Oxford: Ashgate, 1997.
18   Mattingly C, Lawlor M. The fragility of healing. *Ethos* 2001;**21**(1):30–57.
19   Riessman CK. Doing justice: positioning the interpreter in narrative work. In: Patterson W, ed. *Strategic Narrative: New Perspectives on the Power of Personal and Cultural Storytelling*. Lanham, MD: Lexington Books, 2002, pp 193–214.
20   Briggs J. *Never in Anger*. Cambridge, MA: Harvard University Press, 1970.
21   Myerhoff B, Metzger D, Ruby J, Tufte V, eds. *Remembered Lives*. Ann Arbor, MI: University of Michigan Press, 1992.
22   Myerhoff B. *Number Our Days*. New York: Simon and Schuster, 1978.
23   Rabinow P. *Reflections on fieldwork in Morocco*. Berkeley, CA: University of California Press, 1977.
24   DeVault M. Talking back to sociology: distinctive contributions of feminist methodology. *Ann Rev Sociol* 1996;**22**:29–50.
25   Reinharz S, Davidman L. *Feminist Methods in Social Research*. New York: Oxford University Press, 1992.
26   Zola IK. *Missing pieces: a chronicle of living with a disability*. Philadelphia: Temple University Press, 1982.
27   Bell SE. Experiencing illness in/and narrative. In: Bird CE, Conrad P, Fremont AM, eds. *Handbook of Medical Sociology*, 5th edn. Upper Saddle River, NJ: Prentice Hall, 2000, p 186.
28   Bury M. Illness narratives: Fact or fiction? *Sociol Health Illness* 2001;**23**(3):263–85.
29   Skultans V. Editorial: Narrative, illness and the body. *Anthropol Med* 2000;**7**(1):5–13.
30   Bruner J. *Acts of Meaning*. Cambridge, MA: Harvard University Press, 1990.
31   Holstein JA, Gubrium JF. *The Self We Live By: Narrative Identity in a Postmodern World*. New York: Oxford University Press, 2002.
32   Narrative Identity. Special Issue. *Narrative Inquiry* 2000;**10**(1).
33   Bury M. Chronic illness as biographical disruption. *Sociol Health Illness* 1982;**4**(2):167–82.
34   Charmaz K. *Good Days, Bad Days*. New Brunswick, NJ: Rutgers University Press,1991.
35   Frank A. *The Wounded Storyteller: Body, Illness, and Ethics*. Chicago: University of Chicago Press, 1995.
36   Williams G. The genesis of chronic illness: narrative re-construction. *Sociol Health Illness* 1984;**6**(2):175–200.
37   Williams G. Chronic illness and the pursuit of virtue in everyday life. In: Radley A, ed. *Worlds of Illness: Biographical and Cultural Perspectives on Health and Disease*. New York: Routledge, 1993, pp 92–108.
38   Williams G. Review article: bodies on a battlefield: the dialectics of disability. *Sociol Health Illness* 1999;**21**(2):242–52.
39   Bamberg M. 'We are young, responsible, and male': Form and function in 'slut-basing' in the identity construction of 15-year-old males. *Human Dev* (forthcoming).
40   Langellier KM, Peterson EE. *Storytelling Matters: Performing Narrative in Daily Life*. Philadelphia, PA: Temple University Press, 2003.
41   Goffman E. *Forms of Talk*. Oxford: Blackwell, 1981.
42   James D. *Dona Maria's Story: Life History, Memory and Political Identity*. Chapel Hill, NC: Duke University Press, 2000.
43   Young K. Gesture and the phenomenology of emotion in narrative. *Semiotica* 2000;**131**(1/2):79–112.
44   Bauman R. *Story, Performance, and Event: Contextual Studies of Oral Narrative*. Cambridge: Cambridge University Press, 1986.

45 Capps L, Ochs E. *Constructing Panic: The Discourse of Agoraphobia.* Cambridge, MA: Harvard University Press, 1995.
46 Patterson W, ed. *Strategic Narrative: New Perspectives on the Power of Personal and Cultural Storytelling.* Lanham, MA: Lexington Books, 2002.
47 Mishler EG. Models of narrative analysis: a typology. *J Narrative Life History* 1995;**5**(2):87–123.
48 Broyard A. *Intoxicated by my illness: and other writings on life and death* (compiled and edited by Alexandra Broyard). New York: Clarkson Potter, 1992, p 21.
49 Labov W. Speech actions and reactions in personal narrative. In: Tannen D, ed. *Analyzing Discourse: Text and Talk.* Washington, DC: Georgetown University Press, 1982, pp 219–47.
50 Riessman CK. *Narrative Analysis.* Newbury Park, CA: Sage, 1993.
51 Charon R. Medicine, the novel, and the passage of time [personal time]. *Ann Intern Med* 2000;**132**(1):63–8.
52 Bourdieu P, Accardo A, Balazs G, Beaud S *et al. The Weight of the World: Social Suffering in Contemporary Society.* Stanford, CA: Stanford University Press, 1993, pp 124, 127.
53 Radley A. Style, discourse and constraint in adjustment to chronic illness. *Sociol Health Illness* 1989;**11**(3):230–52.
54 Sarangi S, Roberts C. The dynamics of interactional and institutional orders in work-related settings. In: Sarangi S, Roberts C, eds. *Talk, Work and Institutional Order: Discourse in Medical, Mediation and Management Settings.* New York: Mouton de Gruyter, 1999, pp 1–57.
55 Behar R. *The Vulnerable Observer: Anthropology That Breaks Your Heart.* Boston, MA: Beacon Press, 1996.
56 Good BJ, DelVecchio Good MJ. In the subjunctive mode: epilepsy narratives in Turkey. *Soc Sci Med* 1994;**38**(6):835–42.
57 Andrews M. Memories of mother: counter-narratives of early maternal influence. *Narrative Inquiry* 2002;**12**(1):7–27.
58 Riessman CK. Accidental cases: Extending the concept of positioning in narrative studies. *Narrative Inquiry* 2002;**12**(1):37–42.

19: The role of stories and storytelling in organisational change efforts: a field study of an emerging "community of practice" within the UK National Health Service

PAUL BATE

Background

It has long been the fashion to portray organisational change processes as tense, highly politicised affairs characterised by factionalism, ambiguity, conflict, and struggles for power.[1,2,3] The dominant image is one of a "contested terrain", full of pitfalls and dangers, obstructions, and hard climbs. The words that accompany such an image are correspondingly dark, drawing upon the vocabulary of coercion, competition, tyranny, hegemony, control, subjection, engineering, manipulation, domination, subordination, resistance, opposition, diversity, negotiation, obedience, and compliance. Conspicuous for their absence are antonyms like cooperation, convergence, coherence, integration, and consensus, which seem to have been driven out of the vocabulary by their hard-headed cousins.

Until recently, I never had reason to challenge this version of the reality, in fact I may have played some small part in creating it.[4,5] My writings on the subject of organisational and cultural change processes have made frequent reference to the multi-voiced world of the professional organisation (my work being mostly in healthcare), and the "friction", "conflict", "disharmony" and "embittered relations" between different professional groups as they struggled for control of the change agenda (see Bate[6] and Bate et al[7]). Time after time, my research has described how these dynamics play themselves out in an infinite variety of ways, yet offering little by way of challenge to the dominant pluralistic view of the organisational process as "politics with barbs".

However, the purpose of this chapter is to tell a very different story, one that has refused to fit either the perspective or the pattern described. It is about a less adversarial, altogether milder, form of organisational politics, driven by community and a coming together not by contestation and conflict. It describes a major organisational and cultural change process in a UK hospital in which a highly diverse group of healthcare professionals became fellow travellers on the change journey and who, not unlike the motley band of pilgrims in Chaucer's *Canterbury Tales*,[i] were able by way of personal stories and storytelling to construct a shared identity and deep sense of purpose that sustained them on their journey and finally carried them to where they wanted to be.

I wish to draw on the "narrative" and "communities of practice" literatures to offer an interpretation of what I observed, and in so doing offer a different reading on the nature of organisational politics and the process of change from the usual one. Following Wenger,[8] Brown and Duguid,[9,10] and others, I define a community of practice as a loose-knit informal group of people who voluntarily come together because of common interests and shared experiences to solve problems and help drive forward change, and who over time acquire a cultural identity, a shared sense of mission, and a strong in-group coherence and solidarity – "communitas", to use Durkheim's classic term. The ethos of the group is characterised by the constant search for an underlying consensus that might unite and keep them together through thick and thin, by amiability and a willingness to be flexible, accommodating, even selfless in outlook. Of course, the politics and the tensions do not go away; it is just that "change" and simply "getting there" become a more powerful motive than "control" or being the first across the line.

The key to this milder form of organisational politics lies in the personal stories that people recount to each other during the period of change, and the unifying master narrative that emerges from the interweaving of these stories over time. As the weft and warp of social interaction, it is these stories that define and establish "community", and community that ultimately defines and establishes the direction and nature of cultural change. Following Boyce[11] and others (see Boje[12] and Shaw[13]), as well as a number of healthcare writers (see Brown,[1] Bailey,[14] Greehalgh,[15] and Mattingly[16]), I want to show through one example followed over time how the stories told in organisations offer researchers and organisation development practitioners a natural entry point to understanding and intervening in the change – particularly cultural change – processes of an organisation.

Context

First a brief word on context. The UK National Health Service (NHS), the setting for this study, has in recent years embarked upon a major programme of modernisation and reform. The NHS Plan of 2000[17] set out a bold and ambitious agenda for a "quality revolution in healthcare and a step change in results", imposing an obligation on organisations in the front line of care delivery – acute hospitals, primary care trusts – to change their structures, systems, cultures, and behaviours in such a fundamental way as to make such a revolution possible. The particular focus of this study is a large hospital in the north of England where the author has been involved for a number of years as an "ethnographic action researcher"[18] and Organisation Development adviser.

Four years on from the Plan, there are almost as many different modernisation models as there are organisations in the NHS. In this case, people were firmly of the mind that any attempt to bring about major (second order) change through the existing (first order) management processes would be seriously undermined by the day to day pressures to deliver on short term government targets, such as reductions in waiting lists and times, and the time-consuming form-filling and box-ticking that went with this. "Delivery" and "development" were seen as competing pulls, the first always more likely to get the attention because of the greater urgency that surrounded it.

Recognising the tensions between service delivery and service development, a bold decision was taken to step outside the normal organisation and create an alternative transitional structure, a "temporary system"[19] or "parallel learning structure".[20] Through this, people could begin to feel their way towards new ways of thinking and working together, testing and trying things out as they went along, ultimately rolling them out to the rest of the organisation. Above all, this enabling structure would cut some "slack", and provide protected time for those involved in the longer term effort for change and reform. Locally, this came to be known as the "left lung, right lung" model for modernisation, the latter continuing to focus upon the day to day delivery of government and NHS targets, the former starting to engage with the huge developmental agenda at the individual, team and organisational levels.

A top level "Modernisation Team" was established to oversee the development of this transformational process, its membership consisting of 18 staff drawn from different parts of the organisation who were not normally active at senior management levels and mostly from the front line of delivering care: the chief executive, senior managers, surgeons and clinicians, nurses and nurse managers, junior and middle managers, medical secretaries, systems analysts, and technical and ancillary staff. Staff were approached and asked to be members (although membership was clearly stated as being voluntary), based on the skills, knowledge, experience and personal qualities[ii] they brought to the table, not on the occupational roles or positions they occupied within the Trust – sapiential (what you know) rather than positional (where you sit).

The role of the Group, most of whose members had not worked together before, was broadly stated as "assisting the process of modernisation", and later elaborated by the Group itself to include (in the original words): creating a vision for change and providing leadership to take this forward; promoting new ways of working and creative problem solving to help staff make radical, sustainable change; service reconfiguration; sharing good practice and learning within the Team and across the Trust, and working with staff to engage people with change; fostering enthusiasm and motivation for change; and maintaining an overview of modernisation activities across the Trust and within local areas in a dynamic and proactive way, celebrating success and acting as an "early warning system" where necessary. From the outset, the chosen emphasis was to be "big" cultural change, although most confessed to not knowing precisely what that meant or quite how it was to be achieved.

This chapter presents snatches from the Group's journey over a period of 18 months.

Travellers' tales

The Chief Executive's Tale

The first meeting of the Group took place at a small hotel some 15 miles distant from the main hospital site, lasting a full day. Early morning coffee, taken whilst watching the otters playing in the adjoining stream, had done little to quell the nerves of those present. Mike, a surgeon by background, and medical director before his recent appointment to the CEO post, opened up the proceedings. His "Tale" was to come as a surprise to those expecting something more sure-footed of their chief executive.

He began hesitantly, eyes down, mouth clearly dry.

Can I begin by welcoming you and thanking you for coming here today ... I would like to say I am clear why we are here and what I want us to achieve, but I am not. This is new ground for us all and that makes us all learners, including me. In my search for somewhere to start, I have been talking with Paul [author] a lot over the past few weeks, much of our conversation focusing upon the need for some kind of vision for the future that will give us a broad steer. I wasn't exactly sure what was required – am still not, to be perfectly honest – which means I have probably failed the first test of a leader!

As today approached, my anxiety began to increase. I didn't sleep too well last night, and even this morning I was still not exactly clear what I was going to say to you today. Not being able to sleep, I got up early and drove in to the hospital before coming over here. For reasons of which I am not entirely sure, I found myself in the hospital Chapel.

Have any of you ever read the hand-written book in there? It contains entries written by the relatives of our patients, many of them having recently lost friends and loved ones. I want to read you one of these entries. It is written by Mr Richard Smith, whose father was being treated at the hospital for bowel cancer. It reads: "My family and I always believed that the NHS provided the best treatment in the world. We now know that this is not the case. David, my father, died late last night in your hospital after his long fight against cancer. He was admitted three days ago to be operated on to alleviate his symptoms. He was starved for twenty four hours in readiness for the operation. The operation was cancelled on the first day and then again the day after that. You simply cannot starve cancer patients for days on end in the hope that their operation might be carried out. Is this any way to treat a person in the last three days of their life on this earth? I am shocked and amazed that you consider the management of my father's case and the administration of his treatment to be of a good standard."

By the time Mike had reached the end of his story the room had become silent. He looked up, visibly touched by what he had just read, as were those in the room. Suddenly, almost as an afterthought, he threw the paper from which he had been reading on to the table in front of him and said quietly: "No more Mr Smiths. That is my vision for this hospital and this Group. That's the best I can do for now, I'm afraid."

The group began to talk. They all had their own Mr Smith stories to tell …

"No more Mr Smiths" was to become part of the ethic of the group, a point to which they would return on a number of occasions whenever they sensed they were losing their way. As with all symbols, David Smith acquired a "more-than" quality within the change programme. People talked about "passing the Mr Smith test", thereby giving the quality improvement process a real and personalised quality. Over time, linguistic embellishments grew like a vine around the original Mr Smith story, giving it a mythical quality and elevating it to an almost supra-individual, cultural level.

Fern, the complaints manager, said she had seen hundreds of letters like Mr Smith's son's, though not forgetting all the good ones as well. She said she had brought along a sample, and could she read out some extracts from these as part of her story?

The Complaints Manager's Tale

The reading went on for nearly an hour, and only a small sample of the letters Fern read to the Group is included here, but hopefully sufficient to convey the sombre mood her story created.

"When I arrived I was very worried, but the receptionist and other staff around her were making comments amongst themselves. I have a speech impediment but the receptionist told me to hurry up and give her my name."

"During my husband's recent stay at the hospital, I was appalled my husband's lung biopsy was cancelled three times in four days. On complaining to a weekend doctor I was referred to as an "unhappy bunny", very insulting phrase I think, in fact I am still very angry. I do not agree that sick patients should be spoken about in this way."

"Throughout his stay the patient was moved to different wards on four occasions: Ward 21, Ward 32, Ward 12, and Ward 15. When he was moved from Ward 32 to Ward 12 his family were not informed, and it had not been entered officially on the information log. This resulted in his family coming to the hospital and not knowing where their father had been transferred. Staff on Ward 12 were not aware that the patient was already on the ward and they denied all knowledge of the patient when they were asked if he had been moved to Ward 12, even though he was on the ward."

"On several occasions, I asked staff whether I should have a gown for the operation. Eventually, I was told that there was one on the windowsill that I could use if it did not belong to anyone else. By this time, I was feeling very anxious, angry, and upset by the absolute lack of care from the nursing staff. It was very clear that the priority for their day was to discuss Christmas and associated social functions. Indeed, one member of staff spent in excess of twenty minutes on a personal phone call."

Fern said she found it unbelievable these things were happening in her hospital. Sometimes it made her sad, sometimes angry. That was why she had joined this group – to get it sorted out. She wanted the group to ask how care professionals sometimes did things to patients that were callous and uncaring. It would be easy just to say we are the "hospital from hell", and all would be explained, but the evidence didn't bear this out. This was the irony: how a hospital near to the very top of the league could sometimes fail at the basics. Interestingly, she said, one of our patients had asked the same question:

"I would like to make a few more points before I finish this letter, starting with one that comes to mind as I read the hospital website. According to this, the Trust has been awarded "beacon" status within the NHS for its groundbreaking initiative in directly booking patients for treatment – the "booked" scheme. I am also led to believe that the Trust delivers best value for money of all hospitals in the Region. Well!

Again, I'm inclined to wonder whatever value for money the others are offering ... And finally, it's a simple concept I know, but a friendly face letting people know what is happening is always welcome, and reassuring as well – and costs nothing at all. Just a thought."

Others tell their tales

Other members of the Team took turns to tell their stories, for example, the **Dermatologist's Tale**, the **Intensive Care Unit Nurse's Tale**, many of them also about failures in delivering basic care. Whilst some cases were the result of major systems failures (referrals, IT), others could be put down to bad "attitude" or just not thinking. For example, the **Clinical Director's Tale** consisted of him showing examples of posters in patient areas that were likely to cause offence: "If you were an anxious patient," he asked, "How would you feel if you were confronted by one of these?" Not all of the stories involved putting on the proverbial hair shirt; for example the **Ward Sister's Tale** was about the emergency pressures caused by the recent "flu" epidemic, and how people had stood shoulder to shoulder trying to deal with patients on trolleys in walkways and corridors – a tale that was as dramatic as it was heroic. Yet again, it revealed the extremes of care being provided within the hospital.

Discussion naturally turned to the question, *what* are these stories saying about us and our hospital, and how *do* you explain how an apparently outstanding hospital is capable of providing such poor patient care on occasions? Obviously (they agreed), there were "bad behaviours" that had to stop and new behaviours that needed to be nurtured and encouraged. One particular exercise involved hanging four large blank flipchart sheets in each corner of the room: "Stop Doing", "Do Less", "Start Doing", and "Do More", with each group member walking around sticking on Post-Its with one line suggestions for improvement (see Figure 19.1, which shows the original words and team classification).

Although a simple device, the matrix enabled the group to construct a joint diagnosis of what was wrong and what needed to change in the organisation – in their own words. The members also accepted that if they were to "model the way" for the rest of the organisation then it had to be a framework or code for them and how they conducted themselves within the Trust from now on. (They seemed to like the words I had quoted from Ghandi: "If you want to see change, then be the change you want to see.")

It was perfectly natural to move on from this and ask *why* these problems existed, and more importantly why they persisted. Plausible answers were not easy to find, and ranged from "systems" and "structure" problems to "bad apples in the barrel". Inevitably, attention came to rest on the "culture" of the organisation. People

STOP DOING	DO LESS

Bureaucracy
Taking work home
Reinventing the wheel
Reporting for reporting sake
Quality Control delays
 	
Patient Care
Cancellations of operations/appointments
Moving patients to several wards
Flexibility of wards/winter pressures
Opening endoscopy
Crisis management
 	
Blaming
Each other
Patients
Being victimised
Excuses for bad practice
Individuals for not delivering
Dictating
Acknowledging things not good at
	Bureaucracy
	Paperwork/duplication
	Reports to people who don't work for
	  the Trust
	Less "hands-off my patch"
	Too many meetings
	Moaning
	Putting up barriers
	Harking back to the past
	More flexible hours
	Pressurising staff to deliver to tight
	  timescales
	Changing decisions
	Blind adherence to government policy
	Pretending that you know everything

START DOING	**DO MORE**
Strategic Planning Focus more on long term planning Rethink way in which we deliver services Prepare to take risks **Empowerment** Helping staff take responsibility Supporting individuals **Back to Basics** Cleanliness Making time to treat patients as family Give them dignity and respect Individualised care **Communication** Improve interaction between departments Smile/say thank you Value staff Understand other people's perspective **Benchmarking** External collaboration Share good practice Internal collaboration Ask advice from people who know Work out what's in it for me	Talking to patients and staff Communications: to patients, staff and others Time: give staff more time to listen to patients More staff, fewer patients Forward thinking and planning Thinking laterally Giving incentives Planning across Directorates Smiling! Praising good staff Site development Clinical governance Highlighting new incentives Using staff already there Looking more at the long term strategy

Figure 19.1 "Start doing, Stop doing, Do more, Do less" matrix

were at one on this: "The culture in this organisation has to change. We must get a handle on that. This is going to have to involve a new way of thinking."

Bad habits of thinking

Blame culture	Not looking at cultural needs of patients
Not apologising for bad behaviour	Clinically doing things not qualified to do
Fear of admitting to mistakes	"Attitude" towards patients
Not good at praising people	Taking credit for others' work
Bullying	Not looking for new ways of working
Not listening	Not devolving responsibility
Not giving help when required	Lack of equality
Meetings culture	Need to empower people more
Jobs worth attitude	Insensitivity – talking about patients as
Not learning from our mistakes	objects
People being made scapegoats	Relatives and patients' abuse of staff not
Procedures not consistent – receive	acceptable
conflicting advice	

Figure 19.2 Cultural "bad habits of thinking"

The stories began to take a different turn, with temperatures rising perceptibly as people recounted their personal bruisings at the hand of "the culture". Again, everyone had a story to tell. Specific examples related to autonomy and the need to empower people. If people were given a job to do then they should be trusted and if they get it wrong then they should not be blamed. Another example related to financial management; it was felt if a manager could demonstrate they were able to manage their budgets, they should be allowed to make decisions with those resources, but this was not happening at the moment. A particular point was made about the "bullying culture" within certain parts of the Trust, and a management style that put people off taking responsibility and trying to effect change: "Form bullying" is a bit strong but in some parts of the hospital there is a 'your P45 [termination] is on the line' kind of language". "The consequence of this is that taking risks is harder. You have to have a lot of confidence or you package your failure in a way that is less than honest."

As before, the group began to draw up a list of the "bad habits of thinking" (their word for culture) that would need to be eliminated if patient care and staff well-being were to be improved. These are presented in Figure 19.2, again in the original words.

"Tribalism" and the lack of cross-boundary working was a major problem, they said, causing all kinds of hold-ups and bottlenecks on the patient journey: "Tribalism, yes, very much so. One of our weaknesses is there is an incentive to protect your own area and not be open and share things – there's not a sharing approach to solving problems." "Horizontal integration is appalling." "There's still a case of 'it's mine, you're not having it. If you want it you are going to have to fight me for it'." They talked about the "culture of blame": "The culture of blame and shame is always just under the surface. It's a blame culture no matter what the rhetoric might say." And the "culture of secrets": "It's all about how clever you are at spotting what people are doing – sure as hell they won't tell you."

As the stories and comments unfolded, the area of focus for the Modernisation Team became clearer: "culture change" (they said) had to be made the number one priority for the group. The question was how – a question that had defeated most theorists and practitioners up until now. The team had very much liked a paper I had circulated on complex adaptive systems approaches to change, especially the notion of creating "attractors" and "simple rules" for complex processes. Rather than get bogged down in detail and mountains of paperwork (for which the Trust was well known) they decided on some simple rules that would apply to any group anywhere in the Trust that wanted to undertake an improvement project. It meant that so long as people followed these simple rules, they could basically go off and do what they liked; they didn't have to wait for management approval. The "musts" included (original words):

- delivered by a multidisciplinary team committed to cross-boundary working;
- explicitly focused on improving service quality to patients and enhancing the quality of staff's experience of work: must make a difference;
- likely to have an impact across the Trust as well as the host individual clinical directorate;
- leads to major redesign and big change (people "thinking and doing things differently");
- involves sharing learning and good practice across the organisation;
- has direct patient and user involvement;
- will make a visible and demonstrable impact on the culture.

The theory of cultural change was disarmingly simple: don't set up a special project on cultural change or try to change culture directly, which will almost certainly fail. Instead, set some rules (cultural protocols) such as those above that involve people "acting out" – enacting – the kind of culture you want to create (cross-boundary, non-hierarchical, sharing learning, etc.), with cultural change naturally falling out from this process of "being the change you want to see". Hence, service change and cultural change would occur together, the latter as a residue or by-product of the improvement process. Two tales in particular were important to this new line of thinking: my tale (the **Author's Tale**) about similar cultural change programmes in which I had been involved with other organisations, and the **Ophthalmologist's Tale** in which he talked about a successful clinical governance project he and his colleagues had carried out in their area. Both tales enabled the group to reflect on the "dos and don'ts" of change and the necessary antecedents of successful change programmes.

By this point, and by way of the chain of stories, the group had reached a fairly advanced stage in their journey: they had succeeded in constructing a joint diagnosis of the problems and their causes, some definitions of what constituted a modernisation project, some norms and a model for the change process itself (what, why, how), and a theory about how to bring about change, especially cultural change. All that now remained was the actual "doing" of change – making it happen. The difficult part! At this point things began to speed up, for within a very short period of time a number of big modernisation projects had been launched and got under way, one to improve communication with patients and staff (which included among other things "breakfast" and "supper" meetings with the Chief Executive, and an overhauled intranet), and two others to radically redesign emergency medicine and radiology services. The latter in particular really took off, ultimately attracting national support and the attention of the Secretary of State himself. Later, on the strength of these early pioneering projects, the Trust was invited to become a founding member of the NHS Modernisation Agency "Associates" scheme, receiving additional support to pilot and develop new approaches to change in the areas of process redesign and clinical governance. The "delivery-development" approach was also to become quite well known within the NHS, often recommended as a model or template for modernisation.

The team had nearly reached journey's end, or at least the point where they could begin to hand their horses over to others for their own modernisation journeys. However, the storytelling was far from over. As the team became more and more involved in "real" change projects, the more the stories themselves became the real-life, real-time stories – running commentaries – of the change itself. Hence, not surprisingly, the **Pathologist's Tale** was about the ups and downs of the pathology project as it unfolded, as was the later **Nurse's Tale** about the introduction of "modern matrons" into the Trust. It was from these that the team learned most about the nature of change processes – about the unpredictability of it all, the obstacles and the blockages, the need for bold strokes and long marches on the journey, leadership as a team not a solo effort, the need for simple rules, and much more – stories that were no longer historical confabulations but stories from real life, no longer personal narratives but collective narratives of an experience they had shared together.

Discussion

Stories, storytelling, and change

Change is a journey, albeit one that often lacks any clear direction, destination or known balance of advantage.[21,22] Pettigrew[23] develops the engaging metaphor of "change journeys as wagon trains", comparing the organisational change journey to the traditional story of the nineteenth-century US wagon train heading westward to California from the relative safety and security of the eastern seaboard. His purpose is to draw attention to the hazards and uncertainties lying in wait in the punishing contextual terrain that has to be crossed, the ups and downs of energy and hope, and above all the dramas and politics that get played out between the mixed bag of settlers during their long haul towards the land of milk and honey: the enthusiasts (daydreamers, adventurers, missionaries, and zealots), career opportunists and malcontents, resource providers (product champions, political umbrella people and financiers), scouts (internal change agents and external consultants), and the innocent and not-so-innocent bystanders who observe this band of travellers but mostly choose not to participate in the journey themselves:

As the journey proceeds there is a sense of emotional relief as landmarks are reached. But there are ups and downs of energy as obstacles are rounded and blind canyons and other deadlocks encountered. For some (the lost and bewildered) there is journey's end, but not where anticipated. For the fortunate there is the prospect of a new life in California now that this particular stage in life's long journey has come to a successful end[23] (p 275).

Attractive though these images are, they fail to mention one thing: the crucial importance of stories and storytelling to that change journey – hence my allegorical switch from the Pioneers to the Pilgrims in Geoffrey Chaucer's *Canterbury Tales*. Stories may simply be one way of whiling away the time, but they also serve a much deeper social and cultural purpose. They are essential to group formation and development, in this case providing the mechanisms through which a motley collection of individuals, and the "carnival of voices" they represented, was able to metamorphose into a goal-directed community with a common identity and a single voice.[24] In such a community of purpose, people were able to deal with tasks more efficiently with less suspicion of hidden agendas, and a genuine desire to reach consensus on solutions to problems.[25]

Peck,[26] one of the pioneering writers on community, has a definition of community that describes our band of hospital travellers particularly well. He describes it as:

A group of individuals who have learned how to communicate honestly with each other, whose relationships go deeper than their masks of composure, and who have developed some significant commitment to make others' conditions our own. (p 59)

Similarly, Maynard and Mehrtens[27] describe community in the workplace as a situation where "barriers between people are brought down", and this again is very much what happened within the Modernisation Team. On one occasion a senior NHS figure visiting the group confessed afterwards to not being able to tell "who was who" (clinician from manager, senior from junior), adding that had she not known the chief executive beforehand she would also never have guessed his identity from his behaviour alone. The dialogue, she suggested, had been "person to person rather than position to position". A recent UK healthcare study[28] has used the "two-way windows" metaphor to describe how professional boundaries between clinicians and managers have become more permeable, allowing people to occupy each other's cognitive space and work simultaneously with each other's ideas. The crucial significance of stories in this regard is that they can transport people naturally and effortlessly between such thought-worlds.

The case study suggests that community unification and identity are established primarily through language, or rather the use of language ("parole" or script). As I have written elsewhere,[4] "Language is the key, for it is language that gives birth to meaning; and if people share a language they will also share meaning: as Crescimanno observes, words are the wings of meaning" (p 22). Viewed from a symbolic interactionist perspective, the participants' stories provided a unifying voice for the group, and the means through which individual meanings were forged into joint meanings, and ultimately joint acts,[29] where *mine* and *yours* gradually – often touchingly – became *ours*.[30]

"Community" is only one step removed from "social movement", and it is here where importance of stories and storytelling has been most eloquently articulated to date:

Social movements are constituted by the stories people tell to themselves and to one another. They reflect the deepest ways in which people understand who they are and to whom they are connected … They are constructed from the interweaving of personal and social biographies – from the narratives people rehearse to themselves about the nature of their lives … The construction of collective action, therefore, is inseparable from the construction of personal biography, from the ways, that is, we experience the imprecation of our individual and social selves.[31]

Stories might therefore be said to help find a place for the *me* in the *us*, and the us in the me. They are the mechanisms and means through which multiple identities get together under a common social vision (particularly significant in inter-professional organisations like health care). The above quotation also draws attention to the fact that stories are not only about talk but action. They are the springboard for construction of "collective action" and to this extent are not just a telling thing but a doing thing.

Apart from this social psychological dimension, there is also a political dimension to stories and storytelling which is expressed in the notion of *counter*-narratives.[31] (Buckler and Zien[32] have a similar concept of "maverick stories" which are said to give users a licence to break the rules.) We have illustrated how participants in the Modernisation Team would engage in the day-to-day construction of counter-narratives, highlighting the failures of the service and stigmatising the organisation culture that caused these, in so doing putting the case for radical counter-cultural change and playing out a kind of "anti-role" within the organisation. In this sense, stories could be said to be operating as the mechanisms of mobilisation, the means whereby personal experience and biography were forged into some kind of collective movement for action.

The case study shows that stories and storytelling are therefore not only crucial to establishing group identity; they are equally crucial to implementing change, especially cultural change:

> Language is also the key to change. If you want to change the way people think, start by changing the way they talk. You need to encourage them to devise new scripts and participate in new language games. You endeavour to shape intellectual and symbolic structures by giving people new topics of conversation to debate, gossip and fight about; and you give them new stories to tell and retell each other. The theory of change is therefore actually quite a simple one: if you can unfreeze and restructure language you can unfreeze and restructure thought ... Stories and storytelling are a crucial aspect of organisational life ... the narrative to tie experiences, views and interpretations together, something that has sequence, logic, flow and direction, that represents a coherent version of the emerging reality.[4] (pp 258–9)

The type of story varied according to which stage of the journey the Modernisation Team were on, and the main focus of concern at the time. Early stories tended to concentrate on substantive problems and issues, the vision and direction, the task itself, and the behavioural norms of the group – all very much the "whats" of the change journey. Mid-stage stories shifted the focus of attention to the "why" – collective interpretations of why the problems existed (and persisted), such as the cultural interpretation the group constructed to explain the failures and shortcomings in hospital care. Later stories, the **Ophthalmologist's Tale** and the **Pathologist's Tale** for example, addressed the methodology or "how" of change and improvement, the former reporting on a previously successful change attempt, the latter reflecting on the results of a change project initiated by the Modernisation Team itself. These were not so much snapshots as enactments, that is to say not so much pictures of that part of the journey as the very definers of the reality itself – reality as constituted by the stories people tell to themselves and one another.

As previous writers have observed, there is a particularly strong connection between storytelling and *cultural* change (see Boyce[11] for a critical review), Weick and Browning's aphorism summing it up very effectively:

> Stories are not a symptom of culture, culture is a symptom of storytelling.[33]
> (p 249)

What has not been clear, however, is how that relationship works. This case offers some insights into this process, suggesting that the accumulation and coalescence of stories over time gives participants a clearer collective sense of "present culture" (that is, helps them make sense of the "now", especially its more dysfunctional aspects) and from that a picture – and more importantly shared feeling – of the kind of culture to which they wish to move. Stories and storytelling therefore help participants to find a common voice, acting as the medium through which different languages are converted into different dialects of the same language (the notion of communal narrative).

More specifically, it would seem that stories play a crucial role at every stage of the change journey, from conception through to implementation, including:

- building personal awareness and understanding, and finding a place for one*self* on the change journey (personal narrative);
- becoming aware of alternative perspectives and overlapping values, aims and purposes; merging personal and collective identities and building a community of practice (communal narrative);
- critiquing and stigmatising "the present", and building a shared "felt need" and vision for change (counter-narrative);
- translating joint commitments into joint actions; moving forward together, and, most importantly, keeping going (mobilising narrative).

"Communities of practice": a new form of politics in organisational change efforts?

Writing as observer and fellow traveller with this hospital group, the concept that brings the whole experience into focus for me is that of the "community of practice" (CoP). The term "community of practice", though very fashionable today, was used as long ago as 1991 by Etienne Wenger and Jean Lave in their book *Situated*

Learning.[34] The theory and philosophy shaping this view of social learning and knowledge management have been progressively elaborated in later publications by them[35] and numerous others, Brown and Duguid[9,10] in particular. Definitions abound. Wenger himself defines a CoP broadly as one where people share their experiences and knowledge in free-flowing creative ways so as to foster new approaches to problem solving and improvement, help drive strategy, transfer best practice, develop professional skills, and help companies recruit and retain staff. On the other hand, de Merode[36] refers to three elements of a CoP – strategy, trust (ethos), and processes – using these, and the degree of fit that exists between them, to define the features of a successful community of practice.

However, the definition I have adopted for the purposes of this paper comes from Gabbay and Le May,[37] who define a CoP as a group of people who

- may not normally work together
- but who are acting and committed to learning together
- in order to achieve a common task (common action-related interest)
- whilst acquiring and constructing appropriate knowledge
- purposefully constructed but voluntarily attended.

That is to say, a group of people brought together to do a job they all have a keen interest in doing.

This definition fits the hospital Modernisation Team very well, suggesting that what I have been observing has indeed been a nascent and emerging community of practice – not a "network", not a "work group", not even a "team", but a distinctive organisational form/process in its own right: what I would describe idiomatically as a *social group with a job to do, a "mini-movement" for change*. In this sense, I would strongly concur with the distinctions drawn by Wenger and Snyder[35] between communities of practice, networks and teams, highlighting in particular the unique passion and commitment that propel a community of practice forward (the inner emotional drivers).

For a phenomenon that has received so much attention it is surprising how little is known about the internal processes and workings of a community of practice, not least its political nature and dynamics and its role in the change process. My study suggests there are four contexts in particular which shape the ethos, character, and politics of a community of practice, and ultimately its role in the change process: the emotion context, the culture context, the leadership context, and finally the structural context.

First, the *emotion context*. As Wenger and Snyder state,[35] feeling and emotion infuse almost every part of a community's being, providing the background for a unique form of politics to emerge:

This concept refers to the mood or consensually acknowledged presence of emotions that are influencing situational interactions. Emotions, considered at the contextual level, differ from other properties of negotiation contexts, because they can permeate or take over the situation at hand.[38] (p 280)

It is difficult to imagine how the Modernisation Team could have functioned in the way that it did without the strong emotional context set by moments like the **Chief Executive** and **Complaints Manager's Tales**, and the cast of thousands who appeared in them like Mr Smith and all the many other "ghosts" that came to occupy the same socio-emotional space. Not only did stories like his become the main currency of communication between the team members, they also provided the main energising or mobilising force for the group, the thing that kept them going on their journey even, and especially, when the initial vision began to fade. So powerful were these emotions that, to use Sugrue's phrase, they sometimes "took over the situation at hand", enabling participants to transcend the different "life worlds" that separated them, to set their face to the wind and find the strength to inch another step forward towards their goal.

Emotions were the very life-blood of the community of practice that I studied and its change process, and in this the role of stories and storytelling – the other element of our analysis – was pivotal. The role of the stories was to transpose personal feelings into social emotions, and in so doing to help turn and bind a motley group of individuals into a community:

Feelings can be kept to oneself and remain privatized throughout all or part of a negotiation encounter. Those feelings, once incorporated into the interactions become emotions. They become linguistically tagged or categorized as anger, fear, love and so forth ... emotions are aspects of and influences on patterned human conduct.[38] (pp 281, 291)

Listening to each other's stories, people got angry, they got sad, they laughed and they cried, and in so doing they discovered at a deep level how they connected with each other, and why they were there – more so than any document, plan, or programme could ever have done. One of the Chief Executive's favourite sayings was from the old TV advert: "Shake the bottle, wake the fizz." Clearly the stories performed this function of putting life and vitality back into the group and organisational change process. In this respect, it is worth expressing a note of disappointment that the wider change literature, which over the years has become increasingly preoccupied with the "re" prefix – revitalisation, renewal, reframing, revolution and so on – has done little to establish a connection between these large scale change challenges and the emotional dimension of change that was so powerfully revealed in this study.

Social movement theorists talk about tapping into people's "sentiment pools" in order to mobilise the change effort,[39] using the energy within them to drive change. Our case revealed sentiment pools in abundance, and shows how stories and storytelling provided a naturalistic and effective way of locating and tapping into these.

As noted above, up until now most of the change models and approaches proposed in the literature have made little or no reference to emotion or affect. However, recent writings, notably Kotter's latest book *The Heart of Change*,[40] have begun to signal a switch from the "analysis–think–change" model to the "see–feel" model, underscoring the findings of this study that emotion is a – if not the – most powerful "driver" and energiser of change. This could not have been better illustrated than by the hospital modernisation group itself, one of whose favourite phrases became, "You don't need an engine when you've got wind in the sails."

The *culture context* was also crucial to the everyday processes of this particular community of practice. Despite its diverse and multi-professional nature, one of the great achievements of the Modernisation Team was to create a culture that was high on both sociability and solidarity[41] – this being reflected in its self-appended nickname, "The Mod Squad": solid and ready for action. Though undoubtedly pleasant and agreeable in its own right, this quality was more significant for its impact upon group effectiveness, particularly knowledge transfer and group learning. Szulanski[42] has talked about the ease of knowledge transfer depending on the *quality* of the source–recipient relationship and the *strength* and denseness of that relationship, while Yoo and Kanawattanachai[43] have also said that for knowledge exchange (particularly tacit knowledge) and learning to take place, there needs to be strong personal connections, a high degree of cognitive interdependence among participants, a shared sense of identity and belongingness with one's colleagues, and the existence of cooperative relationships. On all of these things the community of practice scored highly.

The *leadership context* is the third framing feature of a community of practice. Surprisingly, leadership receives little attention in the CoP literature, yet this case study underlines its importance in shaping the whole way in which a CoP develops, indeed whether a group develops into a CoP at all. Mike, the CEO, must take credit here for recognising that a community of practice cannot be "directed" as such, otherwise it just becomes another project group or management team. Learning communities such as these cannot be directed, only enabled, facilitated, and supported. As one person in the private sector who led community of practice development at both the US National Securities Administration and Buckman Laboratories remarked: "I had to learn that these learning communities are more like volunteer organisations. They simply cannot be managed like a project or team".[44]

In Mike's "Mr Smith story" we also have powerful confirmation of the notion of "leadership as storytelling". Buckler and Zien[32] have a wonderful summary of this idea, pointing out that like all great leaders of the past, organisational leaders tell parables:

> Leadership through storytelling emphasises the more empowering parts of an organisation's past and brings them into the present for all members of the enterprise. Storytelling is an act of creating future opportunities. Communicating through teaching parables, that serve life as it is configured today, yet are grounded in the organisation's founding experiences ... is part of leading creatively. In this sense the stories are not old, but take an experience from the past ... and create a living "collective memory" of the lessons learned, even for newcomers. The stories provide a continuous thread to bond all in the organisation with the energy and learnings derived from invigorating experiences ... The role of top management is to invent and give form to a transformational story for the organisation. (p 405)

Finally, it is difficult to imagine how any of the processes described could have occurred had there not been the space and protection afforded by the new "temporary", organisation for modernisation. It was within this particular *structural context*, created specifically for the purposes of the organisational change process, that people found themselves able to think the unthinkable, tell their personal stories, develop counter-narratives (many of them risqué, radical, and subversive), rehearse and try out different scripts and ways of working with each other, and generally talk about things other than targets. Employing a dramaturgical metaphor, Mangham and Overington[45] have used the phrase "out-of-town-try-out" to refer to the idea of trying out the Play (change script) in the Provinces before taking it to and mainstreaming it in the West End of London, and it is my view that the Modernisation Team meetings provided similar opportunities for rehearsal and fine-tuning before launching the ideas on the wider organisation. This metaphor adds the further suggestion that the temporary organisation is able to help people reduce the sense of personal risk, thereby increasing their propensity and resilience for change. This also calls to mind Hirsch's powerful notion of organisational "havens",[46] face-to-face settings isolated from people in power in which people can speak freely about their hopes and concerns. This study strongly suggests that organisational change processes need such havens – another neglected area in the literature and not the same as the concept of "slack" that is often referred to.

Above all, this temporary organisation represented a "definitional vacuum" within the structure, an empty vessel into which people could begin to generate and pour "new" meanings, at the same time avoiding the risk of being drowned by the "old" ones. In the social movements literature this would be similar to the notion of "free spaces"[47] and "opportunity structures",[31] both of them shown to be essential for mobilisation and change. McAdam's notion of "cognitive liberation"[48] is also relevant here, when people discover that what they had always assumed to be immutable may not in fact be the case; the realisation that things can actually be changed, that one might, just might, be able to make a difference. Looking back over all these features of the temporary organisation, there is clearly a strong connection between "restructuring" and "reframing" that has yet to be explored in the wider change literature.

Concluding remarks

So what about the wider significance of our story, if indeed there is any? Clearly we cannot say how typical our Modernisation Team is of the NHS or organisations generally, but what we do know is that the community of practice, of which this is but one example, is extremely widespread today, and therefore that processes similar to what we have observed may be at work elsewhere, particularly within organisational change programmes. For example, we know that companies such as Xerox have chosen to base almost their entire change agenda upon "communities of practice" rather than any kind of formal change programme, which they claim rarely delivers anything of significance. For them, such "communities of practice", much more than formal management structures, are vital to how people share experiences, learn about new ideas, coach one another in trying them out, and share practical tips and lessons over time. This is why Xerox commissioned a major ethnographic study to search out natural, informal communities of practice upon which the change programme would come to be based.[49]

Xerox is not exceptional in this regard. Mainly as a consequence of the growing interest in knowledge management, a number of other private sector companies have also come to acknowledge the importance of such communities for learning and change:

> The subject of communities in the business environment has recently taken on heightened interest among some of the world's largest companies. Organisations such as BP Amoco, Royal Dutch Shell, IBM, Xerox, the World Bank and British Telecom have all undertaken significant community development efforts in an attempt to leverage the collective knowledge of their employees.[50]

All of this prompts us to consider whether the community of practice may mark a shift in the way organisational change processes are being played out today, away from adversarialism and contestation towards a form that is generally milder and more communal than before. We examine this proposition briefly below.

Sceptics will no doubt argue that what we are seeing is yet another form of control, another cunning ruse thought up by management in order to maintain its legitimacy and exploit (in today's parlance) the "knowledge labour" of their employees – and in some circumstances this may well be the case. However, in the case of my study it is hard to discern this in the motives or actions of either the Chief Executive or the hospital senior management (who were mostly excluded anyway), and it has to be said that, having observed this process close-to, there have to be easier ways of gaining control and legitimacy than this.

As far as one can best tell, the dominant motive was not management control but improving services for patients, change not order or control, and in this respect the group was actually challenging the existing order. Certainly, a number of the managers not directly involved in the Modernisation Team perceived it as such, which would explain why they spent so much of their time resisting and, on occasions, bad-mouthing it. With membership of a community of practice being voluntary there is a built-in safeguard against management domination. People can walk out on the group at any time, and will only remain if they perceive their needs and interests are being adequately addressed by the group.

One other thing to add before leaving this issue of management control is that the approach adopted by the Modernisation Team allowed previously "silent voices" within the organisation (junior staff) and outside it (patients) to be heard, some for the first time, and to this extent was a wider, more inclusive form of politics than had existed before.[51] The final point on this, again too big to be taken up at any length here, but fortunately already taken up by others,[52] is that the community of practice may be there because it is filling an emotional or spiritual gap. People are looking for more meaning and spirituality in their working lives, more collectivity, and a more intense sense of shared moral purpose, and in some cases the community of practice, as is indeed was the case with the Modernisation Team, may be able to provide this. In the face of such a rich social experience, it is therefore difficult to write the whole thing off as a cynical act of manipulation on the part of management.

We also need to revisit the current cultural paradigm as described in the introduction to this chapter, since its traditional core idea is of culture as a contested process of meaning-making.[53] This has been allowed to go unchallenged for more than a decade, and arguably is stronger today than it has ever been. The contribution of the storytelling and communities of practice literatures is again to challenge this and to suggest that the issue of modern organisational politics may be more one of *construction* than *contestation*, with "power" taking a back seat to "knowledge" – knowledge sharing not knowledge withholding as would typically be found in a negotiation context. This is also the conclusion of Newell *et al*'s fascinating study of another community of practice within the NHS, which like my own highlights the importance of language and narration in the community of practice:

> In a community of practice, knowledge is constructed as individuals share ideas through collaborative mechanisms such as narration and joint work. Within such communities shared means for interpreting complex activity are thus constructed, often out of conflicting and confusing data. It is this *process* of constructing meaning, which provides organisational members with identity and cohesiveness.[54]

Therefore, to conclude: stories and storytelling and the communities of practice lie at the very heart of the change process – in both a literal and metaphorical sense. People "get to know each other" by telling and retelling organisational – in this case quality-related – stories, and from this they construct shared meanings and understandings, and develop trust relationships and emotional ties. As a collective identity emerges they effectively turn into a "unit of action", moving in roughly the same direction of change and connected to the same inspiring purpose. This study therefore offers a timely reminder that cooperation, consensus, and commonality of outlook may not have entirely deserted the modern organisation, indeed may even be making a comeback in the change arena. The convivial travellers in Chaucer's *Canterbury Tales* would no doubt be pleased to hear this, though probably not surprised.

Acknowledgement

An earlier version of this chapter was presented at the 18th EGOS Colloquium, Organizational Politics and the Politics of Organisation, 4–6 July 2002, Barcelona, Spain (Sub theme 23: Anthropological Perspectives on Power, Performance and Organisational Politics). A different iteration of the story and analysis appears in *Intervention. Journal of Culture, Organisation and Management*, **1**(1), September 2003. I wish to thank Routledge for granting permission to use some of that material here.

Endnotes

i   *The Canterbury Tales* (by Geoffrey Chaucer, 1342–1400), said by some to be indebted to Boccaccio's Decameron, is the story of a group of 30 people who travel as Pilgrims to Canterbury (England). The Pilgrims, who come from all layers of society, tell stories to amuse each other and kill time while they travel to Canterbury. No single literary genre dominates. The tales include romantic adventures, fabliaux, saint's biographies, animal fables, religious allegories, and even a sermon, and range in tone from pious, moralistic tales to lewd and vulgar sexual farces.

ii The intriguing list of qualities included: "commitment and a willingness to invest time, enthusiasm, 'thinking out of boxes', 'sparky, switched on people', ability to deliver, sceptical, credibility, opinion leaders, hunger for change, communication ability, comfortable with ambiguity, spirit of experimentation, risk taking, personal vision, prepared to work out of comfort zones."

References

1   Brown A. Narrative politics and legitimacy in an IT implementation *J Manag Stud* 1998;**35**(1):35–58.
2   Mangham IL. *The politics of organisational change*. London: Associated Business Press, 1979.
3   Parker M. *Organisational culture and identity*. London: Sage, 2002.
4   Bate SP. *Strategies for cultural change*. Oxford: Butterworth Heinemann, 1994.
5   Bate SP, Mangham IL. *Exploring participation*. Chichester: Wiley, 1981.
6   Bate SP. Changing the culture of a hospital: from hierarchy to networked community. *Publ Admin* 2000;**78**(3):485–512.
7   Bate SP, Khan R, Pye A. Towards a culturally sensitive approach to organization structuring: where organisation design meets organisation development. *Org Sci* 2000;**11**(2): 197–211.
8   Wenger E. *Communities of practice*. Cambridge: Cambridge University Press, 1998.
9   Brown JS, Duguid P. Organising knowledge. *Calif Manag Rev* 1998;**40**(3):90–112.
10 Brown JS, Duguid P. Balancing act: how to capture knowledge without killing it. *Harvard Bus Rev* 2000;May–June:73–7.
11 Boyce ME. Organisational story and storytelling: a critical review. *J Org Change Manag* 1996;**9**(5):5–26.
12 Boje DM. Stories of the storytelling organisation: a postmodern analysis of Disney as *Tamara*-Land. *Acad Manag J* 1995;**38**(4):997–1035.
13 Shaw P. *Changing conversations in organisations. A complexity approach to change.* London: Routledge, 2002.
14 Bailey P. Storytelling and the interpretation of meaning in qualitative research. *J Adv Nurs* 2002;**38**(6): 574–83.
15 Greenhalgh T. Narrative and the primary care consultation. In: Greenhalgh T. *The academic study of primary health care*. London: BMJ Books (in press).
16 Mattingly C. *Healing dramas and clinical plots: the narrative structure of experience*. New York: Cambridge University Press, 1998.
17 Department of Health. *The NHS Plan: a plan for investment a plan for reform*. Issued by the Department of Health, July 2000.
18 Bate SP. Synthesising research and practice: using the action research approach in health care settings. *Soc Policy Admin* 2000;**34**(4):478–93.
19 Doz Y, Thanheiser W. Regaining competitiveness: a process of organizational renewal. In: Hendry J, Johnson G, eds. *Strategic thinking: leadership and the management of change*. Chichester: Wiley, 1993.
20 Bushe GR, Shani AB. *Parallel learning structures*. Reading, MA: Addison–Wesley, 1991.
21 Marshak RJ. Managing the metaphors of change. *Organisational Dynamics* 1993;**22**(1):44–56.
22 Inns D. Organisation development as a journey. In: Oswick C, Grant D, eds. *Organisation development: metaphorical explorations*. London: Pitman, 1996, pp 20–32.
23 Pettigrew AM. Success and failure in corporate transformation initiatives. In: Galliers RD, Baets WRJ, eds. *Information Technology and Organisational Transformation*. Chichester: Wiley 1988, pp 271–89.
24 Judge WQ, Fryxell GE, Dooley RS. The new task of R & D management: creating goal-directed communities for innovation. *Calif Manag Rev* 1997; **39**(3):72–85.
25 Borei JM. Chaos to community: one company's journey toward transformation. *World Bus Acad Perspectives* 1992;**6**(2):77–83.

26 Peck MS. *The different drum*. New York: Simon & Schuster, 1987.
27 Maynard HB, Mehrtens SE. *The Fourth Wave: business in the 21st century*. San Francisco, CA: Berrett–Koehler, 1993, p 13.
28 Llewellyn S. Two-way windows: clinicians as medical managers. *Org Stud* 2001;**22**(4):593–623.
29 Blumer H. Sociological implications of the thought of George Herbert Mead. *Am J Sociol* 1966;**71**:535–48.
30 Turner RH. The self in social interaction. In: Gordon G, Gergen K, eds. *The self in social interaction*. New York: Wiley, 1981, pp 93–106.
31 Kling J. Narratives of possibility: social movements collective stories and the dilemmas of practice. Paper presented to the *New Social Movement and Community Organising Conference*, University of Washington School of Social Work, November 1–3 1995.
32 Buckler SA, Zein KA. From experience: the spirituality of innovation: learning from stories. *J Production Innovation Manag* 1996;**13**:391–405.
33 Weick KE, Browning LD. Argument and narration in organizational communication. In: Hunt JG, Blair JD, eds. *Yearly Review of Management, Journal of Management* 1986;**12**(2):243–59.
34 Wenger E, Lave J. *Situated Learning*. Cambridge: Cambridge University Press, 1991.
35 Wenger E, Snyder WM. Communities of practice: the organisational frontier. *Harvard Bus Rev* 2000;Jan–Feb:139.
36 de Merode L. demerode@WorldNet.att.net
37 Gabbay J, Le May A. Knowledge management on multi-agency communities of practice. Paper presented to *NHS Knowledge Management Colloquium*, Southampton, March 6–7 2002.
38 Sugrue NM. Emotions as property and context for negotiation. *Urban Life* (special issue on The Negotiated Order, ed. DR Maines) 1982;**11**(3):280–91.
39 Snow DA, Rochford EB, Worden SK, Benford RD. Frame alignment processes micromobilisation and movement participation *Am Sociol Rev* 1986;**51**:464–81.
40 Kotter JP. *The heart of change*. Boston, MA: Harvard Business School Press, 2002.
41 Goffee R, Jones G. *The character of a corporation*. London: HarperCollins, 1998.
42 Szulanksi G. Exploring internal stickiness: impediments to the transfer of best practices within the firm. *Strat Manag J* 1996;**17** (Winter special issue): 27–43.
43 Yoo Y, Kanawattanachai P. Developments in transactive memory and collective mind in virtual teams. Paper presented to the Annual Meeting of the Academy of Management, Washington, DC, 2001.
44 Allee V. Knowledge networks and communities of practice. *OD Practitioner Online* 2000;**32**(4): www.odnetwork.org/odponline.
45 Mangham IL, Overington MA. Performance and rehearsal: social order and organisational life. *Symbolic Interaction* 1992;**5**(2):205–23.
46 Hirsch EL. *Urban revolt: ethnic politics in the nineteenth century Chicago labour movement*. Berkeley, CA: University of California Press, 1989.
47 Evans SM, Boyte HC. *Free spaces: the sources of democratic change in America*. New York: Harper and Row, 1986.
48 McAdam D. *Political process and the development of black insurgency 1930–1970*. Chicago: University of Chicago Press, 1982.
49 Turner C. What are communities of practice? In: Senge P and associates, eds. *The dance of change. A fifth discipline resource*. London: Nicolas Brealey, 1999, pp 477–80.
50 Lesser EL, Fontaine MA, Slusher JA. *Knowledge and communities*. Oxford: Butterworth–Heinemann, 2000.
51 Czarniawska B. *Narrating the organization. Drama of institutional identity*. Chicago: University of Chicago Press, 1997.
52 Turnbull S. Quasi-religious experiences in a corporate change programme – the roles of conversion and the confessional in corporate evangelism. Department of Management Learning, Lancaster University Management School, 2002.
53 Wright S. The politicization of "culture". *Anthropology Today* **14**(2):2–17; RAI Online. http://lucy.ukc.ac.uk/rai/AnthToday/wright.html.
54 Newell S, Edelman L, Bresnen M, Scarborough H. The inevitability of reinvention in project-based learning. Paper presented to 17th EGOS Colloquium, 'The Odyssey of Organizing,' Lyons, 5–7 July.

20: Meta-narrative mapping: a new approach to the systematic review of complex evidence

TRISHA GREENHALGH

This chapter tells the story of how a research team, grappling with a difficult project, discovered that looking for stories enabled them to make sense of a vast, chaotic, and seemingly contradictory set of data. It explores how the key characteristics of narrative as set out in many of the other chapters in this book – its placing of events in historical time, its inherent emplotment (in which one action or event *leads to* another), its inclusion of metaphor and imagery, and, most importantly, its sense-making potential – inspired and drove the search for meaning in a research study where meaning seemed particularly hard to find.

In this chapter, I will introduce the term "meta-narrative mapping" to denote the work of plotting how a particular research tradition has unfolded over time and placing this dynamic tradition within a broader field of enquiry. I will argue towards a controversial new hypothesis: that the science of systematic review should routinely take a narrative perspective, because a *summary* of a set of papers is an impoverished approach compared to giving an account of *how, why,* and *in what order* a research tradition unfolded. Finally, I will propose what I hope will prove to be a transferable schema for applying narrative techniques more generally to the systematic review of complex evidence, and I will invite others to test it out.

The study described in this chapter undoubtedly took the course it did because of my own wider interest in narrative-based research (and especially because I was editing this book while the work was in progress). But it owes much to the input of my fellow researchers Glenn Robert, Paul Bate, Fraser Macfarlane, Olympia Kyriakidou, Richard Peacock, Anna Donald, and Frances Maietta, and to the peer reviewers whose candid feedback took us back to the drawing board on more than one occasion.

Systematic review: its origins and contribution

A working definition of a systematic review is "an objective and dispassionate summary of all the published research on a particular topic area". The task of meticulously tracking down and checking dozens (or, in some cases, hundreds) of primary research studies, and rejecting (with careful justification) those that were methodologically flawed, is a challenging technical task known as secondary research, for which sophisticated evaluation and synthesis methods have now been developed.[1]

The International Cochrane Collaboration, established in the early 1990s, has set itself the task of indexing and summarising all high quality clinical research studies in health care. Their Reviewers' Handbook[1] sets out some key principles for the systematic review of biomedical evidence: (a) be very clear about what you want to find out, and in particular, pose a tightly focused question to exclude material of marginal relevance; (b) search methodically in a defined field of literature (most usually, in the vast electronic databases of biomedical papers such as Medline and Embase); (c) select the best quality research designs (for example, when evaluating a treatment, give preference to large, well-conducted randomised controlled trials); (d) use predefined quality criteria to reject flawed studies (for example, reject a randomised controlled trial if more than a certain proportion of participants "dropped out"); and (e) express results in terms of a clear "bottom line" (for example, in terms of how many patients would need to take the contraceptive pill to produce one thrombosis).

Scholars in fields related to biomedicine (such as nursing, sociology, social psychology, and medical anthropology) have begun to develop a comparable science of qualitative synthesis – that is, finding, evaluating, and combining studies whose data comprises behaviours, statements, and impressions rather than quantities and probabilities. The different approaches to the synthesis of qualitative evidence are beyond the scope of this chapter, but the interested reader might like to consult the references on such techniques as cross-case analysis,[2,3] meta-ethnography by reciprocal retranslation,[4] grounded theory applied across studies,[5] and meta-study (incorporating meta-theory).[6,i] In qualitative synthesis there is no attempt to produce a "grand mean" (a single number with a narrow confidence limit that encapsulates all the results of the separate primary studies). The task of the qualitative systematic reviewer is meaningfully to compare and combine the findings and interpretations of different authors who have approached a single, clearly focused research question in pretty much the same way, thereby achieving higher-order interpretive insights.[ii]

In parallel with these emerging traditions in quantitative and qualitative research, researchers in more applied fields of enquiry (such as health policy, social policy, education, and management) have also taken on the challenge of producing comprehensive, objective, and (as far as possible) unbiased summaries of research evidence relevant to aspects of their work. As Box 20.1 shows, the enquiries of educators, policy makers, and managers often embrace both quantitative biomedical research (trials, surveys, etc.) and "pure" qualitative research (interviews, focus groups, ethnographic observation, etc.) as well as more service-focused designs such as audits, annual reports, satisfaction surveys, market research, secondary analysis of data collected for a different purpose, process description, and so on. Achieving rigour in the synthesis of evidence for policy making is one of the key challenges of secondary research.

Box 20.1 Policy questions that require systematic reviews of complex evidence

How can we prevent childhood accidents?
How can we improve the proportion of working class children who get a university degree?
What should we do about teenage pregnancy?
How can we reduce the growing epidemic of obesity?
What is the best way to care for people with schizophrenia in the community?
How can we disseminate the findings of research so that people actually take notice of it?

I discovered several years ago that in informal spaces such as email lists or the coffee queues of academic conferences, researchers tended to use metaphors like "nightmare", "swamp" or "bottomless pit" to describe their efforts to review systematically the literature on questions of public policy and management such as those listed in Box 20.1.[iii] The work was widely recognised to be demanding, frustrating, and unfulfilling. There was a prevailing belief, rarely articulated in print, that such projects were never adequately funded, and that the task of wading through mountains of "grey literature" that lacked a unitary theoretical coherence was a labour of love properly reserved for the PhD student or geek. Published reviews almost always included the three statements "the research literature was ambiguous and contradictory", "we rejected most studies as methodologically flawed", and "more research on this topic is needed". All in all, producing a coherent account for one's sponsor (and especially for the policy making community) was generally held to be a bit of a fudge. Worse, the more one attempted *not* to fudge (that is, the more stringently one followed the principles of conventional systematic review set out above), the more impossible and frustrating the task seemed to get.

There is a reason for this paradox. All the examples in Box 20.1 – and indeed most other questions in policymaking, management, education, and other complex applied fields – have five important features in common: (a) they have an open-ended stem (that is, they start with phrases like "what should we do about ..." or "how could we change ..." rather than words like "how many", "what is the probability of" or even "what is the experience/perspective of"), and as such are inherently "unfocused"; (b) they are cross-disciplinary in nature (that is, relevant research evidence is likely to come from a multiplicity of separate bodies of literature, including a substantial fraction from "grey" sources); (c) there is rarely a single, self-evident optimum research design to address these sorts of question (indeed, the most useful summary will generally draw on a range of different types of research from interview surveys to formal intervention trials); (d) so-called "flawed" studies (for example, data collected for a different purpose and only subsequently treated as research) may have a critical bearing on the problem; (e) there is very rarely a simple, universal "bottom line"; and (f) it is often extraordinarily difficult to differentiate "is" from "ought" – that is, to define what is a matter of science and what a matter of values. In other words, systematic reviews that are likely to inform policy are not conventional systematic reviews writ large: they are reviews that *break all the fundamental rules of conventional systematic reviewing.*

There has recently begun to emerge a methodological literature that recognises the inherent epistemological paradox of producing systematic reviews of complex evidence.[9-11] There are already some well-established general principles, such as that secondary research in complex fields of evidence should be multidisciplinary, exploratory, flexible, and reflective,[12] and that researchers who use a formulaic, checklist-driven approach to evaluation and synthesis will produce findings of dubious validity.[13] Much of the advice so far published boils down to: take a broad and inclusive rather than narrow and dismissive approach, bear in mind the audience for your findings, use your interpretive faculties and your common sense, and be prepared to defend your judgements.[9] It was against this background that we took on the project described in the next section.

The research question: how do you spread good ideas?

In 2002, the UK Department of Health (via its Service Delivery and Organisation Programme) sought bids for a systematic review on "Diffusion, spread and sustainability of innovations in health service delivery and organisation". The brief for the project was to inform the modernisation agenda for UK health services set out in the white paper *The NHS Plan*[14] and led by the NHS Modernisation Agency. The pragmatic question was: "If hospital X develops a good way of running service Y, how can we best transfer that idea to hospital Z in a way that takes proper account of its different context, history, available resources and current situation?"

My own team were pleased to get the contract, both because we genuinely wanted to answer the question[iv] and because it offered an unparalleled opportunity to develop the methodology of synthesising complex evidence. But even in the early stages, we recognised that the work would indeed be a "nightmare", a "swamp", and much else besides. For one thing, there were no easy definitions of many of the key terms in the project title such as "systematic review",[v] "innovation",[vi] "spread",[vii] and "sustainability".[viii] Although I have revealed our final definitions in the Endnotes on page 376, at the time of planning the project we were working with much fuzzier and contested definitions of our key terms, whose very ambiguity made it almost impossible to define tight inclusion criteria for the primary studies. For another thing, quite frankly, we had no idea where to look for the "good research studies on spreading good ideas" – or even how to spot a good study on this enticing but elusive topic area.[ix] Thirdly, it was clear from the outset that if we kept a very narrow focus to our study (for example, if we restricted our review to research undertaken in public sector health care), we would miss studies from non-health-care sectors and/or from the private sector – which might well prove the best source of original ideas for our client, since the best "new ideas" are very often from initiatives *unlike* one's own!

Faced with what we now know to be the standard headaches of the SODDHS reviewer,[iii] we agreed to each explore a different area of "possibly relevant" research and report back to the team at our next meeting. Each of us asked around our colleagues, sent emails, wandered through libraries and bookshops, sifted through our personal collections of journal reprints, as well as sitting down with a blank piece of paper and a pencil.

I began with the literature on evidence-based medicine (EBM) and guideline implementation ("getting research into practice"),[15] but soon discovered a large literature on health promotion campaigns (especially AIDS prevention and heart health),[16] for which transferring a "good idea" (about healthy lifestyles) was the central theme of most research studies. One member was directed by a colleague towards work on technology transfer to developing countries, and discovered a huge "grey literature" in the databases of international development agencies. The social scientist on the team had previously completed a PhD on social networks and social influence.[17] The organisation and management literature included several "camps" (is the effective diffusion of innovations in organisations fundamentally about having certain critical features of the organisation's structure,[18] or about the operational detail of implementing innovations at different levels,[19] or about teamwork and human relationships,[20] or about the brokering and construction of knowledge?[21]). And so on.

We each brought to our first interim review meeting a number of examples of "good primary research papers", with the initial aim of sorting them first into "relevant or irrelevant" and "methodologically robust or not", and then into half a dozen topic-based piles to which we could then allocate a reviewer. But there were three problems: we could not agree which studies were relevant, which were methodologically flawed, and (perhaps worst of all) which belonged in what topic pile! We all felt to some extent that the other team members had become distracted into marginal fields, and that everyone should help more with the more "mainstream" literature. The trouble was, the definition of "mainstream" was clearly a matter of perspective.

An important early finding of our research was the near-impossibility of sorting the studies into any coherent theoretical taxonomy. We designed a data extraction sheet that sought the underpinning theory for each piece of primary research, but found that fewer than 20% of studies had an explicit theoretical basis, though in many more, a theoretical mechanism was implicit. There was also a highly inconsistent approach to research design. For example, whilst many papers from the social sciences took it as given that studies evaluating the implementation of a programme should be based on in-depth qualitative enquiry, several previous systematic reviews on the implementation of evidence-based practice had classed as "flawed" any primary study that was not a randomised controlled trial (see below, p 369).

At around this time, we presented our emerging results to a group of external peer reviewers drawn from health services research and policymaking in a seminar we called the "fishbowl". Our peers fed back to us the uncomfortable message that our work, while superficially appealing, did not make sense! They did not understand what we were trying to find out, and they criticised us for being too "purist" in our search for theoretical rigour. They were not particularly interested in the focused question we had narrowed ourselves down to ("What are the best worked-up models of dissemination and implementation of organisational innovations in health care?"). They favoured a more pragmatic and descriptive approach that embraced the diversity of the research field and addressed the general question "What research has been done that would help us understand the spread of innovations in organisations; what questions did the various research teams ask; and what did they find?". We returned to the drawing board.

"Normal science", paradigms, and research traditions

In 1962, Thomas Kuhn, a physicist-turned-historian of science, published a book called *The Structure of Scientific Revolutions* in which he proposed a new conceptual model for how progress occurs in science[22] (though, as he acknowledged, others before him had sown the seeds). Science is conventionally assumed to progress by accumulation – that is, like building a wall out of bricks. The history of science might be thought of as the history of new bricks being added to the wall. In this model, the interesting bits in the history of science are the particular delays and frustrations in the *rate* of accumulation of new scientific facts.

Kuhn challenged this view by introducing three important concepts. First, the concept of *normal science* – that most science, most of the time, is conducted according to a set of rules and standards which are considered self-evident by those working in a particular field, but which are not universally accepted. Secondly, the concept of *paradigms* – that any group of scientists views the world through a particular "lens" (paradigm or world view), which privileges and prioritises certain questions, techniques, and procedures at the expense of others.[x] Paradigms have the important characteristic of incommensurability – that is, you can look at the world rationally through one paradigm or another but not through both at the same time. Thirdly, the concept of *scientific revolution*, which occurs when a critical mass of scientists adopts a new view of what counts as "the important stuff to investigate", "the key research questions" and "the best studies to answer these questions", and old theories and models are accordingly dismissed as "unscientific". Such revolutions, incidentally, may only be evident in retrospect.

Kuhn offered (with some caution) an empirical example from gestalt psychology to illustrate what it is like to look at the world through a particular paradigm. Imagine a rogue pack of cards in which some of the hearts are black and some of the spades are red. An unbriefed research subject, exposed to a rapid sequence of cards turned over from the pack, will "see" only red hearts and black spades. Even when he or she is made aware of the trick, these anomalous cards are experienced not as neutral oddities but as highly uncomfortable and even distressing perceptions. Kuhn pointed out that "new paradigm" science is generally introduced either by the very young or by scientists newly introduced to a field – because these are the least well schooled in the prevailing "normal science". They take less for granted, ask more questions, and – most crucially – have made less personal investment in traditional ways of seeing the world. To them, a black five of hearts is not the impossibility it is to their more senior colleagues.

Perhaps Kuhn's most radical and enduring proposition, and certainly the one that will interest us most in this chapter, is the notion that a scientific paradigm is a necessary (though arbitrary) meaning-system without which scientific endeavours *cannot* be focused. This underpins his widely cited principle that it is impossible to understand one scientific paradigm through its successors. Thus, if you are going to explain (for example) Galileo's physics, you must do so not by reference to the "normal science" of twenty-first century physics, but by reference to the concepts, theories, methods, and instruments used by scientists – as well as the ideologies and cosmologies prevalent in wider society – in Galileo's time. Kuhn took pains to point out that a paradigm is *not* a set of rigid, inflexible rules. On the contrary, scope for further development of the paradigm is one of its most critical features. As he said, *"To be accepted as a paradigm, a theory must seem better than its competitors, but it need not, and in fact never does, explain all the facts with which it can be confronted"*[23] (p 17).

The vocabulary that Kuhn used to present his theory of scientific progress did not include any explicit reference to narrative, emplotment, literary devices or genre. But a contemporary reading of his book finds an implicit "storying" of many of the key concepts. He defined "normal science", for example, as *"research firmly based upon one or more past scientific achievements, achievements that one particular scientific community acknowledges for a time as supplying the foundation for its further practice"*[23] (p 10). As note 10 in this chapter shows, his central concept of a paradigm was a "model from which a research tradition springs" (note the metaphor – research does not merely "happen": once the seminal paper has loaded a group of young scientists with momentum and direction, the tradition actually *springs* – and therein lies the excitement of the story).

Kuhn emphasised that the progress of any scientific paradigm in any field follows a very predictable pattern (I would call it "plot") – from pre-paradigmatic through paradigmatic to replacement with a new paradigm. The pre-paradigmatic phase is characterised by near-random exploration. Scientific imagination is at its most unfettered; there is a prevailing atmosphere of "messing around" and "anything goes" in terms of methodology. However, perhaps because the rules of good practice are yet to be defined and the instruments of investigation invented, the data gathered tend to be of poor quality and/or imprecise. The paradigmatic phase, which is where most conventional scientific careers are built, can be said to have arrived when one model of reality becomes accepted as the basis of further work. At this point, fact-gathering becomes highly directed and increasingly refined. Specifically, scientific enquiry in this phase is aimed at *extending the knowledge of those facts that the paradigm displays as particularly revealing*, and also in further articulating the paradigm itself.[xi]

Kuhn described the paradigmatic phase as "puzzle solving", in which every competent scientist pursues with impressive enthusiasm and rigour the task of "finding the missing piece of the jigsaw".[xii] In this phase, the accepted rules, standards, methods, and instruments of normal science are taught in a highly consistent way to students and apprentices and conveyed in a somewhat stereotyped and sanitised form (and using particular language in a particular codified way) in textbooks and university curricula. Importantly, these "rules of the game" and group language (technical vocabulary, jargon) are considered so widely known that they are rarely articulated when a new scientific discovery is reported (hence making much of science inaccessible to the lay person).[xiii] Finally, in the phase during which the paradigm gets replaced, which very often begins when key refinements occur in equipment or methods of analysis, anomalies appear in the collected data which demand new concepts and theoretical models (rather than simply refinements of the prevailing paradigm) to explain them fully – thus setting the stage for the next scientific revolution.

If research unfolds historically over time (with one study leading directly, though never with mechanistic predictability) to the next study; if research traditions often (and perhaps always) follow a common plot; if the unfolding of the tradition depends on a cast of different characters (with experimenters, gurus, faithful footservants, obsessional puzzle-solvers and doubting Thomases all having their accorded parts to play in different phases); if negotiated (and, necessarily, shared) meanings and models are a prerequisite for focused, directed scientific activity – we surely have the makings of an important new hypothesis: that no research field can be understood without attention to the over-arching storylines that describe its progress. About half-way through the nine-month study period of our systematic review on "spreading good ideas", at a time when we were still reflecting on the response of the "fishbowl" participants (who had failed to see sense in our accumulating mass of data), I decided to stop looking at individual primary studies and start looking for stories.

Meta-narrative mapping: developing the technique

One of the most striking features of the vast literature we had identified on "spreading good ideas"[xiv] was the wide time frame during which research had been published. Everett Rogers, whose book *Diffusion of Innovations* (whose first edition was published in 1962) is arguably still the most authoritative and comprehensive text on the subject, himself hailed from the discipline of rural sociology, in which

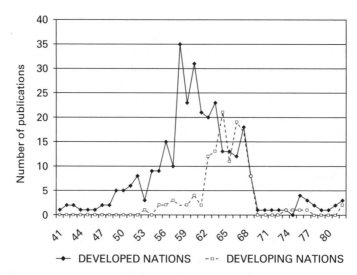

Figure 20.1 Emergence and decline of two research traditions on diffusion of innovations in rural sociology (data from Rogers,[24] reproduced by permission{?})

diffusion of innovations was the focus of considerable research activity in the two decades from 1945.[24] Figure 20.1, based on Rogers' own data, shows the number of papers published per year in two largely separate research traditions within rural sociology: developed countries and developing countries.

As Rogers and his colleague Valente argued,[25] the two curves in Figure 20.1 are explained by the life cycle of a research tradition: (a) publication of an initial "breakthrough" paper that provided model problems and solutions to a particular community of scholars; (b) a sharp increase in intellectual effort as promising young scientists were attracted to the new field;[26] (c) a steady accumulation and exchange of ideas within the field, leading to a recognised body of knowledge and refinement of the research methods; and (d) a decline phase, in which exciting new findings became less and less common and the interest of young scientific blood was directed elsewhere.[26]

I decided to try to replicate the mapping of publications on diffusion of innovations within the health sciences, and found a similar rise and fall pattern (Figure 20.2). Because of the classificatory and methodological problems alluded to earlier, this exploratory exercise produced only an approximation of the accumulation of publications within particular traditions, but nevertheless (and somewhat to my surprise), the trajectory predicted by Rogers and Valente was closely mirrored in each of the four medical sub-traditions shown in Figure 20.2. In early 2003, when I undertook this

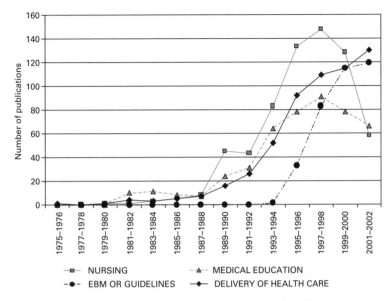

Figure 20.2 Publications indexed on Medline as having "diffusion of innovations" as a central focus within different branches of health sciences, 1975–2002[xv]

search, research activity on diffusion of innovations in both guideline development and delivery of health care appeared to be reaching a peak, whereas that in both nursing and medical education was already declining.

Having demonstrated that research on diffusion of innovations indeed seemed to wax and wane within different disciplines, I felt it was worthwhile to try to *take the research tradition as the initial unit of analysis* for our systematic review. In other words, rather than identifying, counting, indexing, and evaluating primary research studies (as is standard practice for most Cochrane systematic reviews), I wanted to collect and compare the separate stories of the rise and fall of diffusion research within the many separate fields of enquiry that we judged relevant to our policy question.

It was a fairly straightforward task to describe in broad terms the different mental models of "spreading good ideas" implicit in research undertaken by teams from different primary disciplines (Table 20.1), though the interdisciplinary studies proved more of a challenge, and some disciplines (such as psychology) embraced several different models of how ideas might spread. In order to tease out coherent research traditions (as opposed to a more simplistic taxonomy based on academic disciplines), I had to develop a method of demonstrating how one "landmark" piece of research had *led to* a revision of the scientific mind-set on the topic area and set the stage for further

359

Table 20.1   Different conceptual models of diffusion of innovations (informed by various sources)[27,28,29]

Primary discipline	Definition and scope	"Diffusion of innovations" explained in terms of
Anthropology	The study of human cultures and how they have evolved and influenced each other	Changes in culture, values, and identities (includes organisational culture, professional culture, and so on)
Communication studies	The study of human communication, including both interpersonal and mass media	Structure and operation of communication channels and networks. Interpersonal influence (for example, impact of "experts" vs "peers" on decision making)
Economics and marketing	The study of the production, distribution and consumption of goods and services	Affordability, profitability, discretionary income, market penetration, media advertising, supply, and demand
Education	The study of teaching and learning – in particular, of practices that promote understanding, use and valuing of knowledge by individuals	Traditionally, transmission of knowledge from teacher to student. Increasingly, learner motivation and active acquisition of knowledge
Epidemiology (and clinical epidemiology)	The study of the spread of diseases in populations (and the management of individual patients using population derived data)	Social contagion (cf. spread of infectious disease)
Geography	The study of the earth and its life, including the spatial distribution of individuals and the impact of geographical and land structures on human behaviour	Impact of spatial proximity on rate of uptake of ideas
Health promotion (draws on communication studies)	The study of strategies and practices aimed at improving the health and well-being of populations	"Reach" and "uptake" of positive lifestyle choices in populations targeted by health promotion campaigns
Knowledge utilisation	The study of how individuals and teams acquire, construct, synthesise, share, and apply knowledge	Transfer of knowledge – both explicit (formal and codified as in a guideline) and tacit (informal and embodied as in "knowing the ropes")

(Continued)

Table 20.1 (Continued)

Primary discipline	Definition and scope	"Diffusion of innovations" explained in terms of
Political sciences	The study of government structures and their function in developing and implementing policy	Impact of different political structures on the effectiveness of policy-making (includes "modernisation" of urban bureaucracies, citizen involvement)
Psychology	The study of mind and behaviour. Factors that influence human beings to act, particularly cognitive and emotional influences	Motivation, incentives, rewards, emotional needs
Sociology	The study of human society and the relationships between its members, especially the influence of social structures and norms on behaviours and practices	Organisational, family, and peer structures. Group norms and values. In medical sociology, the norms, relationships and shared values that drive clinician behaviour (for example, adoption of guidelines)
Structural organisational studies	The study of the structure of an organisation influences its function	Organisational attributes influencing "innovativeness" – for example, size, slack resources, hierarchical vs decentralised lines of management
Technology transfer	The study of the adoption, adaptation, and use of technology, especially in a development context	Barriers to the uptake of more advanced technologies (for example, labour saving machinery, computers)

studies in the same vein. For this task, I enlisted the help of a librarian, Richard Peacock, who taught me much about tracking research publications through time.

The data in Figures 20.1 and 20.2 were derived from a raw count of publications year by year (in the former case by a hand search of journals and in the latter by searching an electronic database). But the graphs do not actually show that earlier publications *led to* work for later ones. To test for an explicit historical link, a reviewer would need either to manually track *backwards* from the reference lists of the later studies (to see whether these authors had referenced the earlier ones), or track *forwards* from the earlier studies to see which subsequent papers cited them (a technique known as "citation tracking", developed by informaticist Eugene Garfield, and made possible through sophisticated indexing systems on certain electronic databases, notably Science Citation Index, Social Science Citation Index, and Web of Science).[xvi]

As Table 20.2 shows, we made extensive use of both reference tracking and citation tracking in this review, and indeed, these approaches identified more high quality empirical studies than simple searching of databases for index terms. But in order to use these tracking methods effectively, we had to incorporate a quality control mechanism on the papers we found. After all, "lightweight" scientists are ubiquitous and may tend to cite other lightweights while the core business of the tradition follows a largely separate trajectory, so simply tracking papers with no account of their quality will produce a superficial and misleading picture of the meta-narrative. Furthermore, citation tracking is, of course, a quantitative technique that takes no account of *why* someone has cited a particular source – they may have done so to flatter someone in a powerful position or even to show how bad they thought the work was!

An important – and perhaps controversial – feature of our method was that we did not use a single set of "quality criteria" to evaluate all the 6000 publications that our searches uncovered. Rather, we first sought out the key theoretical sources in particular traditions using three very generic criteria (Box 20.2). Once these papers and/or textbooks had been identified, we used them to distil the "unwritten rules" of the paradigm (core concepts, theoretical models, and preferred methods and instruments), from which we extracted – separately for each tradition – a set of quality criteria for primary studies.

Box 20.2 Inclusion criteria for theoretical papers and reviews

1 Is the paper part of a recognised research tradition – that is, does it draw critically and comprehensively upon an existing body of scientific knowledge and attempt to further that body of knowledge?

2 Does the paper make an original and scholarly contribution to research into the diffusion, dissemination or sustainability of innovations?

3 Has the paper subsequently been cited as a seminal contribution (conceptual, theoretical, methodological or instrumental) by competent researchers in that tradition?[xvii]

Reassuringly, we found that studies with comparable *design* tended to be judged by similar quality criteria whatever the research tradition (for example, a survey of organisational attributes in the management literature would be judged by similar methodological criteria as a survey of consumer views in psychology – namely, appropriateness of sampling

Table 20.2   Sources of the papers included in our systematic review of diffusion of innovations in health service delivery and organization

	Empirical research studies	Theoretical or "overview" papers	Total
Electronic database search[a]	75 (35%)	51 (18%)	126 (26%)
Hand search	12 (6%)	12 (4%)	24 (5%)
Tracking references of references	86 (41%)	125 (44%)	211 (43%)
Citation tracking[b]	26 (12%)	8 (3%)	34 (7%)
Sources known to research team[c]	15 (7%)	68 (24%)	83 (17%)
Social networks of research team[d]	4 (2%)	23 (8%)	27 (5%)
Serendipitous[e]	2 (1%)	3 (1%)	5 (1%)
Raw total including double counting[f]	220 (104%)	290 (107%)	510 (105%)
Total papers in final report	212 (100%)	272 (100%)	484 (100%)

[a]Eleven electronic databases were searched in medical, social science, and organisation/management fields. Details are given in the full report.[31]
[b]Using electronic search methods to track forwards a particular paper to identify subsequent papers that cited it in the reference list.
[c]Books and journal articles of which the research team were aware before the study began.
[d]Passed on by a colleague in response to a personal or email request for relevant books or papers.
[e]Finding a relevant paper for this study when looking for something else.
[f]Numbers add up to more than 100% because some sources were located by more than one method. The proportion of sources "double counted" is probably an underestimate since (for example) we did not flag a paper identified in a reference track if we already had it on file

frame, validity of questionnaire items, completeness of response, and so on). Furthermore, whilst all traditions whose methodological toolkit included the survey classified this as a high quality method, those traditions whose toolkit did *not* include surveys were dismissive of any work based on this method, regardless of the research question being considered! We uncovered similar bitter paradigm wars between qualitative and quantitative researchers (see below).

Some examples of meta-narratives on the spread of innovations

I describe below three examples of very different meta-narratives, which, once exposed, allowed us to make sense of the primary research papers within those separate traditions.[xviii] For each tradition I have (a) identified the landmark empirical study or studies that formed a model for further work within that tradition; (b) used Kuhn's framework to outline the core scientific paradigm (conceptual, theoretical, methodological, instrumental) of the tradition; and (c) commented on the aspects of the meta-narrative that appeared to be driving the research – some of which had "literary" qualities (the wider social and historical context that formed the backdrop for this particular meta-narrative; the unfolding "plot" of the research as set out in key publications; and the prevailing language, metaphor, and imagery used by scientists in the field).

Meta-narrative 1: spreading good ideas in rural society

Rural sociology is the study of the social structures, networks, and customs of rural communities. The classic study of the spread of an idea in this field – and probably the most widely cited diffusion of innovations study of all time – was Ryan and Gross' painstaking investigation of the adoption of hybrid corn by Iowa farmers in the 1930s.[32] Iowa is a large state in central USA, composed almost entirely of isolated corn farms, whose proprietors had few social contacts except with one another and the representatives of seed companies. Traditional corn seed gave reasonable crops and re-grew every year by open pollination. A new, hardier hybrid had been developed that gave reliably higher yields and withstood drought better, but this seed (first marketed in 1928) had to be replanted every year – hence an initial buy-in to the idea was needed.

A core concept of the emerging paradigm was interpersonal communication and influence, and the underpinning theoretical model was that people adopt a new idea by copying others who have already adopted it (usually, those who often hold privileged social status – a group subsequently given the label "opinion leaders"). The preferred method was the mapping of social networks (who knows whom, and who views whom as influential), for which the preferred instrument was the sociological survey. Ryan (a recent PhD graduate) and Gross (an impecunious MSc student who had sought a summer job) conducted face-to-face interviews with all Iowa corn farmers in the early 1940s, recording basic demographic information (such as age, income, and years of education), social information (notably how frequently they visited the state's main town of Des Moines), and what year the farmer recalled first becoming aware of, and using, the hybrid corn. The innovation adoption curve is shown in Figure 20.3 below.

Overall, it took 20 years for 99% of farmers to adopt the new seed for 100% of their crops; some – the "innovators" and "early adopters" – adopting

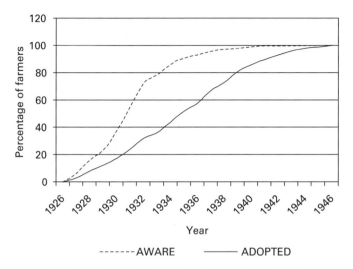

Figure 20.3 Percentage of Iowa farmers classified as (a) aware of hybrid corn and (b) using it on all fields from 1926 to 1945 (data from Ryan and Gross[32,33])

it only a year or two after first encountering it via the seed reps.[24,32] Most (the early and late majority) took between four and nine years, usually trying it out on a small field before switching to it for the entire crop. A few delayed the switch for over a decade, and two (out of a sample of 259) never switched at all. This observation, and the discovery that early adopters were richer, better educated, more cosmopolitan (that is, they visited Des Moines more frequently) and had wider social networks, led to a couching of adoption decisions in terms of personality type – with "late adopters" and "laggards" presented in stereotypical and somewhat disparaging terms (uneducated, socially isolated, and so on).

Ryan and Gross' research, and the spate of similar studies that followed in the rural sociology tradition, occurred in a very particular historical and political context. In the USA in the 1940s and 1950s, fears of a national food shortage had made it a political priority to modernise remote farming communities and improve the nation's crop yields. Colleges of agricultural innovation were established, and were closely linked to academics who were charged with studying how to spread the innovations efficiently from the agricultural colleges to the practitioners in the field – a linkage that was termed "agricultural extension". Innovations, emanating from government-funded centres of excellence, were widely viewed as "progress".

Ryan and Gross' landmark study had a powerful influence on the methodology of subsequent diffusion research, especially within the wider discipline of sociology. The "one-shot research interview", in which respondents were asked to recall decisions made months or years earlier, worked well enough for the Iowa corn study and was adopted somewhat uncritically in later studies (when recall and contextual biases might well have been more influential).

The Iowa hybrid corn had a clear advantage over the previous product and produced, as predicted, both private benefits (to the farmer) and public benefits (to the local economy). But many other agricultural innovations of the day, whose roll-out was planned along similar communication lines, did not produce the same benefits and sometimes had unanticipated consequences elsewhere in the system (for example, "miracle" crops that consumers found unpalatable; labour-saving devices that put farm labourers out of a job; and new technologies that farmers could not afford or did not understand[24,34]). The negative findings of these later studies helped to rock the prevailing paradigm, which was gradually revealed as being couched in a powerful meta-narrative of growth, productivity, domination of the rural environment, and "new is better".[xix]

Everett Rogers, reflecting some 40 years later on the unconscious pro-innovation bias that had prevailed in his discipline, describes how political ideology and scientific priorities were subsequently revisited when agricultural overproduction, rather than food shortages, became America's key farming problem.[24] His description of his first piece of fieldwork – at a time when the meta-narrative of rural sociology had changed to one of conservation and sensitivity to natural processes – is particularly telling:

> Back in 1954, one of the Iowa farmers that I personally interviewed for my PhD dissertation research rejected all of the chemical innovations that I was then studying: weed sprays, cattle and hog feeds, chemical fertilisers, and a rodenticide. He insisted that his neighbours, who had adopted these chemicals, were killing their songbirds and the earthworms in the soil. I had selected the new farm ideas in my innovativeness scale on the advice of agricultural experts at Iowa State University; I was measuring the best recommended farming practice of that day. The organic farmer in my sample earned the lowest score on my innovativeness scale, and was categorised as a laggard.[24] (p 425)

Meta-narrative 2: Evidence-based medicine and guideline implementation

Evidence-based medicine (EBM) – the attempt to get health professionals consistently to base their decisions on the results of scientific research studies – has its roots in rationalist science, and particularly epidemiology (the study of diseases in populations). The mathematical basis for the S-shaped diffusion of innovations curve (illustrated in Figure 20.3) is a fundamental law of nature relating to growth or spread in a closed system. When a bacterium divides, or when one person with influenza coughs on two others, a doubling phenomenon begins. One becomes two, two becomes four, and so on until a point of saturation is reached, at which point the rate of growth slows and the curve levels off at maximum saturation.

Interestingly, epidemiologists sometimes use the language of contagion to talk about the spread of ideas as well as the spread of disease. They talk, for example, of "susceptibility" of individuals to a new idea, the corresponding "contagiousness" of that idea. The term "viral marketing" has even been coined to describe the powerful influence of social movements on individual adoption decisions. Such metaphors implicitly play down the notion of individual agency (after all, you can't *decide* whether you catch a cold!) and prompt a mental model of adoption "just happening" once contact has been made.

It is hardly surprising, then, that research on the spread of EBM was predicated on a highly rationalist conceptual model that saw adoption of the idea (in this case, new scientific knowledge about drug treatments or surgical procedures) as the final stage in a simple linear algorithm (research → published evidence → change in doctors' behaviour). It is noteworthy that the "contagion" metaphor (at least in the traditional use of the word) implies adoption without adaptation. The problem of "getting evidence into practice" was initially couched in terms of an innovation gap (lack of high quality research evidence). Research activity focused on producing the evidence (for example, the UK's extensive Health Technology Assessment Programme which began in the early 1990s – see http://www.hta.nhsweb.nhs.uk/) and on developing methods and systems for packaging and distributing the results of such programmes to fill the evidence gap and make it available in the clinic and at the bedside.

A theoretical paper by Haines and Jones (cited by 148 subsequent papers in the EBM tradition) illustrates how the link between *provision* of best evidence and the *making* of an evidence-based decision was at one stage considered unproblematic by leading medical scientists,[36] though both authors subsequently moved on from this position. Objective and context-neutral evidence was seen to "drive" the evidence-into-practice cycle by a mechanism described by Williams and Gibson (cited in Dawson[37]) as "like water flowing through a pipe". It did not, of course, take much empirical work to demonstrate that research evidence did not "flow" into practice like water!

As the EBM tradition developed, the paradigm shifted slightly and the problem of getting evidence into practice changed from being framed as an "innovation gap" (lack of evidence on what works) and became a "behaviour gap" (doctors' failure to seek out or use this evidence). Research activity focused on finding ways to fill the assumed knowledge gap (via mass media[38] or formal education[39,40,41]) and the motivation gap (for example, using the social influence of opinion leaders[42]), and on providing a variety of behavioural incentives,[43] with the ultimate goal of changing clinician behaviour in line with the evidence.[44] As the systematic reviews referenced above show, although the empirical research drew variously on a host of theories of communication, influence and behaviour change, almost all were designed as randomised controlled trials (RCTs), for which the model study to set the paradigm was Sibley and Sackett's RCT of educational interventions for doctors published in 1982[45] and cited by 149 subsequent papers. Many of these RCTs (including the early work done by Sackett's team) had surprisingly low success at prompting doctors to implement the innovations supported by the evidence.

An overview by Grol, which might one day earn the status of a paradigm-shifting commentary (in the Kuhnian sense), summarises the reasons why intervention studies to promote implementation of "evidence-based" innovations were so ineffectual:[46] many "evidence-based" guidelines were ambiguous or confusing; the guideline usually only covered part of the sequence of decisions and actions in a clinical consultation; they were often difficult to apply to individual patients' unique problems; they generally required changes in the wider health-care system; and their implementation was rarely cost-neutral. In other words, the mental model on which the paradigm was built (research $\rightarrow$ evidence $\rightarrow$ implementation) was critically flawed and needed more than just reframing: there simply is *no causal link* between the supply of research evidence and the implementation of evidence in clinical decision making.

Methodologically and instrumentally, the EBM "diffusion of innovations" trials are something of a curiosity. The EBM community, trained to undertake controlled experiments of disease treatments on populations of patients, had transferred this conceptual model and research methodology wholesale to the new problem of spreading good ideas: their new "population" was the doctors whose behaviour needed to change; their "experimental intervention" was some sort of incentive or educational package to prompt the following of a guideline; and their anticipated "outcome" was adoption of the guideline or other behavioural protocol deemed by the researchers as desirable.

It is one of the hallmarks of traditional epidemiology that RCTs are considered "best evidence" for evaluating interventions. But few scientists from other traditions would support the notion that RCTs are the most appropriate design for exploring the practicalities of implementing new ideas (including those concerned with clinical decision making).[12,47,48,49] The argument might be framed thus: whilst the RCT simulates "laboratory" conditions and minimises the effect of bias, hence making the outcomes of a particular experimental study highly *reliable*, such conditions often exclude the very things that influence implementation in the real world, hence producing little or no data on complex processes or contextual variables and thereby reducing the *validity* of findings.

This deep methodological tension is summed up by two opposing "mission statements". The first, from a wide-ranging systematic review on the dissemination and implementation of health technology reports undertaken by members of the Cochrane Collaboration, which was based on a strict hierarchy of evidence (with RCTs explicitly privileged as "best evidence"), states: "Experimental studies are the most reliable designs for evaluating the effectiveness of dissemination and implementation strategies."[50] This reflects mainstream EBM thinking of the mid-1990s. The second statement, from a senior policy researcher in the complex field of community based mental health, and a clear dissenter from the EBM tradition, states: "The RCT model is unable to control for the effect of social complexity and the interaction between social complexity and dynamic system change."[47]

If we look for the underlying metaphor for change in the meta-narrative of diffusion of innovations in EBM in the 1990s, it is surely the experimental scientist interjecting a clever intervention, and then standing back to measure the impact of his or her work! As Figure 20.2 indicates, the rationalist model linking evidence to implementation in EBM has probably had its day. The research agenda on implementing best practice has begun to move into other traditions with quite different key concepts, mental models and "plots" to the over-arching story, and led by scholars who are not from the epidemiological (or even the medical) tradition.[xx] One such example is considered below.

Meta-narrative 3: Knowledge utilisation

As the two previous meta-narratives show, "communication and influence" was for many years the dominant metaphor for researching the spread of innovations in sociology-based traditions,[xxi] and the rational, linear, "contagion" metaphor was until recently dominant in more medically-based traditions. In knowledge utilisation research, scientists use a very different metaphor for depicting the spread of ideas: the creation and transmission of knowledge. Organisations are conceptualised not in traditional terms (as places of work or collections of formal roles and relationships) but as knowledge-producing systems and as nodes in knowledge-exchanging systems.[52,53] In this context, ideas (innovations) are seen as spreading by two mechanisms: organisational learning (defined as a change in the state of an organisation's knowledge resources[54]), and projecting (the embedding of knowledge in an organisation's product and service outputs[55]).

An inherent tension that plagues knowledge utilisation research (perceived in this tradition as the core task of spreading good ideas) is the complex and fuzzy nature of much of the knowledge associated with "ideas" or "innovations". Such knowledge (as opposed to formal, codified *information*) is not easily transferable, because it is often embodied as know-how or practical wisdom in the person and/or organisation that generated it (a phenomenon known as "stickiness"[56]), and also because the person or organisation receiving the knowledge needs to have some prior knowledge and experience for the new knowledge to make sense (a phenomenon known as *absorptive capacity*[57]). Informal, tacit knowledge is costly and difficult to disseminate because it deals with the specific and the particular, consists of various small increments, and is dependent for its meaning on interpretation and negotiation by individuals in a particular context.[58]

There are various mental models in the knowledge utilisation literature that represent *how* complex knowledge is created and exchanged at organisational level. One good example is that of Nonaka and Takeuchi, who hold that both informal and formal knowledge are systematically acquired, transmitted, transformed, and combined in a cyclical sequence through the activities and interactions of individuals (much of it in informal space).[xxi] Similar, but perhaps competing, models include Weick's focus on knowledge as sense-making (that is, fitting the new idea within an existing conceptual schema, with or without concomitant modification of the schema)[59], Leonard-Burton's notion of the problem-solving cycle,[60] and Hansen's emphasis on the need for "personalisation" of tacit knowledge.[61]

Whatever the precise mental model, the creation and transmission of fuzzy and "sticky" knowledge is not an easy area to research empirically – especially in the field of technology-based systems. Knowledge utilisation research has many branches (indeed, I once saw the field described as "a conceptual cartographer's nightmare"), ranging from the design and analysis of the "hard systems" (computers and their connections) for the transmission of formal knowledge to the exploration and illumination of the "soft networks" of individuals through which informal knowledge and organisational wisdom is transmitted, transformed and enhanced.

The latter field of enquiry is located mainly in the wider discipline of organisational anthropology, and uses predominantly in-depth ethnographic methods to build up rich case studies of particular organisations and their various subcultures. One of several seminal works in this area was Brown and Duguid's *The Social Life of Information*, which describes a year-long field study of the men who mend photocopiers for Xerox.[62] The researchers "hung out" with these technical experts and documented *how* they converted codified knowledge (such as the technical manual) into practical action, and also how they exchanged the richer and more elusive tacit knowledge needed for fixing photocopiers (in informal spaces such as canteens via anecdotes and metaphors, by the provision of "personalised" solutions to real-life problems presented by one member to the group, and by semi-official apprenticeship and shadowing schemes).

The "soft systems" research paradigm, in which innovation is viewed as knowledge and knowledge is celebrated for its uncertainty, ubiquity, and unmeasurability (with adjectives such as "plastic", "sticky", "embodied", "shared", and "fuzzy"), contrasts sharply with the rationalist paradigm of traditional EBM, in which innovation is knowledge celebrated for precisely the opposite qualities (focus, clarity, transferability, accountability, and provenance) and with the traditional sociological paradigm in which innovation is viewed as individual behavioural choices transmitted by interpersonal influence.

In terms of a distinct research tradition, the knowledge utilisation literature is difficult to map, since arguably the entire field of knowledge utilisation research is about spreading ideas! A small subset of this literature, on knowledge utilisation in health care, which I mapped using the technique demonstrated in Figure 20.2 (with "diffusion of innovation" and "knowledge, attitudes, and practice" as index terms), suggests that a bell-shaped curve of publications may have begun in the late 1990s and is on the rise. It remains to be seen, therefore, how this tradition will pan out and how the paradigm will be challenged in future years.

The synthesis phase

As well as the examples described above, we discovered 10 other research traditions[xxii] relevant to our research question. Having unravelled and summarised each of these meta-narratives, we then took seven key dimensions of the spread and sustainability of innovations[xxiii] and for each of these, we distilled the relevant messages from each of the 13 traditions. The review process was laborious, since each piece of evidence had to be double-handled – first for constructing the meta-narrative within its own tradition and again for contributing to the "rich picture" of one of the seven dimensions of spread and sustainability. But although I am sure critics will disagree with specific statements or interpretations made in our final report, all the reviewers were agreed on one conclusion: it *made sense.*[xxiv] My own hypothesis is that we made the crucial leap towards sense-making when we made the decision systematically to produce "storied" accounts of the key research traditions.

Meta-narrative mapping: a template for applying it more generally

We are still developing and refining the technique of meta-narrative mapping and placing it appropriately alongside other approaches to the synthesis of complex evidence. I hope that systematic reviewers will begin to test out the hypothesis that story "adds value" to secondary research more generally. I believe that there are five key principles that underpin this technique (and which distinguish it to some extent from other complex synthesis methods).

Principle of pragmatism

Because of the fuzzy and unsorted nature of the literature in the initial phase of synthesis, "what to include" is not self-evident. Searching should initially be exploratory rather than truly systematic (that is, there is much to be gained by browsing); it should have an "emergent" approach and be guided by discussion amongst the project team and negotiation with the funder or client.

Principle of pluralism

If the body of evidence is complex, there will be no simple, formulaic or universal "solution" hidden in the literature awaiting discovery, nor will a single theory explain all findings. However, the research team should be aware that they will all tend to view the problem through their own paradigmatic lens, which will direct them to an "obvious" body of literature with a preferred methodology; they must take steps not to be drawn into privileging this form of evidence and dismissing all others as "methodologically flawed". In our own work on spreading good ideas, we rejected the temptation to seek out a single, over-arching theory that would explain all the different dimensions of diffusion, dissemination, and sustainability of innovations within a single conceptual framework. Rather, we saw as a key challenge of our research to *expose the tensions, value the diversity, and communicate the complexity* of how the various different paradigms drawn upon by different researchers contribute to an understanding of the problem as a whole.

To fulfil the principle of pluralism, research teams should make explicit use of methods to promote interdisciplinary dialogue and cross-fertilisation of methods and approaches. Our own team included members from a wide range of disciplinary and professional backgrounds. We did not attempt to impose a unified synthesis method until relatively late in each phase of the project. Rather, we allowed each researcher to approach a chosen body of literature (with whose disciplinary basis they were broadly familiar) in the way they perceived appropriate. At planned review meetings (a month into the project for the initial search, half-way through the project for data extraction, and towards the end of the project for analysis and synthesis), we pooled our experiences and developed, as far as possible, a common framework for each of these processes.

Principle of historicity

The defining characteristic of a narrative is the sequencing of events in time in such a way that a "plot" emerges, and Kuhn's notion of a research tradition clearly demonstrates the notion of historicity.[23] It is somewhat curious that the commendable work of the Cochrane Collaboration in finding, indexing, sorting, and synthesising large bodies of evidence has taken almost no account of the historical sequence of studies relating to particular research questions. Indeed, the RefMan software used by Cochrane reviewers for statistical meta-analysis defaults to placing primary studies in alphabetical order of authors' names rather than in date order.[xxv] Arguably, the structured reporting format that strips individual studies bare of their historical and social context is what makes systematic reviews so boring and indigestible that few people read them![64]

Principle of contestation

Related to the principle of pluralism is the notion that the heterogeneity of research questions, methods, results, and interpretation is itself data. It is the contestation between the research traditions that allows the researcher to move from simple description (and lamentation that studies are "conflicting") to higher-level analysis that uses similar principles to those applied to the analysis of contradictions and "disconfirming cases" in primary qualitative research.[65] The goal of the synthesis phase of meta-narrative mapping is to find epistemological (and indeed pragmatic and realistic) explanations that might illuminate the differences in the findings and recommendations made by researchers from widely differing traditions on a supposedly common topic area, and help to reconcile them.

Principle of peer review

Critical reflection on one's own work, and invitation of critical comment from others, is an established principle of academic study. Oakley, cited by Mays *et al*, has said that:

> The distinguishing mark of good research is the awareness and acknowledgement of error and [hence] the necessity of establishing

procedures which will minimise the effect such errors have on what counts as knowledge.[12]

In our own study, we recognised the danger of researchers "flying solo" in literature that was diffuse, poorly organised, of variable quality, and not amenable to evaluation using conventional critical appraisal tools. We were also aware of the risk of the "groupthink" phenomenon, in which close-knit project groups develop an unjustified confidence in their own outputs and sense of invulnerability to external criticism.[66] We therefore sought continually to test our emerging findings against the judgement of others both within the research team and outside it.

Where the research field is highly complex and methods emergent rather than predefined, internal and external peer review is even more critical than usual, and such peer review must be formative (that is, intended to feed into the research process) rather than summative (that is, intended to judge its outputs).

An invitation to develop the technique

As a result of the work described in this chapter, I have reached the conclusion that in situations where the scope of a project is large and the literature diverse; where different groups of scientists in this overall research area have asked different questions and used different research designs; where different groups of practitioners and policy-makers have drawn on the research literature in different ways; where "quality" papers have different defining features in different research and service traditions; where there is no self-evident or universally agreed process for pulling the different bodies of literature together, meta-narrative mapping has particular strengths as a synthesis method.

Nevertheless, I am conscious that the method arose in a pragmatic way within the course of a single project. At the time of writing this chapter, it has not yet been tested prospectively or shown to be transferable to all contexts listed above. Indeed, it would be interesting to address the null hypothesis that the method described here has no advantages over traditional "cross-sectional" synthesis methods (that is, over methods that take no account of the historical unfolding of research in different paradigmatic traditions over time) – perhaps using two different research teams given the same policy question at the outset.

Box 20.3 shows suggested key steps for applying meta-narrative mapping more widely. I am open to feedback on how these steps might be refined or changed.

Box 20.3 Suggested steps for applying meta-narrative mapping to synthesis of evidence for complex "open-ended" research questions

1 Planning phase

    (a) Assemble a research team that is truly multidisciplinary and whose background encompasses the key research traditions relevant to the question.[xxvi]

    (b) Outline the initial research question in a broad, open-ended format.

    (c) Set a series of regular face-to-face review meetings including planned input from external peers drawn from academia and service.

2 Search phase

    (a) Include an early exploratory phase in which searching is led by intuition, informal networking and unstructured "browsing"; the goal here is to map divergence rather than reach consensus.

    (b) Search for "landmark" papers in each research tradition using reference tracking and the evaluation criteria set out in Box 20.2.

    (c) Search for later empirical papers in particular traditions by hand searching key journals and forward tracking the citations of landmark papers.

3 Mapping phase

Identify (separately for each research tradition):

    (a) The key elements of the research paradigm (conceptual, theoretical, methodological, and instrumental);

    (b) The key actors and events in the unfolding of the tradition (including main results and how they came to be discovered);

    (c) The prevailing language, imagery, metaphors, and other literary devices used by scientists to "tell the story" of their work.

4 Appraisal phase

Using appropriate critical appraisal techniques:

    (a) Evaluate each primary study for its validity and relevance to the review question;

    (b) Extract and collate the key results, grouping comparable studies together.

5 Synthesis phase

By considering the commonalities and differences between different contributions:

    (a) Identify all the key dimensions of the problem that have been researched;

    (b) Taking each dimension in turn, give a narrative account of the contribution (if any) made to it by each separate research tradition;

    (c) Where there is genuine contestation between research traditions, treat this as higher-order data (see text for explanation).

6 Recommendations phase

Through reflection, multidisciplinary dialogue and consultation with the service client:

    (a) Consider the key overall messages from the research literature along with other relevant evidence (budget, policymaking cycle, competing or aligning priorities);

    (b) Distil and discuss recommendations for practice, policy and further research.

Acknowledgement

I am grateful to Gene Feder, Hasok Chang, Brian Balmer, Allen Young, Jeanette Buckingham, Lewis Elton, Brian Hurwitz, and Vieda Skultans for helpful feedback on earlier drafts of this chapter.

Endnotes

i   I am grateful to Dr Mary Dixon-Woods of Leicester University for introducing me to the subtle but important differences between these approaches.[7]

ii For a good worked example, see Campbell *et al*'s paper which addressed the question "What is the patient's perspective of their diabetes and its care?"[8]

iii During the work described in this chapter, my own team came up with the acronym SODDHS (synthesis of data from diffuse and heterogeneous sources).

iv Arguably, solving how to effectively "spread good ideas" is the ultimate research challenge for any academic, since our ideas so often go unnoticed or get thrown away with the fish and chips.

v   As discussed above, systematic review means something different to qualitative and quantitative researchers, and something different again to policymakers. We defined it as "a review of the literature undertaken according to an explicit, rigorous and reproducible methodology", and distanced ourselves from any attempt at encyclopaedic coverage of the vast field of potentially relevant material.

vi We defined innovation in service delivery and organisation as "a novel set of behaviours, routines and ways of working, which are directed at improving health outcomes, administrative efficiency, cost-effectiveness, or the user experience, and which are implemented by means of planned and coordinated action".

vii We encompassed in the term "spread" the terms diffusion (a passive phenomenon of social influence – as when someone copies an opinion leader), dissemination (active and planned efforts to persuade target groups to adopt an innovation) and implementation (active and planned efforts to mainstream an innovation).

viii We took sustainability to be when new ways of working become the norm, but we quickly identified an ambiguity in the notion (the more a particular innovation is sustained or "routinised", the less the organisation will be open to the next innovation that comes along).

ix This was despite the fact that the research team and its steering group included a number of international experts on this topic area. Until we had completed the study, and arguably even once we had done so, *nobody* could identify with confidence the best places to start digging, and experts remain deeply divided on what counts as the "high quality research".

x   Kuhn[23] defined paradigms as "models from which spring particular coherent traditions of scientific research" (p 10). He highlighted the four dimensions of a paradigm as conceptual (what are considered the important objects of study – and, hence, what counts as a legitimate problem to be solved by science), theoretical (how the objects of study are considered to relate to one another and to the world), methodological (the accepted ways in which problems might be investigated), and instrumental (the accepted tools and instruments to be used by scientists). Note, however, that Kuhn himself, and many others after him, recognised the inherent ambiguity of the notion of a paradigm. At the start of the book, for example, he uses the term paradigm as an "exemplar", but later in his book, he conflates it with "disciplinary matrix". These fine distinctions are of great interest to philosophers, but the arguments in this chapter do not rest centrally on their resolution.

xi Kuhn[23] recognised the critical importance of the scope for further development of the story when he claimed, controversially, that once a research tradition has moved beyond the pre-paradigmatic phase,"the scientist who writes a textbook is more likely to find his reputation impaired than enhanced" (p 20).

xii The jigsaw analogy illustrates well the notion of the paradigm. When normal science is progressing at its best, the rules of jigsaw-solving are already in place, as are many of the pieces of the particular puzzle under investigation. The scientist may adopt increasingly refined methods (for example, sorting off the straight-edged pieces), but he or she may not turn the pieces upside down, cut the edges off, or make a creative abstract collage rather than completing the picture. All these approaches belong to a pre-paradigmatic phase of a different research tradition!

xiii It might even be argued that scientific training is a form of enacted narrative in which the concepts, theories, methods, and instruments are distilled into the embodied knowledge of its apprentice practitioners.

xiv We browsed 6000 abstracts, pulled 1200 books or papers for full evaluation, and included 600 sources in our final report.

xv These graphs were produced by searching the Medline database for diffusion of innovation (MeSH term or text word), and combining this data set respectively with the exploded MeSH terms "Nursing", "Education", "Evidence based medicine" or "Practice guidelines" or "Guideline implementation"; and "Delivery of health care". Searches were repeated in two-year time bands from 1975 through to the end of 2002. A librarian colleague subsequently pointed out that these different MeSH headings were introduced at different times during the 1990s, so I repeated the search using these expressions as title words as well as MeSH headings, which did not change the shape or timing of the curves significantly (though there was more of a "shoulder" on the early part of the curves). This, of course, is because new MeSH headings tend to reflect the new terminology that authors have introduced in their papers.

xvi These techniques are not without their limitations, which are explored in more detail in the main report.[30]

xvii This criterion could not, of course, be used to assess recently published papers, but for papers more than five years old, the technique of citation tracking (see above) proved very useful in identifying papers that had informed their own research traditions.

xviii For a full description of all the traditions included in our review, see the project final report.[31]

xix It is noteworthy that a parallel tradition in medical sociology, in which doctors' uptake of powerful new drugs, followed a very similar meta-narrative during the 1950s to 1970s. The study by Coleman et al on the speed with which doctors began to prescribe the newly developed antibiotic tetracycline, takes a similarly uncritical view of "innovation as progress" and saw innovation as domination of the body by chemicals developed by experts in universities![35] A fascinating claim by Coleman and his team is that they were *not* aware of the theoretical and methodological work of Ryan and Gross – in other words, they had come up with an almost identical theoretical framework, research design, and instrument (and, incidentally, shown an almost identical S-shaped adoption curve) in a different field of enquiry! The common social, historical, and ideological context to these landmark post-war American studies – each of which was paradigm-shifting in its separate tradition – is surely evident.

xx An important programme of work which might be deemed paradigm-shifting in EBM, but which I have not described here because of space constraints, was undertaken by Ferlie *et al*, who challenged the concept of interventions as dichotomous variables (the putative mechanism for promoting the spread of the idea was classed as "present" or "absent"). Rather, they claim, these are complex, multifaceted issues to be explored, understood, contextualised, and richly described.[51]

xxi Most of the sociological traditions take a largely individual focus, but there are parallel traditions in organisational research which (for example) attempt to delineate the characteristics of "early adopting" vs "late adopting" firms, or which identify particular firms as "opinion leaders". Whilst the unit of analysis has shifted from the individual to the organisation, the dominant metaphor of communication and influence remains.[29]

xxii Communication studies, marketing, medical sociology, educational sociology, health promotion, development studies, social psychology, structural organisational studies, organisational anthropology, and "systems-theory" organisational studies. There was some (but not much) overlap between some of these traditions, and we were aware of other important traditions (for example, economics) which we did not cover at all because of resource constraints.

xxiii Innovations, adopters and adoption, communication and influence, the inner (organisational) context, the outer (environmental) context, the dissemination process, and the implementation process.

xxiv Looking back at the feedback provided to us by the "fishbowl" session one-third of the way through the project, it is clear in retrospect (though it was certainly not clear at the time) that our peers were right to demand sense-making above other worthy goals such as "focus" or "rigour". The interested reader might like to consult the final project report, which is book-sized and densely referenced, and which offers many evidence-based options for spreading good ideas. It is downloadable from the NHSSDO website, www.nhssdo.com.[31]

xxv We found (through our academic networks) one previous reference to quasi-narrative systematic review. When undertaking a systematic review on treatments for nausea and vomiting, Herxheimer reflected that the synthesis of studies would be more meaningful if the RefMan software used by the Cochrane Collaboration routinely placed the studies in historical order and the text of the review contained a corresponding narrative to explain the sequence. His review, in contrast to most conventional Cochrane systematic reviews, includes a narrative that sets the studies in historical order, thus highlighting how different research approaches to the study of nausea and vomiting followed on from previous studies.[63]

xxvi The fact that the breadth of different traditions cannot generally be known in advance means that a substantive review based on meta-narrative mapping must generally be preceded by a scoping phase in which one major task is to define the skill mix for the project team.

References

1 Cochrane Reviewers' Handbook 4.2.0 (updated March 2003). *The Cochrane Library.* Oxford: Cochrane Collaboration, 2003.
2 Yin RK. *Case Study Research: Design and Methods.* London: Sage, 1994.
3 Miles M, Huberman AM. *Qualitative Data Analysis: A Sourcebook of New Methods.* Newbury Park, CA: Sage, 1984.
4 Noblitt GW, Hare RD. *Meta-ethnography: Synthesising Qualitative Studies.* Newbury Park, CA: Sage, 1988.
5 Kearney MH. Enduring love: a grounded formal theory of women's experience of domestic violence. *Res Nursing Health* 2001;**24**:270–82.
6 Jensen LA, Allen MN. Meta-synthesis of qualitative findings. *Qualitative Health Res* 1996;**6**:553–60.

7   Dixon-Woods M, Agarwal S, Jones D, Young B, Sutton A. Synthesising qualitative and quantitative evidence: a review of methods. *J Health Serv Res Pol* 2004, (in press).

8   Campbell R, Pound P, Pope C, Britten N, Pill R, Morgan M *et al.* Evaluating meta-ethnography: a synthesis of qualitative research on lay experiences of diabetes and diabetes care. *Soc Sci Med* 2003;**56**:671–84.

9   Mays N, Roberts E, Popay J. Synthesizing research evidence. In: Fulop N, Allen P, eds. *Studying the organization and the delivery of the health services: research methods.* Routledge, 2001, pp 188–220.

10 Pawson R. Evidence-based policy: the promise of "realist synthesis". *Evaluation* 2002;**8**:340–58.

11 Bero L, Grilli R, Grimshaw JM, Mowatt G, Oxman A, Zwarenstein M. Cochrane effective practice and organisation of care review group. In: Bero L, Grilli R, Grimshaw JM, Mowatt G, Oxman A, Zwarenstein M, eds. *Cochrane Library.* Issue 2. Oxford: Update Software, 2003.

12 Mays N, Roberts E, Popay J. Synthesizing research evidence. In: Fulop N, Allen P, eds. *Studying the organization and the delivery of the health services: research methods.* Routledge, 2001, pp 188–220.

13 Popay J, Rogers A, Wiliams G. Rationale and standards for the systematic review of qualitative literature in health services research. *Qualitative Health Res* 1998;**8**:341–51.

14 Department of Health. *The NHS Plan.* London: NHS Executive, 2001.

15 Grimshaw JM, Thomas RE, MacLennan G, Fraser C, Ramsay CR, Vale L *et al.* Effectiveness and efficiency of guideline dissemination and implementation strategies. Aberdeen: Health Services Research Unit, University of Aberdeen, 2002.

16 Green LW, Johnson JL. Dissemination and utilization of health promotion and disease prevention knowledge: theory, research and experience. *Can J Public Health* 1996;**87**:11–17.

17 Van de Ven AH. Central problems in the management of innovation. *Management Sci* 1986;**32**:590–607.

18 Burns T, Stalker GM. *The Management of Innovation.* London: Tavistock, 1961.

19 Meyer AD, Goes JB. Organisational assimiliation of innovations: a multi-level contextual analysis. *Acad Manag Rev* 1988;**31**:897–923.

20 Edmondson AC, Bohmer RM, Pisano GP. Disrupted routines: team learning and new technology implementation in hospitals. *Admin Sci Q* 2001;**46**:685–716.

21 Nonaka I. A dynamic theory of organizational knowledge creation. *Org Sci* 1994;**5**:14–37.

22 Kuhn TS. *The structure of scientific revolutions.* Chicago: University of Chicago Press, 1962.

23 Kuhn TS. *The structure of scientific revolutions.* Chicago: University of Chicago Press, 1996.

24 Rogers EM. *Diffusion of Innovations.* New York: Free Press, 1962, 4th edn 1995.

25 Valente TW, Rogers EM. The origins and development of the diffusion of innovations paradigm as an example of scientific growth. *Sci Communication* 1995;**16**:242–73.

26 Kuhn TS. *The Structure of Scientific Revolutions.* Chicago: University of Chicago Press, 1962.

27 Johnson JL, Green LW. A dissemination research agenda to strengthen health promotion and disease prevention. *Can J Publ Health* 1996;**87**:S5-S11.

28 Furnham A. *The psychology of behaviour at work: the individual in the organisation.* London: Psychology Press, 1997.

29 Rogers EM. *Diffusion of Innovations,* 4th edn. New York: Free Press, 1995.

30 Greenhalgh T, Robert G, Bate P, Kyriakidou O, Macfarlane F, Peacock R. A systematic review of the literature on diffusion, dissemination and sustainability of innovations in service delivery and organisation. London: NHS SDO Programme, 2003.

31 Greenhalgh T, Robert G, Bate P, Kyriakidou O, Macfarlane F, Peacock R. A systematic review of the literature on diffusion, dissemination and sustainability of innovations in service delivery and organisation. London: NHS SDO Programme, 2003.

32 Ryan B, Gross N. The diffusion of hybrid seed corn in two Iowa communities. *Rural Sociol* 1943;**8**:15–24.

33 Ryan B, Gross N. Acceptance and diffusion of hybrid seed corn in two Iowa communities. *Ames, Iowa Agricultural Station Research Bulletin* 1950;**372**:665–79.

34 Hightower J. *Hard Tomatoes, Hard Times: The Failure of America's Land Grant Complex.* Cambridge, MA: Shenkman, 1972.

35 Coleman JS, Katz E, Menzel H. *Medical Innovations: A Diffusion Study.* New York: Bobbs–Merrill, 1966.

36 Haines A, Jones R. Implementing findings of research. *BMJ* 1994;**308**:1488–92.

37 Dawson S. Never mind solutions: what are the issues? Lessons of industrial technology transfer for quality in health care. *Qual Health Care* 1995;**4**:197–203.

38 Grilli R, Freemantle N, Minozzi S, Domenighetti G, Finer D. Mass media interventions: effects on health services utilisation. *Cochrane Database of Systematic Reviews* 2000;CD000389.

39 Freemantle N, Harvey EL, Wolf F, Grimshaw JM, Grilli R, Bero LA. Printed educational materials: effects on professional practice and health care outcomes. *Cochrane Database of Systematic Reviews* 2000;CD000172.

40 Davis D, O'Brien MA, Freemantle N, Wolf FM, Mazmanian P, Taylor-Vaisey A. Impact of formal continuing medical education: do conferences, workshops, rounds, and other traditional continuing education activities change physician behavior or health care outcomes? *JAMA* 1999;**282**:867–74.

41 Zwarenstein M, Reeves S, Barr H, Hammick M, Koppel I, Atkins J. Interprofessional education: effects on professional practice and health care outcomes. *Cochrane Database of Systematic Reviews* 2001;CD002213.

42 Thomson O'Brien MA, Oxman AD, Davis DA, Haynes RB, Freemantle N. Local opinion leaders. *Cochrane Database of Systematic Reviews* 2003;**1**:2003.

43 Grimshaw JM, Thomas RE, MacLennan G, Fraser C, Ramsay CR, Vale L *et al.* Effectiveness and efficiency of guideline dissemination and implementation strategies. Aberdeen: Health Services Research Unit, University of Aberdeen, 2002.

44 Grimshaw JM, Shirran L, Thomas R, Mowatt G, Fraser C, Bero L et al. Changing provider behavior: an overview of systematic reviews of interventions. *Med Care* 2001;**39**(8 Suppl 2):II2–45.

45 Sibley JC, Sackett DL, Neufeld V, Gerrard B, Rudnick KV, Fraser W. A randomized trial of continuing medical education. *N Engl J Med* 1982;**306**:511–15.

46 Grol R. Improving the quality of medical care. Building bridges among professional pride, payer profit, and patient satisfaction. *JAMA* 2001;**286**:2578–85.

47 Wolff N. Randomised trials of socially complex interventions: promise or peril? *J Health Serv Res Policy* 2001;**6**:123–6.

48 Forbes A, Griffiths P. Methodological strategies for the identification and synthesis of "evidence" to support decision making in relation to complex healthcare systems and practices. *Nursing Inquiry* 2002;**9**:141–55.

49 Campbell M, Fitzpatrick R, Haines A, Kinmonth AL, Sandercock P, Spiegelhalter D *et al.* Framework for design and evaluation of complex interventions to improve health. *BMJ* 2000;**321**:694–6.

50 Granados A, Jonsson E, Banta HD, Bero L, Bonair A, Cochet C *et al.* EUR-ASSESS Project Subgroup Report on Dissemination and Impact. *Int J Technol Assessment Health Care* 1997;**13**:220–86.

51 Ferlie E, Gabbay J, Fitzgerald L, Locock L, Dopson S. Evidence-based medicine and organisational change: an overview of some recent qualitative research. In: Ashburner L, ed. *Organisational behaviour and organisational studies in health care: reflections on the future.* Basingstoke: Palgrove, 2001.

52 Kogut B, Zander U. Knowledge of the firm: combinative capabilities and the replication of technology. *Org Sci* 1992;**3**:383–97.

53 Bartlett CA, Ghoshal S. *Managing across borders: the transnational solution.* Boston, MA: Harvard Business School Press, 1989.

54 Garvin DA. Building a learning organization. *Harvard Business Rev* 1993;**71**:78–92.

55 Holsapple CW, Joshi KD. Knowledge manipulation activities: Results of a Delphi study. *Inf Manag* 2002;**39**:477–90.

56 Hippel EV. "Sticky information" and the locus of problem solving. *Manag Sci* 1991;**44**:429–39.

57 Cohen WM, Levinthal DA. Absorptive capacity: a new perspective on learning and innovation. *Admin Sci Q* 1990;**30**:560–85.

58 Malhotra Y. From information management to knowledge management. In: Srikantaiah TK, Koenig MED, eds. *Knowledge Management for the Information Professional*. Medford, NJ: Information Today, 2000.

59 Weick KE. *Sensemaking in Organizations*. Thousand Oaks, CA: Sage, 1995.

60 Leonard-Burton D. *Wellsprings of Knowledge*. Boston, MA: Harvard Business School Press, 1995.

61 Hansen MT, Nohria N, Tierney T. What's your strategy for managing knowledge? *Harvard Business Rev* 1999;106–16.

62 Brown JS, Duguid KP. *The social life of information*. Boston, MA: Harvard University Press, 2000.

63 Herxheimer A. Drugs to prevent and control nausea and vomiting: A survey of trial reports published since 1950. In: Blum RH, Heinrichs RL, Herxheimer A, eds. *Nausea and vomiting: overview, challenges, practical treatments and new perspectives*. London: Whurr, 2000.

64 Loke Y, Derry S. Does anybody read "evidence-based" articles? *BMC Medical Research Methodology* 2003;3:14.

65 Denzin M, Lincoln Y. *Handbook of Qualitative Research*. London: Sage, 1994.

66 Janis IL. *Groupthink: Psychological Studies of Policy Decisions and Fiascoes*. Boston, MA: Houghton Mifflin, 1982.

21: How narratives work in psychiatric science: an example from the biological psychiatry of PTSD

ALLAN YOUNG

Narratives are ubiquitous in psychiatry. They are part of the process of diagnosis and assessment, the basis for most kinds of psychotherapy, and the means by which patients and clinicians talk about the process of falling sick and being sick. But in addition to clinical narratives, there are also narratives of psychiatric science. The typical journal article contains three narratives: a narrative that justifies a puzzle and a hypothesis (introduction), a narrative of the current research (methods, results, discussion), and a revised version of the opening narrative, incorporating the data and findings described in the middle narrative.

In this chapter I focus on a set of scientific narratives concerned with post-traumatic stress disorder (PTSD) and abnormalities in the hypothalamic–pituitary–adrenal (HPA) axis. These narratives are products of a network of researchers, connected through ties of collaboration and co-authorship which has undertaken a series of linked experiments oriented to a condition called "hypocorticolism". I will refer to this stream of research and writing as "the hypocorticolism programme".[1-13] This programme is not concerned with the phenomenology of PTSD and has no obvious clinical applications. As I will indicate, its value to psychiatry lies elsewhere.

A puzzle and its solution

The PTSD classification dates to 1980 (DSM-III).[14] Psychiatric literature focuses on the chronic form of PTSD. Only a minority of people who are exposed to trauma-level events develop PTSD, and only a minority of this minority develop the chronic form. Nearly all of these chronic cases are associated with co-morbid psychiatric disorders. What makes these people special? Before attempting an answer, one must consider two possibilities: (1) PTSD is a unitary disorder, characterised by a distinctive aetiology and pathogenesis, or (2) PTSD is a syndrome, an idiom of distress expressing either an endogenous disorder (depression, generalised anxiety disorder, etc.) or a pre-existing psychiatric condition such as neuroticism (a personality factor associated with instability, vulnerability to stress, and proneness to anxiety).

The existence of a traumatic memory is the key to diagnosing PTSD and the only way to differentiate between possibilities 1 and 2. It is the motor that drives PTSD's symptoms: distressful re-experiences, avoidance behaviour, emotional numbing, and physiological arousal. However, authentic traumatic memories are easily confused with memories that become "traumatic" after the fact, as a consequence of diagnosis or treatment:

Possibility 1:   traumatic event → traumatic memory → disorder
Possibility 2:   a pre-existing disorder → diagnosis → traumatic memory

The task of distinguishing between the two possibilities is complicated by another factor: PTSD can be a source of significant secondary gain, including compensation, and patients may have strong conscious or unconscious motives for finding appropriate memories, that are unpleasant but not pathogenic. The bottom line is that it is frequently difficult to know whether a patient's distressful memory is the cause or the effect of her current condition, and especially difficult in cases of chronic PTSD.[15] This difficulty is a source of several problems: diagnostic (differential diagnosis), therapeutic (choice of treatment), forensic (decisions relating to entitlements), and epistemological (the underlying nature of PTSD and in particular, the commonalities between all those who suffer from the condition).

The hypocorticolism programme offers a coherent epistemology for PTSD, in the form of a disorder-specific surrogate for traumatic memory and a matching theory of pathogenesis. This surrogate is a biological marker obtained by measuring cortisol excreted in blood, urine, and saliva. Unlike memory, it is unaffected by diagnostic practices or the patient's interest in secondary gain.

Narratives of normality

The hypocorticolism programme began with a research hypothesis.[16] The patient's re-experiences (intrusive images, symptomatic dreams etc.) are frightening, the anticipation of further re-experiences is a source of anxiety, and the symptomatic adaptations and physiological arousal are stressful. The hypothesis: Vietnam War veterans diagnosed with chronic PTSD will have elevated levels of catecholamines and cortisol, consistent with our understanding of the physiology of fear, anxiety, and stress. The hypothesis was tested and produced a "puzzling dissociation": catecholamines conformed to expectations but cortisol was *lower* in the PTSD patients than in the comparison groups. The researchers considered three paths for future research. One, investigate the possibility that the catecholamines and cortisol are tuned to different neurophysiological pathways. Two, focus on the potential clinical utility of the dissociation (diagnostic sensitivity of around 90%). Three, take the Gordian knot solution, forget about the catecholamines and explore the connection between PTSD and cortisol. The programme took the third path.[13]

The findings seemed to suggest that cortisol is initially elevated in PTSD and then falls to a point lower than the original steady state (homeostasis). Animal experiments and evidence from other clinical conditions (Cushing's syndrome) indicate that chronically high levels of cortisol cause neuronal death, atrophy, and a loss of synaptic plasticity in the brain. (The hippocampus, a key element of the memory system, is especially vulnerable.) Thus the evolution of the emergency response (fight–flight–freeze) would have favoured the emergence of a negative feedback loop to protect the brain. This, the researchers concluded, explained the puzzling dissociation: in PTSD patients, the evolutionary adaptation is imperfect, there is an overswing in the homeostatic feedback loop, and cortisol excretion falls too far.

The programme's self-defining moment is the point at which the cortisol levels detected in the PTSD veterans are defined as "abnormal".[9] If "normal" means the average value obtained for a sample of normal people (those without psychiatric disorders), then the PTSD levels *are* abnormal. This is a nominal and uncontroversial use of the term: "abnormality" resides in a statistically significant difference between the mean values for the two samples. For the programme's researchers, "abnormality" meant much more. It implied pathology.

Having solved one puzzle (via the Gordian knot solution), the programme created another, since the cortisol levels detected in PTSD veterans are not pathological in any obvious way. They are not associated with disability, pain, or distress, nor with any problems or damage downstream. Excessively low levels of cortisol *do* cause serious problems. This is what happens in Addison's disease, a disorder associated with weakness, fatigue, weight loss, changes in pigmentation, and physiological effects that can be detected by laboratory tests for hypoglycaemia and elevated levels of serum potassium. But cortisol levels in PTSD, even though "significantly" (in a statistical sense) lower than those in normal individuals, fall completely within the range defined as "normal" by endocrinologists.

On the other hand, there is a way in which this "abnormality" might be considered pathological – if it were shown to be the effect, rather than the cause, of a pathology. This is how the programme connected abnormality to pathology, through a presumed dysfunction (defective negative feedback loop) in the HPA axis. The explanation is circular, since the effects provide the only direct evidence for the existence of the cause. Yet the circularity is not obvious to the programme's researchers/writers or their colleagues and readers. Why? The answer is in the programme's narratives. Before I actually get to these narratives, however, I want to say something more about the phenomenon of abnormality.

By the early 1990s, the hypocorticolism programme had erected a conceptual structure, consisting of an abnormality (a statistically significant difference between mean values), a pathology (a putative dysfunction), and procedures for making the abnormality visible (measuring cortisol circulating in blood and excreted in urine, measuring cortisol following a dexamethasone challenge, counting glucocorticoid receptors, and so on). And the structure had been given a name, "hypocorticolism" (explicitly differentiated from clinical hypocorticolism).

This structure is predicated on the notion of abnormality. Subtract abnormality and the structure collapses. But *whose* abnormality is it? A naive answer would be that abnormality is an attribute of the individuals in the PTSD group. At this point, it is important to distinguish between visible attributes and attributes known by inference. In the case of PTSD, abnormality is a visible attribute of a group (a mean value) but an inferred attribute of the individuals involved. For example, in one study researchers compared urinary cortisol in 16 veterans with PTSD and the same number of healthy veterans.[8] There was substantial variation within each group and substantial overlap between groups. Two PTSD patients were marginally lower than the lowest normal, and two normals were outliers (high excretors) and contributed to pushing the inter-group difference over the threshold of statistical significance. The published research redescribes this difference as "chronic cortisol suppression" originating in a "dysfunction" in the HPA axis. All of the PTSD patients are assumed to have the dysfunction, even though each of these individuals has a statistically indistinguishable counterpart in the normal group. To go from group mean to individual characteristic, one must presume that there is an underlying mechanism (affecting the negative feedback loop), and that it expresses itself not as a diagnosable symptom or feature (a visible attribute of individuals) but rather as a tendency. The source of this presumption is narrative, as we shall see.

Interest in normality and abnormality predated the programme. In DSM-III,[14] PTSD is described as *a normal response to abnormal events.*

The definition was tailored for a specific patient population, Vietnam War veterans. The idea was to construct a diagnosis that would qualify as a "service connected disorder", according to the standards of the US Veterans Administration Medical System (VA). This designation would make veterans eligible for disability pensions and psychiatric care. For the government to assume responsibility however, the new disorder would have to be both exogenous and without a significant precondition (a diathesis, vulnerability). And this is what the term "normal response" was intended to provide. The DSM-III definition passed the test, and the VA quickly established itself as the main source of research into the cause, prevalence, and treatment of PTSD. Its patients doubled as research subjects and its clinicians doubled as investigators. The entire system – intersecting treatment, pensions, and research – was based on the normality thesis.[15,17]

Problems with normality

There is an epidemiological problem with the normality thesis, since only a minority of people exposed to trauma-level events develop PTSD. Research conducted in Scotland and Australia during the 1980s pinpointed the weakness of the normality thesis.[18,19] The research was unusual in that it involved a pre-trauma assessment. Each study concerned a group exposed to a shared event (an oil rig disaster, a forest fire). Prior to exposure, these individuals (police constables, fire fighters) had been given psychiatric evaluations. When psychiatric records were compared with post-event psychiatric work-ups, it became clear that onset and chronicity of PTSD were generally explained by pre-existing psychiatric problems. The research was published in mainstream journals, but attracted no formal response from peers. During this period, most PTSD research was funded by the Veterans Association (VA) and conducted on Vietnam War veterans. Reliable before-and-after comparisons were impossible; there was no way to test the normality thesis and there were political and clinical incentives to accept it.

In 1995, the *American Journal of Psychiatry* published an article by Rachel Yehuda, the leading participant in the hypocorticolism programme, and Alexander McFarlane, author of the Australian PTSD study mentioned above.[9] Their article, "Conflict between Current Knowledge about Posttraumatic Stress Disorder and Its Original Conceptual Basis", proposed to stand the normality thesis on its head. In a brief narrative history of the field, the authors cited evidence of significant "risk-factors" and high levels of co-morbidity in PTSD. The findings had created an "unusual tension" between researchers and people with "a strong allegiance to the social achievements that have been met by the existence of the disorder". The field was fragmented by "competing agendas and paradigms" and "conflict between those who wish to normalise the status of victims and those who wish to define and characterise PTSD as a psychiatric illness".

In reality, the "tensions" and "conflicts" were not recent, but had been ongoing for a century. DSM-III ended the public debate on trauma diatheses, but many clinicians were willing to diagnose PTSD even when aetiological events fell short of the DSM standard (that is, outside the range of normal human experience, certain to produce profound distress in almost anyone) and a diathesis or vulnerability had to be assumed. This practice occurred even in VA hospitals, where the normality thesis was recognised *de jure*. DSM-IV[20] accepted this clinical reality when it shifted the centre of gravity from the objective qualities of traumatic events to the perceptions and subjective experiences of patients.

The bottom line, according to Yehuda and McFarlane, was that a choice has to be made between good science and good intentions. The correct choice is good science: redefine PTSD as an abnormal response to situations that normal people are able to handle. The term "abnormal" could mean two different things. First, people with PTSD are abnormal in a *non-specific* sense, sharing a characteristic that makes them vulnerable to a range of psychiatric disorders. This would explain the epidemiology and co-morbidity associated with PTSD, but would undermine the disorder's validity. The preferred alternative is a pre-existing abnormality *specific to PTSD* – and hypocorticolism fits the bill.

Originally, hypocorticolism was to be the result of a dysfunction caused by a trauma. The abnormality thesis reversed the relationship, by making hypocorticolism a precondition for PTSD. The feedback loop was an important part of the new story, and it remained the source of hypocorticolism's visible marker (a difference between group cortisol averages). But the loop's waywardness was redefined. No longer the consequence of trauma, it became the expression of a previously undetected condition called "hypersensitivity". This is the story line: In a minority of people, the hormonal feedback mechanism that triggers cortisol release is abnormally sensitive to environmental stimuli. Every stressful encounter further sensitises this defective system. In PTSD, the sensitising process is ceaseless, via distressful "re-experiences". The resulting condition, hypersensitivity, is detected in the symptoms of autonomic arousal that the DSM associates with PTSD, and in the characteristic cortisol output.

Here is an example, a research narrative illustrating hypersensitivity. The narrative describes an experiment in which cortisol excretion was measured over a 24 hour cycle.[1,13] Normal individuals were matched with people with PTSD. Peaks and troughs correlated with normal circadian rhythms in both groups. The PTSD group had a lower trough than the normal group, and this is described as a difference in amplitude. This difference (PTSD output has greater amplitude) is then described as evidence of a more sensitive "signal to noise ratio" in PTSD. The signal to noise ratio is then described as evidence that the PTSD nervous system is "exquisitely sensitive" to stimuli and "capable of maximally responding to the environment or at least of mounting a more efficient stress response". In other words, hypersensitivity.

The normality thesis left two puzzles unresolved. The first of these concerned the negative feedback loop. Ongoing high levels of cortisol are characteristic of several psychiatric disorders. Why was natural selection wise in the case of PTSD (providing a negative feedback loop), but unwise in the case of depression and other anxiety disorders? The abnormality thesis eliminated the puzzle by eliminating the evolutionary theme. The other puzzle concerns the high co-morbidity associated with PTSD – the soft under-belly of this diagnostic classification. A solution was now possible, in the form of a multi-diathesis theory that wired PTSD to an unmapped, disorder-specific neurophysiological pathway. According to the new theory, portions of the PTSD pathway are shared with the pathways of the disorders with which it commonly co-exists. This explains similarities between symptoms in PTSD and the other disorders and, so, the apparent co-morbidity. Thus people with PTSD tend to score high on the Hamilton Depression Scale, because the scale is picking up effects produced by shared segments of PTSD and depression pathways.

In choosing good science over good intentions, the abnormality thesis created a moral conundrum. The thesis "de-emphasises the centrality of the trauma as the true cause of post-traumatic symptoms and potentially invalidates the experience of survivors or, worse, blames them for their legitimate reactions to these events".[4] The thesis would not affect the material interests of DSM-III's target population, Vietnam War veterans, for their rights are politically entrenched. However, it might cast a shadow over the *moral distinctiveness* of these traumatised veterans, and also holocaust survivors, rape victims, and certain other clinical populations. Can a diathesis be reconciled with victimhood? One possibility would be to translate the term "vulnerability" into "threshold value" so that normality and abnormality are connected via a continuum. Alternatively, one might produce an additional story, a genealogy that begins with a prior trauma (the cause of the patient's current diathesis) occurring during childhood. In this story, childhood – a period of psychological and biological immaturity – would be a kind of diathesis. A kind consonant with victimhood.

Abductive reasoning

There are interesting similarities between research narratives and fictional narratives of detection. For example, look at the way in which the Sherlock Holmes stories lead the reader from a puzzle to a solution. The stories are not especially clever and they are certainly not believable. Nevertheless many readers, including intelligent people, find the stories to be cognitively satisfying and even worth rereading. The narrative structure of Holmes' adventures contributes to this effect. In the next pages, I want to suggest that a similar structure organises the programme's research narratives.

Every Sherlock Holmes story constructs a puzzle and then solves it. Each solution is the product of a stream of inferences that philosophers call *abduction*, or "reasoning to the best inference". Holmes and Watson claim that their solutions proceed via another kind of inference, namely deduction. The term "abduction" was coined by Charles Peirce, an American philosopher and contemporary of Sherlock Holmes. Abduction is our habitual mode of reasoning and can be defined in the following way:

1 Reasoning proceeds from puzzle to a conclusion via heterogeneous inferences: analogy (a well-understood phenomenon serves as a model for organising and explaining a poorly understood phenomenon), synecdoche (a part identifies a whole), metonym (one feature implicates another feature that is contiguous in time or space), induction (a generalisation inferred from multiple instances), and deduction (inferring a particular instance from general principles).
2 The plausibility of each inference is determined holistically, with reference to the person's stored knowledge of the domain in question.
3 When people are asked to describe the stream of inferences from puzzle to conclusion, their accounts are characteristically "retroductive". They simplify the circumstances, often omitting steps, and narrate the stream of inferences in cognitively and socially satisfying ways.

At this point, I want to exploit an evolutionary argument suggested by Carlo Ginzburg. Analogy, synecdoche, and metonym originated in a "quick and dirty" mode of reasoning employed by our Palaeolithic ancestors. Early hunter–gatherers were able to go from sensory stimuli to behavioural response without a time-consuming search of stored knowledge, classifications, etc. The adaptation worked because the range of environmental stimuli was narrow and stable. There would have been costs: energy wasted on false positives. But even a moderately low hit rate would provide a selective advantage.

Circumstances had changed radically by the time of Sherlock Holmes. A consulting detective with a low hit rate would be a public nuisance. To make his stories work, Conan Doyle had to find a way to improve the effectiveness of Holmes' abductive reasoning. He did this in two ways. Abduction is camouflaged as deduction, as when Holmes tells Watson that, "It is an old maxim of mine, that when you have excluded the impossible, whatever remains, however improbable, may be the truth." Second, Holmes is furnished with a radically stripped down environment. (Its apotheosis is the sealed room that starts *The Adventure of the Speckled Band.*)

Peirce believed that abduction plays an important role in science, by generating hypotheses that will launch experiments that will produce facts. In the Sherlock Holmes stories, abduction is a source of both hypotheses *and* facts (Holmes' conclusions). Real scientists are more like Sherlock Holmes than Peirce's idealised scientist in this regard. This is no criticism, for abduction is not a defective mode of reasoning.

The programme's publications are permeated by abductive reasoning. There are sequences of heterogeneous inferences, in which cortisol serves as a synecdoche for hypocorticolism, glucocorticoid receptors are metonyms for hypocorticolism, and so on. There are radically stripped down environments, in which very complicated things – life events, memories, dreams, existential states – are transmuted via diagnostic protocols, psychometric scales, and biological assays into standardised and commensurable artefacts (data). And there are retroductive narratives, where prior research is stripped of its original ambiguities and equivocations. Thus an article on hypocorticolism mentions in its narrative two earlier publications as confirming its own findings. The first paper, in its original form, mentions that the researchers did not control for alcohol abuse, although it may have affected the outcome. The second cited publication was based on a sample of only four subjects. In the renarration, the equivocation is gone: confirmations are cited without complications.

There is nothing unusual here. This is the way that most science works. Science requires radically stripped down environments in order to isolate factors and determine their contributions. Theory formation and hypothesis testing would be stymied without the help of synecdoche, metonym, and analogy. As for the kinds of simplification that may occur during renarration: *caveat emptor*. One wonders about the experts responsible for the article's peer review, who it might be assumed had begun to get drawn into the developing tale. Whilst they were probably aware on some level of the nature of the original hypothesis (and hence of the discrepancy introduced in later versions), they were also caught up in the narrative – an experience that requires some degree of suspension of disbelief.

Fictive people

If the hypocorticolism programme is special, it is in the matter of *fictive people*. The Sherlock Holmes stories are filled with people – thinking, talking, acting. On the other hand, research narratives appear to be thoroughly depersonalised. Data are portrayed as products of an indifferent technology, rather than handicraft. Time is mere chronology, homogeneous and abstract. Individuals are transmogrified into clinical populations, comparison groups, and constellations of clinical and demographic features. The overall effect is what the philosopher Thomas Nagel called "the view from nowhere". One should not press the point about depersonalisation too far however. Competent readers (many of whom are themselves researchers) understand that there is a difference between doing research and then writing the research, and are aware that there are strategising researchers behind the rhetoric and real people behind the statistics. In other words, research narratives are different from detective stories in that their actors are real rather than fictional, and implicit in the text rather than overt.

The programme's narratives are unusual in this regard. Like other research narratives, they include live actors – the researchers and their "subjects". But unlike most research narratives, they also include fictive characters. The term "fictive" refers to a person who is regarded as being the real thing, but who lacks some feature normally associated with the category in question. For example, fictive kin are found in many societies. People interact with fictive kin as they would with real kin. The difference is in the quality of the connection linking fictive kin: it is different from the link to real kin, for example, through biology, marriage, or legal adoption. The fictive kin are simultaneously fictions and flesh and blood people. The fictive people in the programme's narratives are similarly fictional and real. To be more precise, they are real people who embody two fictive qualities: simple PTSD and metamorphosis.

A few words concerning simple PTSD or, as sometimes described by researchers, "pure PTSD". Most PTSD research, including the programme's, investigates the chronic form of the disorder. The clinical presentation of chronic PTSD is invariably complex. Nearly all patients have diagnosable co-morbid disorders, notably depression, generalised anxiety disorder, panic disorder, or substance abuse. In addition, many PTSD symptoms are polymorphous adaptations to anxiety and easily confused with these same disorders. Where do the symptoms of the co-morbid disorders leave off and the symptoms of PTSD begin?

PTSD researchers manage co-morbidity by following three decision rules:

1   Include individuals in the PTSD group if PTSD is the primary diagnosis – a decision based on clinical judgement. There are two exceptions.
2   Exclude individuals with co-morbid psychotic disorders, bipolar disorder, and organic brain disorders.
3   Exclude patients with co-morbid mood disorders from the PTSD group if the research is intended to isolate or subtract the effect of the co-morbid mood disorder.

Individuals who qualify for an unambiguous PTSD mono-diagnosis – that is, simple PTSD – are exceedingly hard to find, if they exist at all. They are entirely missing from the main research population, veterans of the Vietnam War. To obtain cases of simple PTSD, researchers must extract the pure disorder from the dross of the clinical syndrome, as a chemist must refine an element that naturally occurs only in compounds. This is the function of these decision rules.

The procedure through which PTSD is extracted from a messy syndrome is plausible because of the remarkable qualities that are attributed to traumatic memory. It transforms alcohol abuse into "self-dosing" (symptomatic of PTSD "avoidance behaviour"); ruminations (associated with major depression) into "re-experiencing" (associated with PTSD); irritability, difficulty concentrating, and sleep disturbance (all characteristic of generalised anxiety disorder) into "autonomic arousal" symptomatic of PTSD; and so on.

Earlier in this chapter, I detailed the epistemological and diagnostic problem entailed by the concept of traumatic memory and indicated how hypocorticolism offers a solution by providing researchers with a reliable biological surrogate for an unreliable cognitive mechanism (memory). I made the additional point, that hypocorticolism is a literary product based on a visible difference observed between two average men (the mean values for the PTSD group and the comparison group). The PTSD average man is connected to the flesh and blood PTSD subjects via a theoretical tendency, hypersensitivity. This is the backdrop for a second fictive quality, metamorphosis.

A comparison with Sherlock Holmes once again. In several adventures, Holmes investigates in disguise, usually as a tramp. This is a clumsy literary device and demands a special effort on the part of the reader who wants the story to work. The programme's average man is also a master of interchangeable identities, and there are occasions when he appears in guises that would seem to have little in common. Here is an illustration from a research article of 2000.[4] The project compared levels of urinary cortisol between the offspring of Holocaust survivors and a control group matched for ethnicity. The research narrative divides the 35 survivor offspring into six sub-groups (Table 21.1)

Table 21.1

Group	No	Lifetime PTSD	A-current psychiatric diagnosis	Parental PTSD	Cortisol level
1	7	yes	no	yes	29·48
2	3	yes	yes	yes	45·03
3	10	no	no	yes	33·88
4	4	no	yes	yes	76·10
5	6	no	no	no	64·59
6	5	no	yes	no	63·44
Controls	15	no	no	no	65·1

"Lifetime PTSD" = at least one occurrence. Cortisol measurements are micromilligrams per day.

Nineteen survivors' offspring were recruited from a group psychotherapy programme for Holocaust survivors and their families, conducted at the researchers' host institution. Twelve offspring were currently diagnosed with one or more of the following conditions: major depressive disorder, dysthymia, eating disorder, obsessive–compulsive disorder, anorexia nervosa, substance use, and PTSD. In 24 cases (70%), parents were diagnosed with PTSD by their own offspring; the remaining cases were diagnosed by the investigators.

Only one participant had current PTSD. However, if PTSD is the consequence of a diathesis associated with an HPA abnormality, then evidence of lifetime PTSD (Groups 1 and 2) should also be associated with hypocorticolism. Groups 1 and 2 are significantly lower than the control group (no lifetime PTSD) and therefore the results are consistent with this supposition and the programme's thesis. However, Group 3 (no lifetime PTSD) is markedly lower than Group 2, when the thesis predicts the opposite. Is this evidence of a parental effect? If so, the cortisol level in Group 4 (parental PTSD) must be explained, since it is substantially higher than in the control group, even though a parental effect hypothesis would predict the opposite. Perhaps this result can be explained by the psychiatric problems affecting Group 4. If so, one expects to find analogous results when comparing Group 5 (no psychiatric diagnosis) with Group 6 (psychiatric diagnosis). But Group 6 is marginally lower than Group 5. The bottom line is that there is no coherent pattern.

At this point, the narrative introduces its fictive average man, by re-aggregating the six groups into three groups:

Group A aggregates 1 and 2 (lifetime PTSD plus parental PTSD) cortisol = 37·25
Group B aggregates 3 and 4 (parental PTSD) cortisol = 55·0
Group C aggregates 5 and 6 (no lifetime PTSD, no parental PTSD) cortisol = 64·0

The results become more or less coherent: cortisol levels correlate with PTSD and hypocorticolism is vindicated. "Offspring with both parental PTSD and lifetime PTSD had significantly lower cortisol levels than either offspring without lifetime PTSD or comparison subjects. Offspring with only parental PTSD, but not lifetime PTSD, had an intermediate level of cortisol ...".

Group B must be clarified however. The 35 offspring completed an index of PTSD symptoms. The correlation between their symptoms and the PTSD diagnosis was not statistically significant. The investigators see this as evidence that "PTSD symptoms were present in offspring even in the absence of a PTSD diagnosis". Thus group B represents some kind of subclinical or partial PTSD, undetected by the standard diagnostic protocols.

The researchers describe the link between parental PTSD and cortisol suppression in groups A and B as being a "risk factor". But what is the underlying mechanism? The possibility of a "nongenomic transmission of stress response characteristics" is mentioned. That is, the parents' PTSD may affect their "child rearing practices" in a way that has neuroendocrinological consequences. Three animal studies are then cited in support of this thesis. The morally delicate possibility of a "genomic" factor (a hereditary diathesis) is not considered.

> The message here is that a variety of intercorrelated factors contributing to risk for PTSD may be associated with different effects on cortisol. Thus our findings represent *the beginning of an exploration of this complex issue*, which should be pursued to more carefully examine relationship among these factors ...[4] [emphasis added]

In the hypocorticolism programme's subsequent retroductive narratives, the complications and tentativeness mentioned in the original vanish.

Conclusion

Psychiatric science is in the business of making and remaking epistemic things, like hypocorticolism. The process includes the preparation of texts. Narration is internal to the process of producing knowledge, and not merely a way of representing facts and findings.

Texts "work" to the extent that they are cognitively satisfying and rhetorically successful. The programme's narratives are permeated by abductive reasoning. Abduction is not a defective form of inference. It is the way that we habitually engage the world and it is fairly efficient. Abduction does have this limitation: a superfluity of possibilities. In order for abduction to be efficient, the possibilities must be limited. Deductive inference does this internally, through monothetic classifications and rules of inclusion, exclusion, necessity, and sufficiency. Abductive inference requires some kind of help, namely "the Conan Doyle solution": create a radically simplified environment within which abductive reasoning operates efficiently. This is how the programme's research narratives work, but only up to a point. Conan Doyle's method guaranteed closure. Each of his puzzles is solved unequivocally (with a famous exception, a narrative in which the author attempts to eliminate Sherlock Holmes). Scientific narratives operate according to a different principle. They are open-ended and they substitute holism for closure – their various solutions, epistemic things (for example, hypocorticolism), and fictive embodiments are vindicated within a continuously expanding matrix of theories and proofs.

References

1 McFarlane AC, Yehuda R. Resilience, vulnerability, and the course of posttraumatic reactions. In: Van der Kolk BA, McFarlane AC, Weisaeth L, ed. *Traumatic stress: the effects of overwhelming experience on mind, body, and society.* New York: Guilford Press, 1996.
2 Yehuda R. Biological factors associated with susceptibility to posttraumatic stress disorder. *Can J Psychiatry* 1999;**44**:343–9.
3 Yehuda R. Neuroendocrinology of trauma and posttraumatic stress disorder. In: Yehuda R, ed. *Psychological Trauma.* Washington, DC: American Psychiatric Press, 1998.
4 Yehuda R, Bierer LM, Schmeidler J, Aferiat DH, Breslau I, Dolan S. Low cortisol and risk for PTSD in adult offspring of holocaust survivors. *Am J Psychiatry* 2000;**157**:1252–9.
5 Yehuda R, Giller EL, Southwick SM, Lowy MT. Hypothalamic–pituitary–adrenal dysfunction in posttraumatic disorder. *Biol Psychiatry* 1991;**30**:1031–48.
6 Yehuda R, Giller EL, Levengood RA, Southwick SM, Siever LJ. Hypothalamic–pituitary–adrenal functioning in post-traumatic stress disorder: expanding the concept of stress response spectrum. In: Friedman MJ, Charney DS, Deutch AY, eds. *Neurobiological and clinical consequences of stress: from normal adaptation to PTSD.* Philadelphia: Lippincott–Raven, 1995.
7 Yehuda R, Kahana B, Binder-Byrnes K, Southwick SM, Mason JW, Giller EL. Low urinary cortisol excretion in holocaust survivors with posttraumatic stress disorder. *Am J Psychiatry* 1995;**152**:982–6.
8 Yehuda R, Lowy MT, Southwick SM, Schaffer D, Giller EL. Lymphocyte glucocorticoid receptor number in posttraumatic stress disorder. *Am J Psychiatry* 1991;**148**:499–504.
9 Yehuda R, McFarlane AC. Conflict between current knowledge about posttraumatic stress disorder and its original conceptual basis. *Am J Psychiatry* 1995;**152**:1705–13.
10 Yehuda R, Resnick H, Kahana B, Giller EL. Long-lasting hormonal alterations to extreme stress in humans: normative or maladaptive? *Psychosom Med* 1993; **55**:287–97.
11 Yehuda R, Southwick SM, Krystal JH, Bremner JH, Charney DS, Mason JW. Enhanced suppression of cortisol following dexamethasone administration in posttraumatic stress disorder. *Am J Psychiatry* 1993;**150**:83–6.
12 Yehuda R, Southwick SM, Nussbaum G, Wahby VS, Giller EL, Mason JW. Low urinary cortisol excretion in patients with posttraumatic stress disorder. *J Nerv Mental Dis* 1990;**78**:366–8.
13 Yehuda R, Teicher MH, Trestman RL *et al.* Cortisol regulation in posttraumatic stress disorder and major depression: a chronobiological analysis. *Biol Psychiatry* 1996;**40**:79–88.

14 American Psychiatric Association. *Diagnostic and Statistical Manual of Mental Disorders of the American Psychiatric Association*, 3rd edn. Washington, DC: American Psychiatric Association, 1980.

15 Young A. *The harmony of illusions: inventing posttraumatic stress disorder.* Princeton, NJ: Princeton University Press, 1995.

16 Mason JW. Urinary-free cortisol levels in posttraumatic stress disorder patients. *J Nerv Ment Dis* 1986;**174**:145–9.

17 Young A. Our traumatic neurosis and its brain. *Science in Context* 2001;**14**:661–83.

18 Alexander A, Wells A. Reactions of police officers to body-handling after a major disaster: a before-and-after comparison. *Br J Psychiatry* 1991;**159**:547–55.

19 McFarlane AC. An Australian disaster: the 1983 bushfires. *Int J Ment Health* 1990;**19**:36–47.

20 American Psychiatric Association. *Diagnostic and Statistical Manual of Mental Disorders of the American Psychiatric Association*, 4th edn. Washington, DC: American Psychiatric Association, 1994.

22: Storying policy: constructions of risk in proposals to reform UK mental health legislation

DAVID J HARPER

It is probably fair to say that much narrative research in the field of health has been focused on developing biographical accounts of patients' personal experiences both of illness and of care systems. Of course, these stories are constructed within particular contexts and those contexts afford not only certain possibilities but also certain constraints. In this chapter I will be examining one set of "meta-narratives" which influence the lives of those who receive, or are threatened with receiving, compulsory psychiatric treatment by analysing a text from the UK government White Paper *Reforming the Mental Health Act*.[1] I want to argue that narrative and discursive researchers can provide valuable insights into the assumptions guiding the development and presentation of policies like these. Ian Parker has commented that "people 'make' discourse, but not in discursive conditions of their own choosing".[2] The legislation and policy which define who gets treated compulsorily (and when) shape the conditions within which psychiatric service users' experiences, stories, and identities are constructed.

"Mental illness", the risk of violence and public anxiety

The lay TV audience and newspaper readership could be forgiven for thinking that we are living at a time of increased risk of homicide committed by those in contact with mental health services, but official statistics tell a somewhat different story. First, there are many more suicides than homicides in the general population, with 20 927 suicides and probable suicides in England and Wales during the four years from April 1996 compared with 1579 homicides during the three years from April 1996.[3] Secondly, the contribution of people with mental health problems is not as high as is commonly supposed. Approximately one-quarter of the people killing themselves and 9%

of those killing others had been in contact with mental health services in the year before, although this figure increased when the contact period was extended – for example 18% of homicide perpetrators had had contact with mental health services "at some time".[3] Thirdly, far from the number of homicides committed by those considered mentally ill increasing, they have stayed relatively consistently low and have, if anything, decreased slightly over the past 40 years.[4] Fourthly, a diagnosis of major mental illness is far less predictive of violence than being "young, male, single, lower class, and substance abusing or substance dependent".[5] Some commentators report that less than 10% of serious violence, including homicide, is attributable to psychosis and that, in these cases only a small proportion of the victims are unknown to the assailant.[6]

Of course the array of articles critiquing the association between mental illness and risk of violence also contribute to there being a violence/mental illness literature and may help to sediment the idea that there is a causal link between them. This serves to obscure that risk often lies in the other direction: people with mental health problems are six times more likely to die by homicide than the general population and are also at a raised risk of dying as a result of suicide and accident.[7] People with mental health problems are also at risk from law enforcement agencies because of anxiety about the possibility of violence – witness the shooting dead of Andrew Kernan, who had a diagnosis of schizophrenia, by Merseyside police in July 2001.[8]

Risk and policies on compulsory psychiatric treatment

Socially constructed notions of mental illness are most pernicious when normative notions of mental health are forced on some people through the use of coercive and compulsory treatment. Compulsory psychiatric treatment has a long history[9] and the proposed reforms to the UK's 1983 Mental Health Act (MHA) come at a time of dramatically increasing rates of compulsory treatment – for example, compulsory admissions to hospital increased by 45% between 1991 and 1995[10] and there were 26 300 compulsory admissions in 2001–2002.[11] Current UK mental health legislation permits compulsory psychiatric treatment when a person is considered to pose a risk to themselves or to others as a result of a mental disorder. The act of "sectioning" transforms a social and political problem into a health problem. Such transformations occur in culture when historical conditions mean that certain discourses (for example, "health" as opposed to, say, "religion") are foregrounded. Moreover, these discourses operate simultaneously, with dominance shifting according to context, speaker and so on.

Box 22.1 Timeline of development of proposals to reform the 1983 UK Mental Health Act

1999

July: Report of the expert committee on reform of the MHA chaired by Genevra Richardson published by the Department of Health. Green Paper *Managing Dangerous People with Severe Personality Disorder* published jointly by the Home Office and Department of Health.

November: Green Paper discussing a number of options for reform of the MHA is published by the Department of Health.

2000

December: White Paper *Reforming the Mental Health Act* published jointly by the two departments. It has two parts: "the new legal framework" and "high risk patients" and is seen as differing from the Green Paper in giving more of an emphasis to risk, possibly as a result of joining the two Green Papers.

2002

June: A draft Mental Health Bill is published with a three month consultation period.

September: The consultation period ends with nearly 2000 responses received by the Department of Health.

October: Home Secretary David Blunkett gives a speech at the Zito Trust conference aiming to allay concerns about the draft bill.

November: The Bill is not announced, as had been widely expected, in the Queen's Speech. This is interpreted by some as a sign that the government has shelved the legislation. Soon after, Alan Milburn, the Health Secretary, announces that the Bill will be introduced in the 2002–2003 parliamentary session.

2004

May: Revised Bill presented to key stakeholders. It is announced that the new Bill will go through a process of pre-legislative scrutiny in the current parliamentary session.

Recent proposals to reform UK mental health legislation have placed a greater emphasis on the need to "protect the public" from the implied risk posed by the "mentally ill individual" (Box 22.1 lists some of the important recent events in the shaping of MHA policy). An issue of public safety is thus transformed into one of health.[12] As someone influenced by critical psychology,[13] I am concerned by these proposals and have sought to influence them in a variety of contexts: through my professional organisation, the British Psychological Society,[14] and through activism, for example within the Critical Mental Health Forum, a London-based group of service users, critical mental health professionals, academics, and others.[15] Some readers might view the following analysis as partisan as a result but an alternative view, as set out by the other authors in this book (see, for example, Chapter 21) is that all researchers have some stake and interest in their research and interpret their findings through a particular lens.

The mobilisation of narratives of risk and dangerousness in the warranting of Mental Health Act reform

In my analysis I will draw on concepts used in forms of discourse analysis. These approaches are based on the notion that in any account there is variation, contradiction or inconsistency.[16,17] Discourse analysts see such variation as evidence of the construction of different kinds of repertoires which may serve different functions[17] or even different political interests.[18] In particular I will note how certain rhetorical devices are used to enhance the plausibility of factual claims. Box 22.2 contains a list of rhetorical devices which Derek Edwards and Jonathan Potter note are particularly common in factual accounts and tend to enhance the plausibility of claims about reality.[19]

Box 22.2 Rhetorical devices used in fact construction (summarised from Edwards and Potter[19])

1 **Category entitlement:** People in certain positions are expected to have certain kinds of (expert) knowledge.

2 **Vivid description:** The use of lots of concrete detail in an account.

3 **Narrative:** An account that leads "inevitably" in a causal sequence, adding to the plausibility of a report in a context of deniability.

4 **Systematic vagueness:** Vague global formulations with enough essentials to found an utterance but preventing the easy undermining that a lot of detail might allow.

5 **Empiricist accounting:** Objectifying scientific language where phenomena are treated as agents in their own right whereas people are seen as passive agents.

6 **Rhetoric of argument:** Constructing an account in the form of a logical argument so that the outcome is seen as the result of something external to the speaker (that is, the logical outcome of the argument).

7 **Extreme case formulation:** Versions made more effective by drawing on extreme examples (the use of a "straw man" argument is one example of this).

8 **Consensus and corroboration:** Making an account plausible by noting agreement between (ideally independent) witnesses.

9 **Lists and contrasts:** Very effective in oratory. Three-part lists can seem complete or representative – often using "distinctiveness information".

Discourse analysis, in common with many forms of narrative analysis, is a way of reading which involves asking certain questions of, and bringing certain theoretical resources to bear on, texts. Although my analysis is informed by the extensive literature on the MHA reforms, for convenience I have selected one text to analyse in detail. This consists of excerpts (edited for reasons of space and relevance) from the Foreword to the Government's White Paper *Reforming the Mental Health*

Act signed by Alan Milburn (Secretary of State for Health) and Jack Straw (the then Home Secretary). Obviously this is an "artificial" text, the result of a complex process involving negotiation between different ministers and civil servants from different departments but discourse analysts find such texts analytically interesting[19] and I am selecting it precisely because of its performative functions – it tells us what "the government" says is important about its reforms.

Box 22.3 Foreword to the Government White Paper *Reforming the Mental Health Act*

1   The current 1983 Mental Health Act is largely based on a review of
2   mental health legislation which took place in the 1950s. Since then the
3   way services are provided has dramatically changed. The current laws
4   have failed properly to protect the public, patients or staff.
5   Under existing mental health laws, the only powers compulsorily to treat
6   patients are if they are in hospital. The majority of patients today are
7   treated in the community. But public confidence in care in the community
8   has been undermined by failures in services and failures in the law. Too
9   often, severely ill patients have been allowed to drift out of contact with
10   mental health services. They have been able to refuse treatment.
11   Sometimes, as the tragic toll of homicides and suicides involving such
12   patients makes clear, lives have been put at risk. In particular existing
13   legislation has also failed to provide adequate public protection from
14   those whose risk to others arises from severe personality disorder. We
15   are determined to remedy this.
16   Of course, the vast majority of people with mental illness represents no
17   threat to anyone. Many mentally ill patients are among the most
18   vulnerable members of society. But the Government has a duty to protect
19   individual patients and the public if a person poses a serious risk to
20   themselves or to others.
21   These changes amount to the biggest shake up in mental health
22   legislation in four decades. They will strengthen the current laws. They
23   will introduce new safeguards for patients. They will improve protection
24   for the public. The safety of the public and of patients will be enhanced
25   as a result.

26   **Alan Milburn**
27   **Jack Straw**

Warranting reform

One question discursive psychologists have in mind as they read an account is "to what problem is this account a solution?" A key concern for those wishing to change policies is to establish a warrant for reform and it is no surprise that narratives of modernisation are drawn on in order to do this. Who can argue that something that is new and modern is not preferable to something old and outdated? The extract begins by implying that the current (1983) MHA is outdated by describing it as largely based on a review in the 1950s (lines 1–2). Of course, simply because laws are old does not necessarily mean that they are no longer appropriate but the need for reform is emphasised through the assertion that services have dramatically changed since that time (lines 2–3), an assertion bolstered by noting ways in which there is a mismatch between services and the law (lines 5–7).

This first argument for reform is largely implicit with the 1983 MHA constructed as being left behind by the changes in services. However, the argument becomes more explicit in lines 3–4 where it is explicitly stated that current laws have failed to protect "the public, patients or staff". The authority of this statement emanates from the identity of the two signatories (lines 26–27): the ministers heading the Department of Health and the Home Office. This is an illustration of a rhetorical device which Edwards and Potter term *category entitlement* where the truth of a report is warranted by the entitlements or category membership of the speaker – in other words, people in particular categories are expected to know certain things. Thus ministers should know whether or not laws are working properly.

The text goes on to construct a narrative of failure and another rhetorical device, a *narrative form of accounting*, can be seen at work here. This is where the plausibility of an account is increased by linking events together in a sequence that implies causality. The argument runs thus:

> Current laws only allow treatment in hospital > most patients are in the community > patients have been allowed to lose contact > and refuse treatment > lives have been put at risk > especially from those with severe personality disorder > the proposed changes in legislation will remedy this.

This paragraph also constructs a narrative of failure both of laws and mental health services in lines 7–8. Another question discourse analysts might ask is "what might have been said here but isn't?"[2] One could imagine that an alternative argument might be that these failures show that community care has failed. However, this account is structured in a different way by focusing on "public confidence in care in the community". As a result community care policies are seen as unproblematic; rather it is public confidence which is problematic. Similarly, attention is focused then on strategies to manage risk but the basic assumptions of discourse about madness go unchallenged.

"Public confidence" could be said to be manifested in media reporting of mental health issues and, in her study comparing TV news coverage in the summer and winter of 1986 with TV news and other programmes between May and July 1992, Diana Rose has argued that there was a change following the case of Christopher Clunis, diagnosed with schizophrenia, who murdered Jonathan Zito in 1992, leading to a public inquiry.[20] Before 1992/1993, Rose suggests that there were stories linking mental illness with violence or with neglect but few, if any, stories linking violence with neglect. Following this period, however, she notes that blaming the violence of people with mental health problems on neglect as a result of the failures of community care became the dominant category of explanation despite no corresponding rise in the rates of violence.

Interestingly, no evidence is presented in the White Paper to support the claim for lack of confidence and, again, the account works by drawing on the category entitlements of the signatories. Another alternative argument might have been to state that public confidence was misinformed (which might have been accompanied by a call to influence media reporting of such events) or even prejudiced and discriminatory (which might have been accompanied by a call for anti-discriminatory legislation or consciousness-raising policies). The account also works by constructing two groups: the "public" and "patients". "Patients" are, of course, also members of the public – as clinical psychologist and survivor Rufus May has remarked, "We are the public too!" The account therefore functions not only to construct the need for legislative change as necessary but also to obscure alternative constructions of the "problem" and thus alternative solutions.

The discursive management of blame and responsibility

Another interesting aspect of this paragraph of the text is how blame and responsibility are managed. The language used is very passive and responsibility is located in external and abstract structures ("services" and "laws") rather than individuals with agency. For example, in lines 9–10 patients are said to have "been allowed to drift out of contact" with services. Here neither the patients nor the practitioners who work in services are constructed as active agents, instead the word "drift" functions as a non-human agentive causal factor. However, in line 10 patients are constructed as having agency when it is noted that they "have been able to refuse treatment". Here, though, the expression of agency is viewed as problematic and, in part, this effect is achieved through the use of the term "treatment". Such a word implies a whole range of subject positions:[2] doctor, patient, treatment, and cure for example. The notion of treatment implies a willing patient who takes the treatment prescribed by a doctor in order for cure to take place. The refusal of treatment can be seen as a disjuncture from this implicit array of narrative positions.

The word "able" in line 10 functions ambiguously here. It could imply that being able to refuse treatment should be seen in a negative light – there could be an implicit assumption here that treatment is self-evidently beneficial. It could also imply that refusal of treatment is likely unless otherwise prevented. The ability of patients to choose (whether to stay in services and to accept treatment) is constructed here both as problematic and as in need of a solution.

No context is given here so there is no mention of some of the reasons people might refuse treatment (because of, say, serious and unpleasant side effects[21]). But the text does not locate responsibility in the patient; it does not say "patients have refused treatment". Instead, responsibility is placed in an external agent which has allowed the refusal of treatment. No people are held responsible here – if they were this might conflict with popular representations of caring professionals.

From failure to danger and risk

The narrative of failure is also a narrative of danger and risk. Patients are placed in a number of positions here: as "severely ill" (line 9) which, in a mental health context, implies that they are not responsible for their own or others' well-being; as able/likely to drift out of contact with services (lines 9–10); as able/likely to refuse treatment; as putting their own and others' lives at risk (lines 10–12); and as necessitating the protection of the public. This account draws some power from *extreme case formulation*[19] by referring to somewhat extreme cases – in this context the "tragic toll" (line 11) of homicides and suicides.

The media are regularly blamed for exaggerating cases of homicide by people with mental health problems but one factor is the increased number of official inquiries following the Department of Health's decision in 1994 to hold an independent inquiry into every homicide associated with mental health services.[8] The increase can be seen in Box 22.4. Two homicides in particular have aroused particular concern. The first was the killing of Jonathan Zito by Christopher Clunis, discussed earlier. The second concerned the killing of Lin and Megan Russell, a mother and her young daughter, by Michael Stone, who was considered by psychiatrists to have had an untreatable antisocial personality disorder. Jack Straw, the then Home Secretary, publicly clashed with Robert Kendell, the then president of the Royal College of Psychiatrists. Straw said that it was "time, frankly, that the psychiatric profession seriously examined their own practices and tried to modernise them in a way they have so far failed to do".[22] One media commentator has asserted that, as a result, fear has become one of the major drivers of mental health policy.[8]

Box 22.4 Number of independent inquiries into homicides associated with mental health services[8]

1978–1988	1
1988–1996	26
1994–2002	120

In the Foreword to the White Paper patients are constructed as non-agentive, or "automatons".[23] Indeed, even the risk some pose is said to "arise from severe personality disorder" – agency is again located in a non-human causal factor. Similarly, other influential actors (victims, family members, bystanders, the police, friends etc.) not only are not given agency here,[23] they are entirely absent from the account. Since the only actors in the account are patients, diagnostic categories, services, and the law, they are the only place where responsibility can be located and we have already seen how the text works to locate responsibility in services and the law.

Repairing and disclaiming

The account so far in the Foreword portrays a largely negative view of people with mental health problems. Surveys of attitudes towards psychiatric service users commonly report that they are seen as unpredictable and potentially dangerous to others,[24] a view shared, to some extent, even by medical students and doctors.[25] The narrative link between violence and mental illness is widely culturally available, especially in the news and entertainment media which focus primarily on violence against others when addressing issues relating to "mental illness" with these items receiving headline treatment.[26] Negative media accounts can even override positive or neutral personal experience of those with mental health problems.[27] Such portrayals have consequences for users of mental health services, with half the respondents of one survey reporting that their mental health had been negatively affected and a third saying others had reacted negatively towards them as a result of such reports.[28] In contrast, professional accounts of the linking of violence and mental health appear to have become increasingly assertive.

Thus Walsh and Fahy comment that "the scientific literature ... refutes the stereotyping of all patients with severe mental illness as dangerous"[6].

Were the Foreword to end here then the reader might have a fairly negative view of mental health service users and so the next paragraph contains two repairs. Thus it is noted that the "vast majority" of patients represent no threat to anyone (line 16) and that these patients are "among the most vulnerable" in society (lines 17–18). These sentences act as potential disclaimers for the previous largely negative portrayal of service users. If the previous paragraph in the Foreword were to be challenged, government spokespeople could always point to these lines in their defence and so they act as a qualifier and a rhetorical inoculation to such challenges. Of course, there remains an imbalance in terms of the quantity of negative comments and the fact that they come before the more positive descriptions, perhaps implying some priority to the more negative appraisal.

As well as developing a narrative of danger and failure, the text also draws on a moral and legal discourse of duties, rights, and responsibilities. One challenge to the narrative so far might be to say that the risk, such as it is, is a problematic cost of living in a democratic society much as we have to live with other homicides (858 deaths in the UK initially recorded as homicides in 2001–2002[29]) or deaths associated with road traffic collisions (3450 in 2001[30]). Instead, the text notes that the government has "a duty to protect" (line 18). This provides a final warrant for reform and it completes the narrative effect of the historical inevitability and necessity of reform.

The final paragraph of this extract (and also of the original Foreword) consists of five very short sentences. Here we see the use of another rhetorical device: a *list*. Edwards and Potter note that lists (especially three-part lists – a list with three elements) and contrasts are commonly found in political oratory and are regarded as rhetorically effective (like Tony Blair's "education, education, education" 1997 election speech).[19] They also note that such lists can be used to construct descriptions that are complete and representative and they are enhanced if contrasted with a threatening alternative, often formulated in an unconvincing manner. This list seems to have these effects and there is inbuilt protection against challenges since both safeguards for patients and protection of the public are promised. The alternative is implied rather than made explicit: that not to support change would mean that patients were not provided with safeguards and that the public would have less protection.

The final sentence notes that the "safety of the public and of patients will be enhanced as a result" (lines 24–25). What is interesting here is that these two issues are seen as following unproblematically from legal reform. A challenge to this might be that they are contradictory imperatives: that one cannot protect both public and patients' civil liberties simultaneously. However, the word "safety" functions in an ambiguous manner here: the public are to be safe from (protected from) patients whereas the patients are to be "safe" from themselves. This draws on implicit notions that service users are not able to be responsible for themselves or their actions. In a similar way we can note how the word "risk" is used in mental health settings to cover both risk of violence to others but also risk of harming oneself, two sets of behaviours which are very different (one involves only harming oneself whereas the other involves harm to another person), this difference obscured through the use of the word "risk". Some readers may assume that there is a lot of overlap between people engaging in each kind of conduct but, in the general population, there are 25 times more people who kill themselves than kill others. Of the small proportion (9%) of homicide perpetrators who had been in contact with mental health services in the year before the offence, 57% had a "history of self harm", broadly defined.[3]

I have attempted to describe some of the ways in which this text serves to warrant reform by drawing on a range of rhetorical devices and on narratives of failure and danger and I have sought to highlight links to relevant debates in the literature. However, some discourse researchers also seek to analyse how the discursive positions taken up in documents like these are afforded by wider discourses. In the next section I want to develop a further level of analysis, one that attends to the wider effects of such discursive positions, in particular highlighting the effects on mental health service users and professionals.

The effects of discursive positioning in policies on risk and mental health

Effects on service users and survivors

Policymakers' dual concerns to reform mental health legislation and develop a framework to address anxiety about homicides by those with a diagnosis could be said to have shaped not only the MHA proposals but also a raft of new investment in services for those considered to be dangerous and to have a "severe personality disorder" ("D&SPD" in official jargon). The late 1990s saw a rapid growth in research on SPD in the UK as a result of explicit government guidance and funding, leading some researchers to conclude that SPD is a good example of the social construction of a new category of disorder as a result of complex interaction between policymakers, academics, and other professionals despite it not existing as a formalised category in psychiatric classifications like the DSM or ICD.[31]

Nikolas Rose has argued that these policy concerns can be traced back over a long period of time, dating most recently from the nineteenth century assertion that the explanation for apparently unmotivated homicides lay in the pathological mind of dangerous individuals.[10,32,33] However, Castel traces a further shift from a focus on a concrete individual to a combination of factors of risk which lent itself easily to statistical and actuarial procedures to estimate risk.[34]

Gerard Drennan (personal communication) notes that positioning service users as violent obscures their vulnerability to the violence (both metaphorical and real) done to them by others. He also points out that the discourses from which identity is constructed afford certain scripts for behaviour and thus their actions can become decontextualised in the eyes of others so that, for example, acts of aggression are seen as sadistic and unprovoked rather than as, say, understandable (though not, of course, excusable) in the context of their life histories.

In his discussion of the construction of identity, Sampson has described how a "serviceable other" is constructed in accounts which is then contrasted with a (usually implicit) norm or "absent standard".[35] I would argue that texts like this Foreword function to explain bizarre and frightening conduct. Indeed Morrall has argued that there is such intense and disproportionate media coverage of apparently motiveless stranger homicides by those considered to be mentally ill precisely because they are so apparently unpredictable and inexplicable.[36]

In her investigation of TV coverage relating to mental health (from news to soap operas and comedies), Diana Rose has argued that these programmes have diverse and multiple meanings.[20] When individuals seen as having mental health problems are filmed in both factual and fictional programmes, close-up and extreme close-up shots are used and individuals are frequently filmed alone, in contrast to the way others are filmed. She argues that this leads to such individuals being seen as different, as other. Accounts like those seen here may thus provide an explanation for such events by appealing to inferred constructs, seen as agentive (like "mental illness", "personality disorder" and so on). Of course describing actions as "mad" or "crazy" also has the effect of implying that these actions require no explanation since they cannot be understood with reference to, for example, "normal" psychological processes. As Jeremy Laurance notes "we reject people who transgress social norms and above all we feel threatened by unpredictability"[8]. Moreover, such accounts also provide a moral warrant for action taken in response to such events or to prevent them.

However, Sampson's analysis suggests that these accounts serve not only to construct the mentally ill as "other", they also implicitly construct a particular kind of identity for "us" as rational, predictable, and reasonable. Evidence for this assertion can be seen in the summing up of the judge, Mr Justice Sedley, after the conviction of Horrett Campbell, who attacked a group of schoolchildren with a machete. He said:

> In some ways it is a relief to know it was a profoundly sick and deluded individual who committed these offences. To believe such an attack could be carried out by a sane person would shake belief in humanity.[37]

Thus the very existence of a "mad other" helps to reinforce how normal "we" are. Without this category of explanation we might have to find other, possibly more threatening, explanations for such conduct. However, the subtle shift from a discourse of care to one of risk – or, as we have seen here, to one of safety – also has a range of consequences for professional conduct.

Effects on professionals

Nikolas Rose argues that as well as focusing on abstract risk factors the concept of "risk" reshapes the obligations of professionals so that "risk management and risk reduction, as logics for professional action, [have] come to supplement or replace other forms of professional action and judgement"[32]. Government of risk takes place, then, not only through a transformation of the psychiatric subject but also of the professional.

This shift becomes more evident when we consider how the notion of care has been thought about differently in different historical and cultural contexts. Nick Fox, for example, has written about "care as gift" and "care as vigil", which seems to capture this move from care to surveillance.[38] Moreover, the surveillance is not only of the patient by the professional but also of the professional themselves, existing in a panoptical space inhabited by NHS managers, government ministers, inquiry teams, the media, and so on. An effect of this is increasingly defensive and bureaucratic practice. At times the word "risk" is ambiguous since whereas the focus appears to be on risk to or from the patient, the professional is also aware of the medico-legal risk to their employer in a context of rising litigation.

Implications for the relationship between research and policy

This chapter has mainly focused on the value of discursive research in examining policy but, in concluding, I want to look at how research might be used more actively to influence policy itself.

Policymakers are interested in different kinds of evidence in order to answer different research and policy questions.[39] To this one could add that different audiences are likely to be persuaded by different kinds of evidence. This can be framed as a problem but it is also an opportunity, since researchers can seek to influence policy through those other means too. Prilleltensky and Nelson have argued that critical psychologists should seek to reframe social problems and work in partnership with social movements.[40] Weiss' work suggests that we can reconceptualise policy questions by interrogating the assumptions which shape those questions, delineating normative discourses and reporting alternative or marginalised discourses.[41] There are now a variety of ways of working with the major social movement in mental health: the service user movement.[42-46] This study falls more into the category of questioning policy assumptions, though my contact with service users in a variety of contexts suggests that this is also a key concern of theirs.

What implications might this study have for the construction of risk in mental health policy? There are several implications which are consistent with my analysis though they could not be said to flow from it in any direct sense. First, I think that policymakers need to be aware of the exaggerated influence that extreme cases can have on policy development. Rather than simply be driven along by an exaggerated fear of homicide, there is an urgent need to combat discrimination against people with mental health problems. Policymakers need to rethink "anti-stigma" campaigns aimed at encouraging the public to view psychological distress as an "illness like any other" since they appear to have had a very limited effect as even their proponents acknowledge.[24] Indeed, there is some research evidence to suggest that a disease view of distress – as opposed to a psychosocial one – may lead to increased stigma.[47] Some have argued instead for campaigns focused on fighting discrimination rather than stigma[48,49,50] with slogans like "It's normal to be different" or "Crazy? So what?".[49] We do not talk of ending the "stigma" of being black or being a woman; quite rightly we talk of racist and sexist discrimination. Similarly we might have more success in campaigning against discrimination rather than stigma, for example, in the workplace and this is now a possibility with the Disability Discrimination Act.

A second implication is that mental health professionals need to be more open about the contested nature of concepts in mental health and of the constraints within which they work (for example, the trial and error nature of most psychiatric treatments). A recent training manual for mental health professionals includes discussion of key debates, for example about the validity of the concept of schizophrenia.[51] The public need to know that, quite often, "experts" disagree. Since professionals, like anyone else, are not always aware of their blind spots there is also a need for better systems of accountability through the provision of adequately funded and independent survivor-run organisations and advocacy services.

Thirdly, risk assessment in mental health, like risk assessment in other contexts, should, as far as possible, be undertaken within a collaborative partnership relationship rather than an adversarial one. Margaret Clayton, the chairman of the Mental Health Act Commission, has talked of the need for forms of "relational security"[8] and there have been many sensible suggestions about how to make the mental health risk assessment and management process more of a shared enterprise between professional and service user.[52,53]

Acknowledgements

This chapter is dedicated to the memory of Pete Shaughnessy (1962–2002), survivor, activist, and one of the founder members of Mad Pride. Pete made a committed and creative contribution to these debates[54,55,56] – to read more on that contribution visit www. peteshaughnessy.org.uk.

I would like to thank Mary Boyle, Louisa Cadman, Gerard Drennan, Ian Parker, Sim Roy-Chowdhury, Helen Spandler, Sam Warner, Carla Willig, and the editors for their valuable comments on an earlier version of this chapter.

References

1 Department of Health/Home Office. *Reforming the Mental Health Act*. White Paper. London: The Stationery Office, 2000.
2 Parker I. *Discourse dynamics: critical analysis for social and individual psychology*. London: Routledge, 1992, p 32.
3 Department of Health. *Safety first: five-year report of the national confidential inquiry into suicide and homicide by people with mental illness*. London: Department of Health, 2001.
4 Taylor PJ, Gunn J. Homicides by people with a mental illness: myth and reality. *Br J Psychiatry* 1999;**174**:9–14.
5 Hiday VA. The social context of mental illness and violence. *J Health Soc Behav* 1995;**36**:122–37.
6 Walsh E, Fahy T. Violence in society: contribution of mental illness is low. *BMJ* 2002;**325**:507–8.
7 Hiroeh U, Appleby L, Mortensen PB, Dunn G. Death by homicide, suicide, and other unnatural causes in people with mental illness: a population-based study. *Lancet* 2001;**358**:2110–12.
8 Laurance J. *Pure madness: how fear drives the mental health system*. London: Routledge, 2003.
9 Coppock V, Hopton J. *Critical perspectives on mental health*. London: Routledge, 2000.
10 Rose N. Living dangerously: risk thinking and risk management in mental health care. *Mental Health Care* 1998;**1**:263–6.
11 Department of Health. In-patients formally detained in hospitals under the mental health act 1983 and other legislation, NHS trusts, primary care trusts, high security psychiatric hospitals and private facilities. *Press release* 2003; 28 March, 0132.
12 Szmukler G. A new mental health (and public protection) act: risk wins in the balance between providing care and controlling risk. *BMJ* 2001;**322**:2–3.
13 Prilleltensky I, Nelson G. *Doing psychology critically: making a difference in diverse settings*. Basingstoke: Palgrave Macmillan, 2002.

14 Cooke A, Harper D, Kinderman P. An invitation to debate: do clinical psychologists care about the Mental Health Act reforms? *Clin Psychol* 2002;**15**:40–6.

15 Harper D. A summer of protests against the mental health bill. *Asylum: the magazine for democratic psychiatry* 2002;**13**:4–8.

16 Parker I. Discursive psychology. In: Fox DR, Prilleltensky I, eds. *Critical Psychology: An Introduction*. London: Sage, 1997.

17 Potter J, Wetherell M. *Discourse and social psychology: beyond attitudes and behaviour*. London: Sage, 1987.

18 Harper DJ. Poverty and discourse. In: Carr SC, Sloan TS, eds. *Psychology and poverty: emergent critical practice*. Dordrecht: Kluwer, 2003.

19 Edwards D, Potter J. *Discursive Psychology*. London: Sage, 1992.

20 Rose D. Television, madness and community care. *J Community Appl Social Psychol* 1998;**8**:213–28.

21 May R, Hartley J, Knight T. Making the personal political. *The Psychologist: Bull Br Psychol Soc* 2003;**16**:182–3.

22 Warden J. Psychiatrists hit back at home secretary. *BMJ* 1998;**317**:1270.

23 Szmukler G. Homicide inquiries: what sense do they make? *Psychiatr Bull* 2000; **24**:6–10.

24 Crisp AH, Gelder MG, Rix S, Meltzer HI, Rowlands OJ. Stigmatisation of people with mental illnesses. *Br J Psychiatry* 2000;**177**:4–7.

25 Mukherjee R, Fialho A, Wijetunge A, Checinski K, Surgenor T. The stigmatisation of psychiatric illness: the attitudes of medical students and doctors in a London teaching hospital. *Psychiatr Bull* 2002;**26**:178–81.

26 Philo G. Media images and popular beliefs. *Psychiatr Bull* 1994;**18**:173–4.

27 Philo G. The media and public belief. In: Philo G, ed. *Media and mental distress*. London: Longman, 1996.

28 MIND. *Counting the Cost*. London: MIND, 2000.

29 Flood-Page C, Taylor J. *Crime in England and Wales, 2001–2002: supplementary volume*. London: National Statistics, 2003.

30 National Statistics Online. *Passenger death rates by mode of transport, 1981–2001: social trends 33*. www.statistics.gov.uk/Statbase/ssdataset.asp?vlnk=6536&More=Y. Downloaded 10 April 2003.

31 Manning N. Actor networks, policy networks and personality disorder. *Sociol Health Illness* 2002;**24**:644–66.

32 Rose N. Psychiatry as a political science: advanced liberalism and the administration of risk. *History Human Sci* 1996;**9**:1–23.

33 Foucault M. About the concept of the "dangerous individual" in 19th century legal psychiatry. *Int J Law Psychiatry* 1978;**1**:1–18.

34 Castel R. From dangerousness to risk. In: Burchell G, Gordon C, Miller P, eds. *The Foucault Effect: Studies in Governmentality*. London: Harvester Wheatsheaf, 1991.

35 Sampson EE. Identity politics: challenges to psychology's understanding. *Am Psychol* 1993;**48**:1219–30.

36 Morrall P. *Madness and murder*. London: Whurr, 2000.

37 Chaudhary V. School's machete attacker sent to mental hospital. *Guardian* 8 March 1997, p 10.

38 Fox NJ. *Beyond health: postmodernism and embodiment*. London: Free Association Press, 1999.

39 Kane E. The policy perspective: what evidence is influential. In: Priebe S, Slade M, eds. *Evidence in mental health care*. Hove, East Sussex: Brunner–Routledge, 2002.

40 Prilleltensky I, Nelson G. Psychologists and the object of social change: transforming social policy. In: *Doing psychology critically: making a difference in diverse settings*. Basingstoke: Palgrave Macmillan, 2002.

41 Weiss CH. Introduction. In: Weiss CH, ed. *Using social research in public policy making*. Lexington, MA: Lexington, 1977.

42 Faulkner A, Layzell S. *Strategies for Living: The Research Report*. London: Mental Health Foundation, 2000.

43 Wallcraft J, Michaelson J. Developing a survivor discourse to replace the "psychopathology" of breakdown and crisis. In: Newnes C, Holmes G, Dunn C, eds. *This is madness too: critical perspectives on mental health services*. Ross-on-Wye: PCCS Books, 2001.

44 Faulkner A, Thomas P. User-led research and evidence-based medicine. *Br J Psychiatry* 2002;**180**:1–3.
45 Thornicroft G, Rose D, Huxley P, Dale G, Wykes T. What are the research priorities of mental health service users? *J Ment Health* 2002;**11**:1–3.
46 Trivedi P, Wykes T. From passive subjects to equal partners: User involvement in research. *Br J Psychiatry* 2002;**181**:468–72.
47 Mehta S, Farina A. Is being "sick" really better? Effect of the disease view of mental disorder on stigma. *J Soc Clin Psychol* 1997;**16**:405–19.
48 Bracken P, Thomas P. Stigma or discrimination? *Openmind* 2000;**105**:20.
49 Perkins R. Stigma or discrimination? *Openmind* 2001;**112**:6.
50 Sayce L. Stigma, discrimination and social exclusion: what's in a word? *J Ment Health* 1998;**7**:331–43.
51 Bassett T, Cooke A, Read J. *Psychosis revisited: a workshop for mental health workers.* Brighton: Pavilion, 2003.
52 Hird M, Cash K. Power play. *Openmind* 2000;**101**:12–13.
53 Langan J, Lindow V. Risk and listening. *Openmind* 2000;**101**:14–15.
54 Shaughnessy P. July 9th: day of action. Mad Pride view. *Asylum: the magazine for democratic psychiatry* 2001;**13**:7–8.
55 Hart S, Olden M. Radical Mad Pride pioneer mourned. *The Big Issue*, January 2003, p 5.
56 Olden M. Obituaries: Pete Shaughnessy. Campaigner who took the stigma out of insanity. *Guardian* 23 January 2003, p 22.

23: The temporal construction of medical narratives

BRIAN HURWITZ

> Narrative is a doubly temporal sequence. There is the time of the thing told
> and the time of the narrative. One of the functions of narrative is to invent one
> time scheme in terms of another time scheme.
>
> (C Metz, 1968)[1]

The aspect of existence we call time passes automatically. Neither seen
nor felt directly, not heard, tasted or smelt, time permeates
experience, and preoccupies both storytelling and medical practice.[2,3]

Clinical representation of time in case reports and illness narratives
is central to the task of disease and illness depiction. Clinicians
generally show meticulous concern for chronology and for the
temporal relations of succession and association. Clinical encounters
focus typically on temporal sequences, on relations of before and
after, on discussions of beginnings and endings. Some medical
conditions are associated with slow, unfolding awareness of difficult-
to-pinpoint feelings, others with instantaneous, "thunderclap"
experiences, extremes that encompass a spectrum of sensations which
"come" and "go" and move about with unaccountable tempo,
causing feelings that fluctuate in quality, intensity, and rhythmicity.

This chapter examines how the sense of time passing is evoked and
managed in writing case reports and illness narratives. It explores the
limited novelistic techniques employed in the composition of case
reports, which generally recount unfolding facts according to a linear
chronology, and contrasts these with how illness narratives about the
lived experience of ill health are organised around biographically
segmented chronologies, which are more sensitive to the inner
experience of time.

Biological and narrative time

Subjective experience of the passage of time is frequently out of
kilter with objective "clock time". When people are busy and their
lives eventful, time passes quickly, but it passes more slowly when
self-consciousness is heightened but duration apparently empty – as
in the watched kettle experience.[4] Certain mental and emotional

states seem to slow time's passing, such as boredom, unhappiness, pain, and ill health.[5]

Box 23.1 Waiting

Waiting and time

Recently, or was it years ago, my wife found a breast lump which turned out to be malignant. She's 36. Since then, time has become distorted, the objective measures of calendars and clocks becoming meaningless as appointments, results, operations, and treatments have approached and passed. Minutes, hours, and days have become prolonged and compressed ... Six months have sped by ... what about the waiting? What to say to each other at the start and end of each day when there is only one date, and time, and result on your minds? ... as the end of active treatment looms, there is the hardest wait of all. Life is no longer measured in terms of "expectancy" but rather as "survival."[6]

A snippet from a clinical tale

While John is waiting for hospital admission, the 3 of us [patient, his wife, and the author–doctor] meet several times to discuss the situation. Strangely, in these meetings, time seems to have distended, slowed down, become dense with meaning. Words, thoughts, and emotions all condense into the eternal present: Minutes seem like hours, hours like days or even years.[7]

The mysterious immateriality of time is evoked by Paul Ricoeur, when he writes that "time has no being since the future is not yet, the past no longer, and the present does not remain. And yet we do speak of time as having being. We say that things to come will be, that things past were, and that things present are passing away".[8]

Tense alludes to several aspects of time: its "flow", "direction" and the relative position of events and actions within the "flow". Biologically, time seems to flow in the direction of causality, along an axis extending through "before" and "after", providing a temporal matrix not only for the bodily processes of birth, growth, ageing, and illness, but for the development and unfolding of stories of fact and fiction also:

> The foot of Aristion's female slave spontaneously ulcerated in the middle of the foot on the inner side. The bones became corrupted, separated and came off little by little, eroded. Diarrhoea developed; she died.[9]

This snippet of a tale from the fourth century BC treatise *Epidemics* in some ways is typical of Hippocratic narration. Despite its terseness, it displays close attention to observational detail, a clear and linear temporal sequence, and a discrete beginning and end. The narrator is separate from but a close witness to – peers at – the foot (its constituent bones) of a sick woman. As with other Hippocratic case reports (see Box 23.2) the sequence of bodily events referred to in the case of Aristion's slave takes place some time in the narrative past, although time relations in this account are unspecified: how long the observed processes took to unfold remains unclear.

This case report brings a sick slave to the notice of an anonymous, emotionless gaze. We learn nothing of the woman's life, age or relationships, whether she suffered pain or discomfort from the affliction, or how she may have tried to respond to her situation; her death is reported in the same descriptive tone as the onset of a new symptom. If the observer–narrator was a physician – the description matches a physician's focus and attention to detail – then nothing in the account betrays a doctor's sense of clinical responsibility for her welfare as apparently no treatments were tried. This woman's death is the death of an object not a subject.

Here is another Hippocratic case history:

> The man hit on the head by the Macedonian … fell down. On the third day he was voiceless. He heard nothing, was not conscious, nor was he still. But on the fourth day, he showed movement; he had moisture around the forehead, under the nose, and down the chin; and he died.[9]

Compare this tale with the opening to a novel, written in 1927, by American author Thornton Wilder:

> On Friday noon, July the twentieth, 1714, the finest bridge in all Peru broke, and precipitated five travellers into the gulf below. This bridge was on the high road from Lima and hundreds of persons passed over it every day. It had been woven of osier by the Incas more than a century before. The bridge seemed to be among the things that would last for ever; it was unthinkable that it should break. The moment a Peruvian heard of the accident he signed himself and made a mental calculation as to how recently he had crossed by it and how soon he had intended crossing by it again. People wandered about in a trance-like state, muttering: they had the hallucination of seeing themselves falling into a gulf.[10]

The opening of *The Bridge of San Luis Rey* refers to a unique happening located in time and place.[i] Initially, the impression given is of reading a report about the failure of a piece of engineering. How the bridge collapsed – what, for example, happened to the moorings at each end of its span when it broke up and how long the process took – is not described by the author. But the effects of its having fallen reverberate in the imagination of the Peruvian people; just thinking about what happened to the bridge causes them to experience the sensation of being thrown off it.

Time frames

A measurable duration spanning events and actions, Aristotle considered time the "calculable measure of motion with respect to before and afterness".[11] In the unending flow of occurrences marked out by "before" and "after," time provides the framework in which positions, sequences, values, and functions can be compared, computed, and juxtaposed. An important task for clinicians, therefore, is to try to match the temporal order of biological processes to that which troubles patients.

Delineating the order of occurrences along the axis of time's arrow allows key clinical relations to be charted: "For *how long* have you had these symptoms? Were they troublesome *before* (or *after*) your wife died? Do they vary in any way over time? What else did you notice when these symptoms started?" are questions aimed not only at clarifying what is complained of, but at discerning a flux of events and experiences that may be associated with it, perhaps causally.

Thornton Wilder's novel continues:

> It was very hot noon, that fatal noon, and coming round the shoulder of a hill Brother Juniper stopped to wipe his forehead and to gaze upon the scene of snowy peaks in the distance, then to the gorge below him filled with the dark plumage of green trees and green birds. He had opened several little abandoned churches, and the Indians were crawling in to early Mass. Perhaps it was the pure air from the snows before him; perhaps it was the memory that brushed him for a moment of the poem that bade him raise his eyes to the helpful hills. At all events he was at peace. Then his glance fell upon the bridge, and at that moment a twanging noise filled the air, as when a string of some musical instrument snaps in a disused room, and he saw the bridge divide and fling five ants into the valley below.

Although the bridge has already fallen, here in a flashback, we momentarily see the intact bridge in all its splendour, amidst the magnificence of its natural setting. Then (once again) we see it collapse. The collapse is "re-enacted" through the perceiving eyes of a monk who at that moment happened to come into view of it, and who saw (and heard) the bridge break up. To have heard the noise, Brother Juniper must have been quite close to the catastrophe – the bridge made a "twang", indicating the break-up occurred in an instant, as when a thread snaps:

> Anyone else would have said to himself with secret joy: "Within ten minutes myself!" But it was another thought that visited Brother Juniper: "Why did this happen to *those* five?" If there were any plan in the universe at all, if there were any pattern to human life, surely it could be discovered mysteriously latent in those lives so suddenly cut off. Either we live by accident and die by accident, or we live by plan and die by plan. And on that instant Brother Juniper made the resolve to inquire into the secret lives of those five persons that moment falling through the air, and to surprise the reason of their taking off.

The monk had, indeed, been close to the fatal occurrence. Had he been but ten minutes ahead of his journey time (as recounted in the story) Brother Juniper himself would have been a member of that small hoard of ants flung off it into the gorge. This happenstance – viewing and almost participating in the collapse – compels Brother Juniper to consider the cause of the catastrophe and whether, one day, this might be determined.

In the rich interplay of description and association which the story so far has conjured up, a sense of fate looms large: an event (collapse of a bridge) has been linked to the mental life of many Peruvians – imaginatively they identify with those who lost their lives in the collapse. Quite contingently, the catastrophe was seen by a monk (he just happened to be there when it collapsed), who ponders the collapse and resolves to investigate who was on the bridge (and why) when it collapsed, which the novel goes on to recount.

Although the sequence of events related took place in the past – the reader is transported to *being with* the monk when the bridge collapses, so that the reader "sees" (and "hears") what the monk sees (saw then): "five persons that moment falling through the air".

Time sequence, period, duration, and change of pace are facets of narrative organisation. Medical case reports generally restrict the temporal range and reference of their narration to a short segment of a person's life, presupposing the order of happening to be mirrored by the order of appearance in the text. Flashbacks, re-descriptions or re-enactments of events and revisiting processes "as if they were actually happening" rarely form part of medical case reports.[ii] Although, patients are frequently unable to recount the events and experiences which concern them in a clear chronological sequence, case reports frequently recast the sequence of what's been said between patient and doctor, to represent occurrences within the uniform realm of biological time.

Gillian Beer, a literary theorist, notes that: "The story is enacted in narrative time, the story teller in natural time – the time of the body."[12] Narrative time is constructed by the way the teller tells the story, a novelist being generally much freer than is the author of a case report to jump about in time and space (as Box 23.2 makes clear).[13] But although clinical narratives are clearly constrained in ways that fiction is not, case reports could also jump about in temporal sequence, but they rarely do so. They are constrained in their creation of perspectives that could support new understandings and points of view, particularly the point of view of the suffering subject. The proverbial perspective of "medical hindsight" – which stems in part from the completeness conferred on a narrative once closure has been achieved – is rarely to be found in case reports. Other narrative techniques, such as bringing forward in sequence (as foreflashes do in films) later developments in the case story, could be harnessed by the authors of case reports to considerable dramatic (and pedagogical) value. However, in case reports these novelistic devices are not generally employed. "In realistic narratives, the time of the story is fixed following the ordinary course of a life," writes Seymour Chatman, also a literary theorist. "A person is born, grows from childhood to maturity and old age, and then dies. But the discourse-time order may be completely different: it may start with the person's deathbed and 'flashback' to childhood."[14] Such orders are rare in case reports. The discourse sequence of the case report follows the sequence of symptoms, feelings, events, and action in the order (but not at the pace) at which they eventuate in natural time.

Box 23.2 Preface from *To the Hermitage*

This is (I suppose) a story. I have altered the places where facts, data and info, seem dull or inaccurate. I have quietly corrected errors in the calendar, adjusted flaws in world geography, now and then budged the border of a country, or changed the constitution of a nation. A wee postmodern Haussman, I have elegantly replanned some of the world's greatest cities, moving buildings to better sites, redesigning architecture, opening fresh views and fine urban prospects, redirecting the traffic. I've put statues in more splendid locations, usefully reorganised art galleries, cleaned, transferred or rehung famous paintings, staged entire new plays and operas. I have revised or edited some of our great books, and republished them. I have altered monuments, defaced icons, changed the street signs, occupied the railway station. I have also taken the chance to introduce people who never met in life, but certainly should have. I have changed their lives and careers ...[15]

Medical diagnostic processes mirror natural time, "the time of the body". Yet diagnoses usually unfold in twists and turns created by actual and potential clinical leads as a result of questions posed, answers given, and following promising (and dead end) avenues of investigation. Case reports frequently edit out such meandering details to reflect only what the author considers germane to the clinical condition reported. In common with many stories – spoken, written or enacted – the case manipulates time by compressing, omitting or collapsing temporal span, with consequent effects on the story's contents. One purpose of such temporal distortion is to create (in the words of the physician and editor Frank Davidoff) a "bird's eye, after-the-fact version of the diagnostic process".[16]

Clinical case reports are intended to be factual, literal, and objective in the sense of recording accurately what happens during an illness (their subject being the course of the disease as opposed to the life of an individual – see Box 23.3). Particular procedural and documentary techniques are applied in the construction of case reports which ensure a degree of standardisation.[17] Cases are written up from the point of view of the treating physician, in the third person and in the voice of an anonymous, effaced narrator,[18] who sets out a chronology of events, actions, appearances and findings (see Chapter 2 and its account of the SARS epidemic). In this, the modern medical case report is bound by certain narrative conventions: it usually commences with a brief account of the subjective experiences of a patient as picked out by the doctor, refers to what the patient "complained of", sometimes verbatim (if deemed noteworthy). The report proceeds towards "the findings" – first of clinical then of laboratory and imaging examinations, before moving on to diagnosis of a cause and the instituting of treatment. Finally, the case report moves towards closure (a cure, complication or perhaps the death of the patient), relaying progress or deterioration along the way (see Box 23.3).

Box 23.3 A case history from hospital outpatients

A 50-year-old woman was referred to Outpatients Department because of pain in the face for six months. At first for several months the pain had been intermittent, lasting for up to half an hour at a time, but more recently it had been present to some extent continuously with occasional exacerbations. The severity of the pain had also slowly increased so that it now sometimes reduced her to tears. For the last month the pain had been particularly troublesome at night. She described the pain as dull and boring. It came and went slowly rather than abruptly, and occurred for no obvious reason. It did not seem to be provoked by going out into the cold, or by washing the face, and she had noticed nothing herself which either produced or relieved it. The pain was centred around the left eye, and spread when it was most severe downwards into the left cheek.

Over the past year she had felt generally less well. She had felt anxious and depressed on occasion for no obvious reason and her appetite had been poor. She thought that she had lost about a stone in weight but was pleased by this as she was still a little obese. She had also noticed a little epigastric discomfort after meals, but since avoiding fatty food this has seemed better. For the past few months she had also been troubled by dull aching pains in her limbs, unrelated to exercise, which were most noticeable when she went to sleep at night.

On examination she was pale and obviously anxious. The pulse was 110/min regular. The left eye seemed a little prominent and congested but there was no pulsation and no bruit [noise] could be heard. The sclerae [white of the eye] was visible above and below the cornea on the left, but not on the right. Neurological examination was normal except the corneal sensation on the left was blunted subjectively. General examination was normal except for the presence of a soft systolic murmur, heard best a little internal to the apex, and minimal epigastric tenderness.[19]

Case reports are a feature of many disciplines, including ethics, theology, law, medicine, psychotherapy, social work, and police detective work.[20] The narrative work of fashioning case reports involves assembling and relating evidence – often a compilation of text-based renderings of what the clinician has heard, seen, felt (palpated) or uncovered about a particular person. In this way, a narrative of fact – a transcription of events and other non-linguistic phenomena into a linguistic form[21] – is created. This narrative of fact is then related to a theory or body of knowledge (or law), so that a process of reasoning and inference can be supported concerning how to understand (and to act on) a person's situation.

Oliver Sacks, in discussing the strengths and weaknesses of viewing the case history as a narrative, argues that:

> case histories go no further than the historical presentation of disease. They are wholly descriptive, not narrative or dramatic. They do not present "patienthood" but only "eyehood". They do not show us the patient thrust into a role – nor the fateful character of sickness, which imposes on him roles. The idea of fate, hence of existential drama, is missing from case histories. It is only in a fully narrative form – a clinical tale – that the subject has "fate", the drama of his existence in all their fullness and force.[22]

The philosopher Nelson Goodman, in examining how robustly narratives survive re-orderings of their telling, notes that displacements in the order of events as told may frequently leave the basic plot intact. But consider, he suggests, "a psychologist's report which recounts a patient's behaviour chronologically. It is a story, a history. But rearranged to group the incidents according to their significance as symptoms – of, say, suicidal tendencies, then claustrophobia, then psychopathic disregard of consequences – it is no longer a story but an analysis, a case study". A re-telling that involves re-ordering according to principles extraneous to the story, which goes beyond simple re-ordering of incidents, may subdue or entirely nullify its narrative quality. Goodman believes: "The general lesson is that while narrative will normally survive all sorts of contortion, still sometimes when we start with a tale, enough twisting may leave us without one."[23] It may be that the rigid chronology of the clinical case report, its staged organisation and linear sequencing, have evolved precisely to place strict limits on elaborations that would threaten the essentially historical nature of its underlying plot.

The literary analyst Tod Chambers argues that despite the historical and descriptive appearances of case histories, there are no privileged or innocent compositions (or readings) of such histories in a field such as medical ethics. What is required for analysis of ethics cases, he urges, is a sophisticated response to the story of the case, one that enables detailed attention to be paid by readers to its "constructedness".[24,25]

Chambers finds that many of the recognised devices adopted in clinical case composition, such as ellipsis (loss of time), summary, scene setting, and pause (apparent stopping of time sequences so the narrator can add a new element, perhaps a reflection, hypothesis or diagnosis) can be found in bioethics cases, too, although he notes that stretch (where the description takes longer than the events of the story) almost never features. Ellipsis on the other hand – loss of time in the sense of periods unrepresented in the case narrative – is frequently to be found between periods of entrance of the *dramatis personae* into medical settings: "In other words, in an almost Einsteinian manner, the tempo of the narrative expands as the patient enters into the sphere of the health care professional."[18] Likewise, the physical space of the text *enlarges* as characters enter hospital and *contracts* when events take place elsewhere.

The author of the case report mediates happenings and text; he or she is a "star witness" who observes, describes, interprets, and transmits what happens. The assumed veracity of the case report depends, to a large extent, upon the first person nature of the report which announces that what the reader reads is (exactly) what the narrator–observer saw. The richness of a case report, its focus and attention to detail and the disciplined framework brought to bear on its interpretation, are aspects of composition signalling not only verisimilitude but the limited nature of its representation.

Inner temporality

Patients' accounts of illness experiences also carry first person authority. These accounts frequently segment the story told – most usually into medico-biographical eras, such as "before", "at the start", "during", and "at the end" of an illness. However, they adopt less predictable formats than the case report version of what happened. This is not surprising, because illness narratives are textually much longer than case reports and their focus is not generally the biomedical condition – disease minus sufferer – but the inner subjectivities related to illness and treatment as experienced and understood by the ill author.[26]

On July 7, a week after my emancipation [from a 3 year spell as Chairman of the Department of Anthropology at Columbia University], I threw out a heavy old air-conditioner, and the next day I noticed that I had a peculiar muscle spasm in my anus. It was a tightness that would not go away and that seemed to have no special relation to bowel function. My first reaction was to shrug it off, for I was brought up in a tradition that treated illness by ignoring it. This attitude was the product of the Depression-era inability to pay doctors, the value of stoicism in the face of pain, and an unwillingness to face up to an unpleasant fact. Most symptoms do go away, most ailments are self-limiting, and I decided to wait it out for a couple of weeks, convinced that I had simply pulled a muscle when foolishly lifting a heavy weight.

The spasm persisted, however, and one afternoon I had difficulty in urinating. ... The progress of my illness was neither rapid nor dramatic, and its most profound effect was upon my consciousness, my self-awareness, the way I apprehended and constructed the world and my position in it. It was as if a mortgage had been placed on my thinking, as if a great uncertainty, an unspoken contingency, had entered my life. This reaction will sound familiar to anyone who has experienced a serious or chronic illness, but it was totally new to me. My only prior sickness had been occasional colds, and I even enjoyed good health during anthropological field trips to the Amazon and Africa. My body gave me no trouble and I gave it little attention. This was all changed by my altered condition, however, and though I did not brood about my health, my thoughts occasionally would return to it. My problems also introduced a new wedge of anxiety into my general mood. A pall had been cast over my thoughts and into the shadowy area just below thinking, where dwell the things that go bump in the night.

A neurologist once told me that most of his patients came to him with symptoms that were three years old, and I was no exception. As with his other patients, my own delay was the product of misdiagnosis, complicated by my own denial of illness. The operation on the anal sphincter had placed me in a no-man's land of medical territoriality. My internist deferred to the surgeon, and the surgeon had no idea what ailed me.[27,iii]

As this account of symptoms (eventually unravelled as caused by a spinal tumour) shows, the temporal perspective is key to the manner in which the illness narrative is organised. Time is the axis around which biological goings on revolve (and evolve), and against which mental, emotional, and interpretative processes are placed. A sense of inner time connects ideas and memories of past experiences with present experiences, and links knowledge of who Robert Murphy the anthropologist once was with whom he is becoming. "Making sense of one's life as a story is ... not an optional extra," writes the philosopher Charles Taylor, "for in order to have a sense of who we are, we have to have a notion of who we have become, and where we are going".[28]

The subjective sense of time passing (or standing still) is often a major feature of an illness narrative which focuses on disrupted bodily functions and feelings, and on the illness' effects on relationships and assumptions of futurity (see Box 23.1). Illness distorts time's subjective flow[29] and one way in which illness narratives reflect this is in their temporal organisation, in their compressing and stretching of time sequence, in their manipulation of temporal gaps. By contrast, the disruptive, distorting and fragmenting influence of illness on inner temporality is rarely featured in clinical case reports, precisely because the clinical case lacks the inner perspective of the suffering subject.

Medical stories manipulate time for the same sorts of reasons that all narratives of fact manipulate time: in order to transform actual events and experiences into narratable accounts. "Actuality is too rich in sensory materials to be available instantaneously as narrative,"[12] remarks Gillian Beer. The narrative of fact cannot be a simple mirror of events and feelings. Time, itself, is required to distance the subject of experience from actuality, to allow sensory, emotional and intellectual interpretation to take place; to allow views to form about what has happened or is happening in the context of wider frames of reference, be these factual, biographical, temporal or mythic.

Recounting involves shaping and ordering events in ways that go beyond questions of sequence and chronology, to include valuation of significance, ascriptions of causation and above all of meaning. In creating narratives of experience and fact, the work of composition takes place at the interface between experience of the world – what happens – and efforts required to describe it and present its potential polyvalent meanings.

In different ways, stories, case reports, and illness narratives instantiate Ricoeur's view that "to narrate a story is already to 'reflect upon' the event narrated".[8] The end of the story, its closure, is generally not unknown to (has to be within the view of) the author and narrator. It cannot be unknown to re-readers either, whose relationship to the narrative future is radically different from the unknown (undetermined) futures of lives as they are lived. The literary theorist Gary Morson reiterates this point: "Narratives are more successful if they display a structure, which it is hard to find in life. We can stand outside the narratives we read but not outside the lives we live. And stories have real closure, in which all loose ends are tied up; but there is no privileged point in life comparable to the ending of a novel."[30] In the case history, the equivalent of the novelistic ending is diagnosis followed by treatment and treatment outcome, though these may be withheld for pedagogical purposes (see Box 23.3).

Case reports and medical records

Case reports differ from the medical record – that highly telegraphic chronicle from which they arise. The modern medical record seeks to document clinically salient aspects of discussion, examination, investigation, and treatment, selected by the healthcare attendant from consultations undertaken. Written down in chronological form as a dossier, the medical record may feature diagnoses entertained, confirmed or ruled out, together with unfolding listings of reported events, feelings, symptoms, and biological variables. The record is not itself a story but the raw materials for one.

As the narrative theorist Hayden White emphasises, the world of experience does not present itself to perception in the form of well-made stories "with central subjects, proper beginnings, middles, and ends, and a coherence that permits us to see 'the end' in every beginning" as does a good novel. Rather, "it presents itself more in the forms that the annals and chronicle suggest, either as mere sequence without beginning or end or as sequences of beginnings that only terminate and never conclude".[31] But to the extent that the authors of case histories and illness narratives succeed in narrativising their subject matters, they do so in large part by capturing and representing their materials within particular temporal frameworks.

Conclusion

Representation of time in case reports and illness narratives is a central aspect of depiction in medicine. In this chapter I have sought to draw out how case reports and stories reflect, incorporate, and manage temporality. The tales discussed arise from my interest and current reading and not from a representative or systematic survey. Nevertheless, the approach taken highlights the temporal and narrative framing that takes place in representing and communicating the phenomena of illness.

Case histories are narratives of fact, which may appear to model natural occurrences through the "eyenness" of the observer (to adapt Sacks's formulation). Yet, as we have seen, the tense of the telling, tempo of events, and the order and duration of appearances in the text-which-is-the-case can vary in ways that do not match the order of events as they may have happened. For Seymour Chatman, lack of hard gearing between such time frames is a defining feature of a narrative order: a narrative "combines the time of the histoire ('story-time') with time of the presentation of those events in the text, which we call 'discourse-time'. What is fundamental to narrative regardless of medium, is that these time orders are independent."[14]

The narratives of patients, clinicians, and the authors of clinical tales and novels are constrained to differing degrees by representational conventions concerning temporal relations. Case histories are generally organised around a notion of biological time that is linear and sequential, illness narratives around potentially more irregularly sequential biographical time periods, partaking of natural and experiential senses of the flow of time. Clinical tales and fiction, on the other hand, are least constrained by simple chronologies, textual positioning or even by time's direction of flow.[32]

Despite the linearity of their chronology, clinical case reports are part narrative constructions, which manipulate the temporal elements of their subject matter. Appearances to the contrary, they are complex compositions written from a particular point of view that not so much mirrors events and experiences as narratively inflects them. In such inflections, time is a powerful vehicle for meaning.

Acknowledgement

This chapter draws on my chapter "Biological and narrative time in clinical practice" in Elder A and Holmes J, eds. *Mental health in primary care – a new approach*. Oxford: Oxford University Press, 2002, and "Time, a narrative organiser of events and experience", *Br J Gen Pract* 2002;**52**:344–7. Thanks to Neil Vickers for many stimulating discussions about narrative and time and to Andrew Herxheimer for helpful comments on an earlier draft.

Endnotes

i   The paragraphs quoted are abridged by BH from pages 7–9.
ii However, the equivalent of the "flashback" can sometimes be found in case reports, for example, as descriptions offered by the friends or relatives of a collapsed patient detailing what they saw when a patient suddenly fainted or suffered an epileptic fit.
iii Abridged by BH from pages 11–14.

References

1   Metz C. *Essais sur le signification au cinema*, vol 1. Paris: Klincksiek, 1968 (*Film language: a semiotics of the cinema*, trans M Taylor, New York: Oxford University Press, 1974, p 18). Quoted in Genette G. *Narrative discourse: an essay in method* (trans JE Lewin). New York: Cornell University Press, 1980, p 33.
2   Heidegger M. *Being and time*. Oxford: Blackwell, 2000.
3   Elias N. *Time: an essay*. Oxford: Blackwell, 1992.
4   James W. *The principles of psychology*. New York: Holt, 1890.
5   Buetow S. Patient experience of time duration: strategies for "slowing time" and "accelerating time" in general practices. *J Eval Clin Pract* 2004;**10**:21–5.
6   McLeary G. Waiting with time. *BMJ* 2000;**321**:940.
7   Helman CG. Possession. *Ann Intern Med* 2004;**140**:229–30.
8   Ricoeur P. *Time and narrative*. Chicago: University of Chicago Press, 1984, p 7.
9   Hippocrates. *Epidemics V*. In: Smith WD, trans. *Epidemics II and IV–VII*. Cambridge, MA: Harvard University Press, 1994.
10 Wilder T. *The bridge of San Luis Rey*. Harmondsworth: Penguin Books, 1941.
11 Aristotle. *Physics* IV II 219 b1. Quoted in Eco U. Times. In: Lippincott K, ed. *The story of time*. London: Merrell Holberton, 2000, pp 10–15.
12 Beer G. Storytime and its futures. In: Ridderbos K, ed. *Time*. Cambridge: Cambridge University Press, 2002, pp 126–42.
13 Lamarque P. Narrative and invention: the limits of fictionality. In: Nash C, ed. *Narrative in culture*. London: Routledge, 1994, pp 172–98.

14 Chatman S. What novels can do that films can't (and vice versa). In: Mitchell WJT, ed. *On narrative*. Chicago University Press, Chicago, 1981, pp 117–36.
15 Bradbury M. *To the hermitage*. London: Picador, 2000, p xxi.
16 Davidoff F. *Who has seen a blood sugar?* Philadelphia: American College of Physicians, 1996, p 5.
17 Forrester J. If p, then what? Thinking in cases. *Hist Hum Sci* 1996;9:1–25.
18 Downie RS The doctor–patient relationship. In: Gillon R, ed. *Principles of health care ethics*. Chichester: Wiley, 1994, pp 343–64.
19 Beck ER, Francis JL, Souhami RL. *Tutorials in differential diagnosis*. Tunbridge Wells: Pitman Medical Publishing, 1974, p 167.
20 Kennedy MA. A curious literature: reading the medical case history from the Royal Society to Freud. PhD Thesis, Providence, RI: Brown University, 2000.
21 Genette G. *Narrative discourse: an essay in method* (trans JE Lewin). New York: Cornell University Press, 1980, p 165.
22 Sacks O. Clinical tales. *Lit Med* 1986;5:16–23.
23 Goodman N. Twisted tales; or, story, study, and symphony. In: Mitchell WJT, ed. *On narrative*. Chicago: Chicago University Press, 1981,99–115.
24 Chambers TS. *The fiction of bioethics: cases as literary texts*. New York: Routledge, 1999.
25 Chambers T. From the ethicist's point of view: the literary nature of ethical enquiry. *Hastings Centre Report*, Jan–Feb 1996. Reproduced in: Fulford KWM (Bill), Dickenson DL, Murray TH. *Healthcare ethics and human values* Cambridge: Cambridge University Press, 2002, pp 70–5.
26 Hawkins AH. *Reconstructing illness: studies in pathography*. West Lafayette, IN: Purdue University Press, 1999, p 12.
27 Murphy RF. *The body silent*. New York: WW Norton, 1990.
28 Taylor C. *Sources of the self*. Cambridge: Cambridge University Press, 1989, 47–9.
29 Davies ML. Shattered assumptions: time and the experience of long-term HIV positivity. *Soc Sci Med* 1997;44:561–71.
30 Morson GS. *Narrative and freedom: the shadows of time*. New Haven, CT and London: Yale University Press, 1996, p 20.
31 White H. The value of narrativity in the representation of reality. In: Onega S, Landa JAG, eds. *Narratology*. London: Longman, 1996, pp 273–85.
32 Amis M. *Time's arrow*. London: Penguin, 1991.

Index

Note: Entries in **bold** refer to boxes and tables, those in *italics* refer to figures; page numbers with suffix 'n' refer to notes.